Current Drugs
and Methods of
Cancer Treatment

edited by

Georges Mathé, M.D.

Service des Maladies Sanguines et Tumorales
Institut de Cancérologie et d'Immunogénétique
Hôpital Paul-Brousse, Villejuif, France

Enrico Mihich, M.D.

Division of Experimental Therapeutics
Roswell Park Memorial Institute
Buffalo, New York

Peter Reizenstein, M.D.

Karolinska Hospital and Institute
Stockholm, Sweden

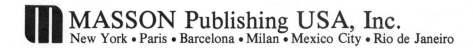

MASSON Publishing USA, Inc.
New York • Paris • Barcelona • Milan • Mexico City • Rio de Janeiro

Proceedings of the Second Annual International Symposium of the Simone and Cino Del Duca Foundation on Cancer Pharmacotherapy in 1982.

Library of Congress Cataloging in Publication Data

Simone and Cino Del Duca Foundation on Cancer Pharmaco-
   therapy. International Symposium (2d : 1982 : Paris,
   France)
   Current drugs and methods of cancer treatment.

   "Proceedings of the Second Annual International
Symposium of the Simone and Cino Del Duca Foundation
on Cancer Pharmacotherapy in 1982" — T.p. verso.
   Bibliography: p.
   Includes index.
   1. Cancer — Chemotherapy — Congresses. 2. Antineo-
plastic agents — Congresses. I. Mathé, Georges,
1922-   . II. Mihich, Enrico. III. Reizenstein,
Peter, 1928-   . IV. Title. [DNLM: 1. Neoplasms —
Drug therapy — Congresses. 2. Antineoplastic agents —
Therapeutic use — Congresses. 3. Clinical trials —
Congresses. W3 SI369 2nd 1982 c / QZ 267 S598 1982c]
RC271.C5S534   1982   616.99'4061   83-12048
ISBN 0-89352-201-5

ISBN 0-89352-201-5
Library of Congress Catalog Card Number: 83-12048 ·

Printed in the United States of America

INTRODUCTION

In 1957, Georges Mathé and I organized at the Hôpital Saint-Louis, under the auspices of the Centre National de la Recherche Scientifique, a Symposium devoted to the classification and treatment of Hodgkin's disease. Domagk, Sidney Farber, Alexander Haddow, Joseph Burchenal, the most renowned specialists of America and Europe, were among the participants. After 3 days of discussion, their conclusions were categorical: no classification is possible; treatment can be only palliative; we must resign ourselves to the fact that the result of Hodgkin's disease will remain forever fatal. These proved to be amazingly shortsighted predictions, for, in 1982, 80% of cases of Hodgkin's disease, all forms included, progressed toward a cure.

In 1947, acute leukemia was a very cruel disease, constantly and rapidly fatal, killing afflicted children and adults within two months. The first two complete remissions were induced in Paris (1947) and Boston (1948), but these were of very short duration. In 1982, cure was obtained in 55–60% of cases of acute childhood lymphoblastic leukemia, and in 10–15% of cases of other acute leukemias.

These two examples may serve as models. Progress in oncology over the last 25 years has made possible at times a nearly total victory, as in the case of Hodgkin's disease, and at other times fruitful but partial successes; however, numerous and grave failures remain.

Chance and reason — such could be the title of this chapter in the recent history of cancer treatment. Certain therapies have a theoretical foundation; others, more numerous, are empiric. We can cure Hodgkin's disease, but we do not understand it. We know neither its cause, or causes, nor its physiopathology. Quite probably, this empiricism no longer suffices, and in order to cure the still incurable cancers, theoretically grounded therapies are necessary. This necessity and this perspective have inspired the research — highly theoretical — presented at this Symposium.

The majority of these studies are devoted to destructive therapies. After all, until now, chemotherapy of a cancer has not been very different from the amputation of a diseased limb. But greater understanding of the mechanisms of carcinogenesis, of the specific characteristics of cancerous cells, allows us to envision differential chemotherapies. It makes possible — to go back to the title itself of certain papers — the "exploitation" of fundamental data, the theoretically based approach to therapeutic applications.

It is often said that medicine fulfills four functions: destruction of diseased tissues, replacement, remedy of disorders, and action on the cause. In cancer medicine, it is above all the first function that has been fulfilled. Replacements, at the present time, are limited to bone marrow transplants. Our habitual ignorance of causes does not allow us to carry out the fourth function.

The hope of restoring to normal a cancerous cell or a cancerous tissue is no longer completely vain. Hormonal treatment of cancer has had until now only limited indications, but it provides useful examples. The progress we anticipate in our knowledge of the relationships between host and tumor should allow rapid development of new immunotherapies. The study of the surveillance (in the broad sense of the term) that the organism exercises, or fails to exercise, on cancerous cells has given rise to fruitful developments.

This volume brings together studies of very high scientific standards and of very diverse origins. Their scientific rigor and their diversity form the basis of their quality.

Biologists engaged in fundamental research, biochemists, biophysicists, pharmacologists, clinicians, endocrinologists, and immunologists have found a meeting ground here for the results of their work. The data they have contributed are important and will surely lead to new progress.

Jean Bernard
Service d'Oncologie Médicale
Hôpital de la Salpetrière
Paris, France

CONTRIBUTORS

J.P. Armand, Service des Maladies Sanguines et Tumorales, and Institut de Cancérologie et d'Immunogénétique, Hôpital Paul-Brousse, Villejuif, France

N. Azarnia, Roswell Park Memorial Institute, Buffalo, New York 14263

M. Barcos, Roswell Park Memorial Institute, Buffalo, New York 14263

E.E. Baulieu, Department of Biochemistry, University of Paris-Sud, Laboratory Hormones, 94270 Bicêtre, France

M. Bayssas, Service des Maladies Sanguines et Tumorales, Institut de Cancérologie et d'Immunogénétique, Hôpital Paul-Brousse, 94804 Villejuif, France

M. Bennoun, Institut de Cancérologie et d'Immunogénétique, Hôpital Paul Brousse, 94804 Villejuif, France

W. Bollag, Pharmaceutical Research Department, F. Hoffman-La Roche & Co. Ltd., CH-4002 Basel, Switzerland

C. Bourut, Institut de Cancérologie et d'Immunogénétique, Hôpital Universitaire Paul-Brousse, 94800 Villejuif, France

Martin L. Brecher, Department of Pediatrics, Roswell Park Memorial Institute, Buffalo, New York 14263

J. Brennan, University of Rochester, Roswell Park Memorial Institute, Buffalo, New York 14263

D. Brouty-Boye, Institut de Recherches Scientifiques sur le Cancer, Laboratoire d'Oncologie Virale, 94802 Villejuif, France

G. Browman, Ontario Cancer Clinic, Roswell Park Memorial Institute, Buffalo, New York 14263

D. Buscaglia, Roswell Park Memorial Institute, New York State Department of Health, Buffalo, New York 14263

H. Calderoli, Service de Radiothérapie, Laboratoire de Cancérologie, CHU- Strasbourg, France

E. Chenu, Institut de Cancérologie et d'Immunogénétique, Hôpital Paul-Brousse, 94800 Villejuif, France

N. Cohen, Department of Medical Oncology, Roswell Park Memorial Institute, Buffalo, New York 14263

O. Michael Colvin, The Bone Marrow Transplant Unit, The Johns Hopkins Oncology Center, Baltimore, Maryland 21205

J. Wayne Cowens, Roswell Park Memorial Institute, Buffalo, New York 14263

P.J. Creaven, Roswell Park Memorial Institute, Buffalo, New York 14263

B. Dadey, Department of Medical Oncology, Roswell Park Memorial Institute, Buffalo, New York 14263

D. Dantchev, Institut de Cancérologie et d'Immunogénétique, Hôpital Paul Brousse, 94800 Villejuif, France

M. Delgado, Institut de Cancérologie et d'Immunogénétique, Hôpital Paul Brousse, 94800 Villejuif, France

T. Dorval, Institut de Cancérologie et d'Immunogénétique, Hôpital Paul Brousse, 94800 Villejuif, France

A.P. Early, Roswell Park Memorial Institute, Buffalo, New York 14263

J.J. Farhi, Institut de Cancérologie et d'Immunogénétique, Hôpital Paul Brousse, 94800 Villejuif, France

A. Fourcade, Institut de Cancérologie et d'Immunogénétique, Hôpital Universitaire Paul-Brousse, Villejuif, France

Arnold I. Freeman, Department of Pediatrics, Roswell Park Memorial Institute, Buffalo, New York 14263

M. Fukushima, Aichi Cancer Center, Department of Internal Medicine, Chikusa-ku, Nagoya 464, Japan

G. Gahrton, Head Division of Clinical Hematology and Oncology, Department of Medicine, Huddinge Hospital and Karolinska Institute, Huddinge, Sweden

J. Gastiaburu, Service des Maladies Sanguines et Tumorales, Institut de Cancérologie et d'Immunogénétique, Hôpital Paul Brousse, 94800 Villejuif, France

J. Goldberg, Upstate Medical Center, Syracuse, New York 13210

E. Goldschmidt, Service des Maladies Sanguines et Tumorales, Institut de Cancérologie et d'Immunogénétique, Hôpital Paul Brousse, 94800 Villejuif, France

J. Gouveia, Service des Maladies Sanguines et Tumorales, I.C.I.G., Hôpital Paul Brousse, 94800 Villejuif, France

Daniel M. Green, Department of Pediatrics, Roswell Park Memorial Institute, Buffalo, New York 14263

I. Gresser, Institut de Recherches Scientifiques sur le Cancer, Laboratoire d'Oncologie Virale, 94802 Villejuif, France

H. Grunwald, Queens Hospital Center, Roswell Park Memorial Institute, Buffalo, New York

T. Han, Department of Medical Oncology, Roswell Park Memorial Institute, Buffalo, New York 14263

M. Hayat, Service des Maladies Sanguines et Tumorales, I.C.I.G., Hôpital Paul Brousse, 94804 Villejuif, France

K. Hellmann, Cancer Chemotherapy Department, Imperial Cancer Research Fund, Westminster Hospital, London, SW1, England

D.J. Higby, Department of Medical Oncology, Roswell Park Memorial Institute, Buffalo, New York 14263

Bridget T. Hill, Laboratory of Cellular Chemotherapy, Imperial Cancer Research Fund, Institute of Urology, Lincoln's Inn Fields, London WC2A 3PX, England

R. Hulhoven, Clinique Saint Luc, Catholic University of Louvain, B-1200 Bruxelles, Belgium

J.L. Imbach, Centre Paul Lamarque, Hôpital Saint Eloi, Laboratoire de Chimie Bio-Organique, Université des Sciences et Techniques du Languedoc, 34000 Montpellier, France

C. Jasmin, Service des Maladies Sanguines et Tumorales, I.C.I.G., Hôpital Paul Brousse, 94800 Villejuif, France

H. Kaizer, The Bone Marrow Transplant Unit, The Johns Hopkins Oncology Center, Baltimore, Maryland 21205

R. Keiling, Service de Radiothérapie, Hospices Civils de Strasbourg, Centre Hospitalier Régional, 67091 Strasbourg, France

E. Kelly, Roswell Park Memorial Institute, New York State Department of Health, Buffalo, New York 14263

M. Koutsilieris, Clinical Investigation in Reproductive Endocrinology, Obstetrics/Gynecology, McGill University Clinic, Royal Victoria Hospital, Montreal, Quebec, Canada

D. Kramer, Department of Experimental Therapeutics and Grace Cancer Drug Center, Roswell Park Memorial Institute, Buffalo, New York 14263

C. Lombardo, Multiscreening Laboratory, Giannina Gaslini Institute, 16148 Genoa, Italy

F.R. Macbeth, CRC Medical Oncology Unit, Southampton General Hospital, Southampton SO9 4XY England

J.S. MacDonald, Cancer Treatment Evaluation, Division of Cancer Treatment, National Institute of Health, Bethesda, Maryland 20014

D. Machover, Service des Maladies Sanguines et Tumorales, I.C.I.G., Hôpital Paul Brousse, 94800 Villejuif, France

R. Maral, Institut de Cancérologie et d'Immunogénétique, Hôpital Paul Brousse, 94800 Villejuif, France

M. Marinello, Department of Medical Oncology, Roswell Park Memorial Institute, Buffalo, New York 14263

J. Marquet, Service Central d'Hématologie-Immunologie, CHU Henri Mondor, 94000 Créteil, France

G. Mathé, Service des Maladies Sanguines et Tumorales, Institut de Cancérologie et d'Immunogénétique, Hôpital Paul-Brousse, 94804 Villejuif, France

Y. Matsumura, Department of Urology, Okayama University, Medical School, Okayama, 700 Japan

B. Michalski, Service des Maladies Sanguines et Tumorales, I.C.I.G., Hôpital Paul Brousse, 94804 Villejuif, France

E. Mihich, Department of Experimental Therapeutics and Grace Cancer Drug Center, Roswell Park Memorial Institute, Buffalo, New York 14263

K. Miller, New England Medical Center, Roswell Park Memorial Institute, Buffalo, New York 14263

J.L. Misset, Service des Maladies Sanguines et Tumorales, Institut de Cancérologie et d'Immunogénétique, Hôpital Paul Brousse, 94804 Villejuif, France

R. Mortel, Milton S. Hershey Medical Center, Hershey, Pennsylvania 17033

M. Musset, Service des Maladies Sanguines et Tumorales, Institut de Cancérologie et d'Immunogénétique, Hôpital Paul Brousse, 94804 Villejuif, France

M. Namer, Centre A. Lacassagne, 06054 Nice, France

C. Ogier, Institute of Cancerology and Immunogenetics, I.C.I.G., Hôpital Paul-Brousse, Villejuif, France

H. Ohmori, Department of Urology, Okayama University, Medical School, Okayama, 700 Japan

R.K. Oldham, Division of Cancer Institute, Frederick, Maryland

M. O'Leary, Department of Medical Oncology, Roswell Park Memorial Institute, Buffalo, New York 14263

K. Ota, Aichi Cancer Center, Department of Internal Medicine, Chikusa-ku, Nagoya 464, Japan

H. Ozer, Department of Medical Oncology, Roswell Park Memorial Institute, Buffalo, New York 14263

M. Paintrand, Institut de Cancérologie et d'Immunogénétique, 94804 Villejuif, France

M. Paganuzzi, Multiscreening Laboratory, Giannina Gaslini Institute, 16148 Genoa, Italy

C. Paul, Division of Clinical Hematology and Oncology, Department of Medicine, Huddinge Hospital and Karolinska Institute, Huddinge, Sweden

Z.P. Paxelic, Roswell Park Memorial Institute, Buffalo, New York 14263

L. Pendyala, Roswell Park Memorial Institute, Buffalo, New York 14263

C. Peterson, Department of Pharmacology, Karolinska Institute, Stockholm, Sweden

I. Pignot, Institut de Cancérologie et d'Immunogénétique, Hôpital Paul Brousse, 94804 Villejuif, France

C. Porter, Department of Experimental Therapeutics and Grace Cancer Drug Center, Roswell Park Memorial Institute, Buffalo, New York 14263

H. Preisler, Roswell Park Memorial Institute, New York State Department of Health, Buffalo, New York 14263

L.A. Price, Head and Neck Unit, Royal Marsden Hospital, London WEN 1AG, England

A. Raza, Roswell Park Memorial Institute, Buffalo, New York 14263

F. Reiss-Eichler, Service de Radiothérapie, Laboratoire de Cancérologie, CHU- Strasbourg, France

P. Reizenstein, Division of Hematology, Karolinska Hospital, Stockholm, Sweden; Visiting Professor, Institute of Cancerology, University of Paris-Sud

G. Renoux, Laboratoire d'Immunologie, Faculté de Médecine, 37032 Tours, France

M. Renoux, Laboratoire d'Immunologie, Faculté de Médecine, 37032 Tours, France

P. Ribaud, Service des Maladies Sanguines et Tumorales, I.C.I.G., Hôpital Paul Brousse, 94804 Villejuif, France

P. Robel, Department of Biochemistry, University Paris-Sud, Laboratory Hormones, 94270 Bicêtre, France

Y.M. Rustum, Roswell Park Memorial Institute, New York State Department of Health, Buffalo, New York 14263

T. Ruzzen, Multiscreening Laboratory, Giannina Gaslini Institute, 16148 Genoa, Italy

G.W. Santos, The Bone Marrow Transplant Unit, The Johns Hopkins Oncology Center, Baltimore, Maryland 21205

A. Sarasin, Institut de Recherches Scientifiques sur le Cancer, 94802 Villejuif, France

C. Sarasin, Ecole des Hautes Etudes en Sciences Sociales, 75006 Paris, France

R. Saral, The Bone Marrow Transplant Unit, The Johns Hopkins Oncology Center, Baltimore, Maryland 21205

P. Schein, Vincent T. Lombardi Cancer Research Center, Georgetown University, Washington, DC 20057

L. Schwarzenberg, Service des Maladies Sanguines et Tumorales, I.C.I.G., Hôpital Paul Brousse, 94804 Villejuif, France

B. Serrou, Centre Paul Lamarque, Hôpital Saint Eloi, Laboratoire de chimie Bio-Organique, Université des Sciences et Techniques du Languedoc, 34000 Montpellier, France

S.A. Sherwin, Division of Cancer Treatment, National Cancer Institute, Frederick, Maryland 21701

H.K. Slocum, Roswell Park Memorial Institute, New York State Department of Health, Buffalo, New York 14263

R.K. Stuart, The Bone Marrow Transplant Unit, The Johns Hopkins Oncology Center, Baltimore, Maryland 21205

H. Tapiero, Institut de Cancérologie et d'Immunogénétique, Hôpital Paul Brousse, 94804 Villejuif, France

D. Thompson, Department of Medical Oncology, Roswell Park Memorial Institute, Buffalo, New York 14263

G. Tolis, McGill University, Royal Victoria Hospital, Montreal, Quebec, Canada

M. Tubiana, Institute Gustave-Roussy, Rue Camille Desmoulins, 94800 Villejuif, France

Peter J. Tutschka, The Bone Marrow Transplant Unit, The Johns Hopkins Oncology Center, Baltimore, Maryland 21205

F. De Vassal, Service des Maladies Sanguines et Tumorales, I.C.I.G., Hôpital Paul Brousse, 94804 Villejuif, France

R. Vogler, Emory University School of Medicine, Atlanta, Georgia 30322

G. Wang, Roswell Park Memorial Institute, New York State Department of Health, Buffalo, New York 14263

V. Weinberg, Department of Pediatrics, Roswell Park Memorial Institute, Buffalo, New York 14263

G. Willoquet, Institut de Cancérologie et d'Immunogénétique, Hôpital Paul Brousse, 94804 Villejuif, France

C. Wrzosek, Roswell Park Memorial Institute, New York State Department of Health, Buffalo, New York 14263

Y. Yoshimoto, Department of Urology, Okayama University Medical School, Okayama, 700 Japan

Charles W. Young, Memorial Sloan-Kettering Cancer Center, New York, NY 10021

Sigmund F. Zakrzewski, Roswell Park Memorial Institute, Buffalo, New York 14263

J. Zittoun, Service Central d'Hématologie-Immunologie, CHU Henri Mondor, 94000 Créteil, France

R. Zittoun, Service d'Hématologie, Hotel Dieu, 75181 Paris, France

G. Zwingelstein, Laboratoire de Physiologie Générale et Comparée, Centre National de la Recherche Scientifique, 69000 Lyon, France

CONTENTS

PART I

New Drugs

CHAPTER 1

CNCC Compared to HECNU, Two New Third-Generation Nitrosourea Analogs: Experimental Oncostatic Screening

R. Maral,[a] G. Mathé,[a] P. Schein,[b] J.S. MacDonald,[c] C. Bourut,[a] E. Chenu,[a] J. Oiry,[a] and J.L. Imbach[a]

Clinicians have been working with two generations of nitrosourea (NU) analogs. The first includes BCNU,[1] CCNU,[19] and MeCCNU,[20] which induce responses mainly in colorectal carcinoma, Hodgkin's disease, non-Hodgkin's lymphomas, and brain tumors.[1] BCNU, CCNU, and MeCCNU produce serious hematologic toxicities, especially thrombocytopenia and accumulated myelosuppression with chronic treatment.[1] They are also mutagenic.[8,13]

The hematotoxicity[1,19,20] and mutagenicity[13] of these available NU analogs were taken into consideration by Johnston et al.[8] in the U.S., and by Montero et al.[14] in France. Glycosidic NU analogs were then synthesized.

Of the second generation of NU, the first, chlorozotocin (CZT), was studied experimentally by Schein et al.,[16] by Mathé et al.,[3,4,7,9,15] and by Vlaeminck.[18] To date, it has proven to be clinically active in pre-viously untreated melanoma,[17] and in hematologic malignancies.[11] The second series of analogs, RFCNU and RPCNU, were studied experimentally[3,4,7,9,15] and clinically by us. RFCNU produced clinical good responses in selected patients with colorectal carcinoma as well as in cases with adenocarcinoma of unknown origin.[12] RPCNU is still under phase II study; its activity for human cancer is still unknown, but it already appears to be more hematoxic than RFCNU.

These data led Imbach et al.[5] to synthesize a third generation of NU analogs. In this article we present the experimental oncostatic study of N,N'-bis(2-chloroethyl)-N-nitrosocarbamoyl)cystamine, or CNCC, or ICIG-1325, which is a mixture of three isomers (Fig. 1).

We compared the activities of CNCC to those of 1-(2-hydroxyethyl)-3-(2-chloroethyl) 3-nitrosourea or HECNU*[2] synthesized by Zeller et al.[21] and also to those of restudied CZT, RFCNU and RPCNU. The rational of the formula of CNCC (Fig. 1) lies in the fact that cystamine moiety may confer unique pharmacologic and toxicologic properties to the

[a]Unité de Pharmacologie Humaine Simone et Cino del Duca, Institut de Cancérologie et d'Immunogénétique (INSERM U 50), Hôpital Paul-Brousse, Villejuif, France
[b]Vincent T, Lombardi Cancer Research Center, Georgetown University, Washington, D.C.
[c]Cancer Treatment Evaluation, Division of Cancer Treatment, National Institutes of Health, Bethesda, Maryland.
[d]Laboratoire de Chimie Bio-Organique (ERA du CNRS 948), Montpellier, France

*HECNU was provided to us by Dr. G. Eisenbrand of the Institute of Toxicology and Chemotherapy, German Cancer Research Center, Heidelberg, F.R.G.

CNCC (ICIG 1325)

N,N'-bis [N-(2-chloroethyl)N-nitrosocarbamoyl]cystamine

```
S-CH2-CH2-R1-CH2-CH2-Cl
|
S-CH2-CH2-R2-CH2-CH2-Cl
```

Isomer	R1	R2
A ICIG 1725	H O NO | || | -N-C-N-	 -N-C-N- | || | H O NO
B ICIG 1952	NO O H | || | -N-C-N-	 -N-C-N- | || | NO O H
C ICIG 1937	NO O H | || | -N-C-N-	 -N-C-N- | || | H O NO

CNCC (ICIG 1325) is a mixture of the three isomers, one of them A (ICIG 1725) in very small amount (<1%) and the two others:
B (ICIG 1952) ∽52%
C (ICIG 1937) ∽47%

FIGURE 1.   CNCC (ICIG 1325), isomers A, B, and C.

new compound; the disulfide bridge can be easily cleaved *in vivo*.[5] CNCC is a liposoluble compound, and it was to be expected that it would cross the blood–brain barrier in effective concentrations.

Methods

TOXICITY, LETHALITY, AND L1210 LEUKEMIA PRIMARY SCREENING

The method used has been previously described and discussed.[10] On day 0, adult BDF_1 mice were inoculated i.p. with 10^5 leukemia cells. On day 1, they received graded doses of CNCC or other compounds at doses of 5–150 mg/kg i.p.; CNCC, RPCNU, and RFCNU were dissolved in olive oil, whereas CZT and HECNU which are hydrosoluble were dissolved in distilled water. On days 5 and 9, drug or solvent injections were repeated

only in those mice which presented no manifestation of toxicity. The mortality of the mice was monitored daily and autopsies were performed to determine whether deaths were due to leukemia or to a toxic action of the drug. The acute LD 50 of each compound was determined graphically. For each compound, the oncostatic effects of specified doses are expressed as a survival index: I = T/C × 100; T = median survival time (MST) in the treated group of mice; and C = MST in the control group.

When I is greater than 125 and the difference between treated and control groups is statistically significant according to the Wilcoxon nonparametric W-test, the agent is considered as active at the given dose. For each compound, a graph is drawn, representing the correlation between the therapeutic effect and the dose. If the curve presents a plateau called "maximally effective dose range" (MEDR), its median is considered as the optimal dose, and the lowest dose of MEDR is the one to be studied for toxicity.

ACTIVITY ON OTHER MURINE TUMORS

Seven other implanted murine tumors, Lewis lung carcinoma, melanocarcinoma B16, mammary adenocarcinoma TM2, fibrosarcoma ICIG-C_1, colon 26 carcinoma, M555 ovarian carcinoma, and glioma 26 were treated with the median dose of MEDR (on day 0).

The drugs were administered i.p. on days 1, 5, and 9 in distilled water solution (HECNU and CZT) or in olive oil (CNCC, RFCNU and RPCNU). The control groups received the same volume of solvent (water or oil). Mortality was noted daily.

Results are expressed according to the above described survival index: I = T/C × 100. They are also statistically evaluated according to the Wilcoxon test.

Results

1) The acute LD50 of CNCC in mice is 75 mg/kg, while it is 25 mg/kg for HECNU.

2) The MEDR of CNCC in L1210 leukemia is broader (a wider dose range) than that of HECNU and those of the other three analogues also studied. Such a large range is considered to represent an advantage for CNCC, since it means greater security in the choice of optimal therapeutic dose without toxicity.

3) The activity on intracerebrally grafted L1210 leukemia and on the other murine tumors was studied using the i.p. optimal dose for each compound.

Table 1 shows that CNCC and HECNU are significantly oncostatic on all the tumors used except fibrosarcoma ICIG-C_1. Their spectrums of activity are almost identical and wider than those of RFCNU, RPCNU, and CZT.

Both CNCC and HECNU are effective against glioma 26, grafted S.C., and leukemia L1210, transplanted intracerebrally.

The efficacy of CNCC for intracerebral L1210 was compared to that of RFCNU (water insoluble) and to that of HECNU (water soluble). With CNCC and HECNU more than 50% of the animals are cured; the effect of RFCNU is only significant when the median is compared to that of the controls, but this analog induces no cure. RPCNU and CZT are inactive.

The *oral route* of administration of CNCC given on days 1, 5, and 9 is also more efficient in the treatment of L1210 leukemia grafted i.p. than is that of RFCNU. A plateau is obtained with CNCC while RFCNU gives only a peak.

Discussion

CNCC has proven to have important biologic activity:

1) The LD 50 in mice of CNCC (mg/kg) is higher than that of HECNU and CZT and is intermediate to those of RPCNU and RFCNU.

2) The oral toxicity of CNCC is lower than that of RFCNU, a nitrosourea which we have studied in a phase II trial,[12] showing that the cystamine congener is more efficient and less toxic than the first generation analogs.[1,19,20]

3) With the method used to compare the dose–effect relationship for oncostatic action on i.p.-implanted L1210 leukemia,[10] BCNU, CCNU, MeCNU presented a peak of activity,[6] while RPCNU, CZT, and HECNU produced a narrow MEDR plateau, RFCNU presented a longer plateau than these analogs on which we have developed human toxicity data[3,7,9,15] and subsequently studied in phase-II trial.[12] CNCC, however, gives the longest MEDR plateau of all these analogs.

4) Both CNCC and HECNU are very active against intracerebrally grafted L1210 leukemia, as well as subcutaneously transplanted glioma 26.

5) CNCC and HECNU are also effective against a large number of subcutaneously implanted solid tumors: Lewis lung car-

TABLE 1. Activity[a] of CNCC on Seven Solid Murine Tumors Including Glioma 26 and in Intracranially Grafted L1210 Leukemia — Comparison with That of HECNU and Those of RFCNU, RPCNU, and CZT

Tumor	CZT 15 mg/kg i.p.	RFCNU 20 mg/kg i.p.	RPCNU 15 mg/kg i.p.	CNCC 30 mg/kg i.p.	HECNU 10 mg/kg i.p.
Leukemia L1210 (grafted intracerebrally)	N.S.[b]	167 S	N.S.	∞	∞[c]
Glioma 26 (grafted subcutaneously)	N.S.	N.S.	127 S	200 S	182 S
Lewis Lung Carcinoma (LLC) (grafted subcutaneously)	N.S.	N.S.	N.S.	∞	∞
Colon 26 Carcinoma (grafted subcutaneously)	∞	N.S.	N.S.	∞	∞
Melanocarcinoma B16 (grafted subcutaneously)	N.S.	144 S	151 S	200 S	198 S
Mammary Adenocarcinoma TM2 (grafted subcutaneously)	N.S.	N.S.	134 S	185 S	165 S
Fibrosarcoma ICIG C$_1$ (grafted subcutaneously)	∞	∞	Not studied	N.S.	N.S.
M55 Ovarian carcinoma (grafted subcutaneously)	∞	N.S.	∞	254 S	210 S

[a]Increase life span (I.L.S. = T/C × 100).
[b]N.S. = Not significant.
[c]∞ ≥ 50% or over of the animals in the treated group are cured.

cinoma (Ca), colon 26 Ca, ovarian M555 Ca B16, while RFCNU, RPCNU, and CZT B16, while RFCNU, RPCNU, and CZT have a narrower spectrum.

ACKNOWLEDGMENT

This work was conducted at the Fondation Simone et Cino del Duca, and in the frame of the French–American Agreement INSERM-NCI.

REFERENCES

1. Carter, S.K.: Cancer Chemother Pharmacol 4(3): 35, 1973.
2. Eisenbrand, G., Habs, M., Zeller, W.J., Fiebig, H., Berger, M., Zelesny, O., and Schmahl, D.: In Nitrosoureas in Cancer Treatment. B. Serrou, P.S. Schein, and J.L. Imbach, eds. Elsevier/North Holland, Amsterdam, 1981, p. 175.
3. Florentin, I., Hayat, M., Kiger, N., Maral, J., Imbach, J.L., and Mathé, G.: Internat J Immunopharmacol (in press).
4. Hayat, M., Bourut, C., Chenu, E., Montero, J.L., Imbach, J.L., MacDonald, J.S., and Mathé, G.: Cancer Chemother Pharmacol 3: 217, 1979.
5. Imbach, J.L., Martinez, J., Oiry, J., Bourut, C., Chenu, E., Maral, R., and Mathé, G.: In Nitrosoureas in Cancer Treatment. B. Serrou, P.S. Schein, and J.L. Imbach, Eds., Elsevier/North Holland, Amsterdam, 1981, p. 123.
6. Imbach, J.L., Montero, J.L., Moruzzi, A., Serrou, B., Chenu, E., Hayat, M., and Mathé, G.: Biomedicine 23, 410 1975.
7. Jasmin, C., Mori, K.J., MacDonald, J.S., and Mathé, G.: In Nitrosoureas in Cancer Treatment. B. Serrou, P.S. Schein, and J.L. Imbach, Eds. Elsevier/North Holland, Amsterdam, 1981, p. 193.
8. Johnston, T.P., MacCaleb, G.S., and Montgomery, J.A.: J Med Chem 18: 104, 1975.
9. Marzin, D., Jasmin, C., Imbach, J.L., and Mathé, G.: In Nitrosoureas in Cancer Treatment. B. Serrou, P.S. Schein, and J.L. Imbach, Eds., Elsevier/North Holland, Amsterdam, 1981, p. 165.
10. Mathé, G. and Jasmin, C.: Cancer Chemother Pharmacol 3: 203, 1979.
11. Mathé, G., Schein, P.S., MacDonald, J.S., Hercend, T., Misset, J.L., Ribaud, P., Gouveia, J., De Vassal, F., Jasmin, C., Machover, D., Schwarzenberg, L., Musset, M., Gastiaburu, J., Tapiero, H., and Maral, R.: Cancer Res (submitted for publication).
12. Mathé, G., Schein, P., MacDonald, J.S., Imbach, J.L., Misset, J.L., De Vassal, F., Ribaud, P., Serrou, B., Gouveia, J., Musset, M., Machover, D., Schwarzenberg, L., Jasmin, C., and De Jager, R.: Eur J Cancer (in press).
13. Moertel, C.H.: Cancer Chemother Rep 4(3): 27, 1973.
14. Montero, J.L., Moruzzi, A., Oiry, J., and Imbach, J.L.: Eur J Med Chemother 12: 397, 1977.
15. Mori, K.J., Jasmin, C., Hayat, M., MacDonald, J.S., and Mathé, G.: Cancer Res 40: 4282, 1980.
16. Schein, P.S., McMenamin, M.G., and Anderson, T.: Cancer Res 33: 2005, 1978.

17. Van Amburg, A., Ratkin, G., and Washington, U.: *Proc Assoc Soc Clin Oncol 21: 354, 1980.* (Abstract C-137).

18. Vlaeminck, M.N., Collyn, M., D'Hooghe, M., Cappelaere, P., Biserte, G., Oiry, J., Montero, J.L., and Imbach, J.L.: *Biomedicine 35: 27, 1981.*

19. Wasserman, T.H., Slavik, M., and Carter, S.K.: *Cancer Treat Rev 1: 131, 1974.*

20. Wasserman, T.H., Slavik, M. and Carter, S.K.: *Cancer Treat Rev 1: 251, 1974.*

21. Zeller, W.J. and Eisenbrand, G.: *Oncology 38: 39, 1981.*

CHAPTER 2

Phase II Study of RFCNU

G. Mathé,[a] P. Schein,[b] J.S. MacDonald,[c] J.L. Imbach,[d] J.L. Misset,[a] F. De Vassal,[a] P. Ribaud,[a] B. Serrou,[d] J. Gouveia,[a] M. Musset,[a] D. Machover,[a] and L. Schwarzenberg[a]

Introduction

Several nitrosourea (NU) analogs have undergone clinical evaluation. The phase II trial results of these drugs have been reviewed by Carter for BCNU,[1] and by Wasserman et al. for CCNU[22] and methyl CCNU (MeCCNU).[23] These three NU have a broad spectrum of antitumor activity in human malignancies and have shown a significant therapeutic effectiveness in Hodgkin's disease (BCNU, CCNU) and in non-Hodgkin's lymphomas (BCNU and CCNU). They are the only class of drugs with consistent activity for CNS tumors.[1] In respect to digestive tract (DT) tumors, Moertel[13] reported an overall 17.5% response rate (complete remissions (CR) + partial responses (PR)) with MeCCNU, but the collected results in the literature suggest the rates of CR + PR for BCNU of only 12.5% in colorectal carcinomas, 0%

[a]Unité de Pharmacologie Humaine Simone et Cino del Duca, Service des Maladies Sanguines et Tumorales, Institut de Cancérologie et d'Immunogénétique (INSERM U 50), Hôpital Paul-Brousse, Villejuif, France
[b]Vincent T. Lombardi Cancer Research Center, Georgetown University, Washington, D.C., in the framework of the French–American Agreement INSERM-NCI
[c]Cancer Treatment Evaluation, Division of Cancer Treatment, National Institutes of Health, Bethesda, Maryland
[d]Centre Paul-Lamarque, Hôpital Saint-Eloi and Laboratoire de Chimie Bio-Organique, Université des Sciences et Techniques du Languedoc, Montpellier, France

in pancreatic cancers, and 12% in overall GI tumors.[1] For CCNU, a 10% response in colorectal cancer and in the overall GI neoplasias has been described.[22] For MeCCNU, an 11% response has been reported for phase II trial of the major GI tumor sites.[23]

Moreover, the use of most NU in cancer chemotherapy has been limited by the delayed and cumulative bone marrow toxicity demonstrated mostly by the long-lasting and often severe thrombocytopenia which necessitates not only shortening of the duration of treatment, but also long intervals between two treatment cycles.

The present study deals with phase II study of a series of second generation NU analogs in the formula of which the cyclohexyl group of CCNU is replaced by a sugar molecule related to ribose, xylose, or glucose. Our aim was to identify one or several analogs, effective not only in DT neoplasias, but also in tumors resistant to the first generation of NU analogs, and which have less myeloid or platelet toxicity.[2]

Thirty-seven analogs[20] produced for us by Montero et al.[14,15] were tested against L1210 Leukemia. Only RFCNU: 3-(2-chloroethyl) 3-nitroso 1-[2,3-isopropyliolene 5-(nitro-4-benzoyl) 1-ribofuranosyl] urea, and RPCNU: 3-(2-chloroethyl) 3-nitroso 1-(2, 3, 4 triacetyl 1-ribopyranosyl) urea, gave a dose–effect relationship with a plateau,[5] called the "maximally efficient dose range" (MEDR). This parameter has been used as a preliminary test to compare NU analogs in regard to their "operational" therapeutic index.[11] Chlorozotocin (CZT) or 3-(2-chloroethyl) 3-nitroso 1 (D_2-glucopyranosyl) urea,[7,19] which we studied in a second experiment, also produced a short MEDR, whereas BCNU, CCNU, and GCNU did not. RPCNU produced a short MEDR, while RFCNU gave the largest range of effective doses.[4,5]

RFCNU had excellent antitumor activity in several transplanted murine leukemias and solid tumors.[4,5] It is only moderately toxic to hemopoietic stem cells (CFUs), and the toxicity is rapidly reversible. Similarly, there is only moderate and reversible acute toxicity on granulopoietic precursors (CFU-c),[16] and the hematological toxicity in the mouse is not cumulative.[6] RFCNU is not immunosuppressive. In contrast, the doses optimally oncostatic on L1210 leukemia were found able to potentiate delayed hypersensitivity and macrophage cytostatic activity.[3] RFCNU is moderately mutagenic,[9] which may be the result of its relatively low akylating activity — 40% of that of choroethyl nitrosourea (CNU); CZT has 64% of CNU mutagenicity and RPCNU 11%. RFCNU (as RPCNU) blocks cells in G_2-M for 24 hours, at doses of 20 μg and 50 μg/ml respectively, while CZT (at 20 μg/ml) blocks them for 72 hours.[21]

Patients and Methods

We report here the treatment results for two categories of tumors — DT and carcinomas of unknown origin. The patients were entered into study according to the general rules for phase II trials.[24] They were in an advanced stage of their disease and had one or more measurable metastases, or a locally recurrent primary localization not amenable to surgery or radiotherapy. Eighteen patients had been previously treated and were resistant to chemotherapy; six had already received a NU analog.

Eligibility criteria were: 1) the histological confirmation of malignancy, 2) the evidence of tumor progression under all previous therapies and/or the absence of any effective therapy, 3) the presence of measurable disease, and 4) the possibility of adequate follow-up.

Fifty-seven patients presenting these criteria were available for evaluation. There were 32 men and 25 women with a mean age of 54 years (range: 26–74 years).

Antitumor response was classified as a complete response (CR) or partial regression (PR). PR was greater than 50% of the sum of the products of the diameters of measured lesions and lasted more than 6 weeks. There could not be a simultaneous increase in size of any other lesions or appearance of new localizations if a PR was diagnosed. Minor responses were also noted, which included regressions between 50% and 30% in objectively measurable lesions.[10,24]

Only the patients with platelet counts superior to 15×10^4 per mm^3, with more than 25×10^2 polymorphonuclears per mm^3 and more than 11 g hemoglobin per 100 ml were considered suitable for the evaluation of hematological toxicity. Thrombocytopenia was considered as significant when the platelet count was less than $10^5/mm^3$, and severe when it was below $5.10^4/mm$; anemia was considered as significant when the hemoglobin level was less than 10 g/100 ml, and neutropenia when the number of polymorphs was below to $15 \times 10^2/mm^3$.

Since RFCNU is not a water-soluble compound, it was given orally. The conduct of the trial was as follows: the patients were treated for 2 days per month. A hematological control was performed the first day. A phase I trial[12] indicated that the optimal dose was between 300–350 mg/m^2/month, which was also the dose designated in preclinical, systematic toxicity study in baboons.[17] We started the phase II trial at this dose and when tolerance was good we further escalated it to 500–600 mg/m²/month in a few patients, and to a maximum of 750 mg/m²/month in one case. Patients with previous bone marrow insufficiency were given less than 200 mg/m²/month. Treatment was delayed when platelets were below 50,000/mm³ and/or granulocytes less than 1,500/mm³ the day before the cycle. It never had to be interrupted for other side effects.

Results

As seen in Table 1, we obtained eight objective responses (14%). Three complete responses were obtained (one of a pancreatic carcinoma with metastasis in the liver, one of an adenocarcinoma of unknown origin with metastases in the liver, and one with a similar tumor, metastatic to the lung). Five partial remissions were also recorded (Table 1). In addition, eight minor responses were found. The disease progressed despite treatment in 41 patients.

The characteristics of the responding patients are: four patients with liver metastases (2 CR), three patients with lung metastasis (1 CR), and one rectal tumor. The median duration of the response was 9 months with a range of 2–44+ months. The lowest effective dose was 275 mg/m² per cycle. There is no clear correlation between the dose administered and the antitumor effect.

TOXICITY

Eight patients (14%) had nausea and/or vomiting. Of 50 patients, 2% had anemia, 4% had neutropenia, 18% had platelets under 100,000/mm³, and 6% below 50,000/mm³. This toxicity was not directly related to the number of cycles administered, but it was directly correlated with prior treatment. No severe hematologic toxicity was thus observed among the 32 previously untreated patients. Severe thrombocytopenia occurred only in those patients previously given chemotherapy. One patient, previously treated with RPCNU, died of thrombocytopenia.

Discussion

The remission rate observed with RFCNU in this trial (14%), is comparable to that reported for BCNU (13%),[1] CCNU (7%),[22] and MeCCNU (11%).[23] Liver and lung metastases seem to be sensitive

TABLE 1.   Therapeutic Activity of RFCNU on Digestive Tract (DT) Tumors and Tumors of Unknown Origin

Diagnosis Primary Tumor		No. of Patients	Major Responses[a]		Minor Responses[b]	Progressive Disease
			CR	PR		
Colorectal		2	—	1	1	—
		7	—	—	1	6
	Liver metas	18	—	—	2	16
	Lung metastases	5	—	2	—	3
Pancreas		6	1	—	—	5
Gall bladder		1	—	—	—	1
Liver		1	—	—	1	—
Esophagus		1	—	—	—	1
Stomach		3	—	—	1	2
Unknown	Adenocarcinoma	10	2	1	1	6
	Undifferentiated carcinoma	3	—	1	1	1
Total		57	3	5	8	41

(Colorectal group total: 32)

,[a]>50% according to WHO/EORTC/NCI Report.[24]
[b]<50%.

targets — four major regressions in 15 patients with liver metastases and three major regressions in six patients with lung metastases. The length of some remissions should be noted — the median duration was 9 months, with one CR lasting more than 44 months.

The toxicity of RFCNU was moderate, which made it easier to use, in our experience, than any classical analog.[1,13,22,23] Moreover, we observed only 14% digestive side effect (nausea and vomiting) compared to 55% reported for CCNU[22] and 58% for MeCCNU.[23] We saw anemia in only 2% of the patients, and severe neutropenia in 4%. RFCNU appears to be less toxic for neutrophils than BCNU, CCNU, and MeCCNU,[1,22,23] but this can only be objectively examined in a controlled comparative trial. Finally, severe thrombocytopenia was found in 18% of patients with RFCNU versus 66–68% for BCNU, 59% for CCNU, and 47–62% for MeCCNU.[1,22,23] Platelet counts below 50,000/mm^3 were found in 6% of patients treated with RFCNU, compared to 41% with BCNU, 28% with CCNU, and 28% with MeCCNU.[1,22,23] One patient remained in CR for 3½ years on RFCNU. In one patient, a dose of 750 mg/m^2 did not result in severe toxicity; platelet counts remained over 100,000/mm^3.

The hematologic toxicity of RFCNU appears not to be correlative with the number of cycles administered. Cumulative bone marrow toxicity is not evident, as is the case for the first generation of NU, despite the fact that 18 of the RFCNU patients had previously been submitted to chemotherapy. Six had received NU analog(s). Thus RFCNU appears to be less hematotoxic and especially less thrombocytotoxic than BCNU, CCNU, and MeCCNU.

In conclusion, this phase II trial suggests that RFCNU is an active drug in colorectal tumors and metastatic carcinomas of unknown origin, with response rates similar to those of classical NU analogs.[1,12,22,23] In addition, a number of minor regressions have been documented. The dose-limiting toxicity appears to be late bone marrow depression. This toxicity is not strictly dose-dependent, possibly because of incomplete and variable absorption of RFCNU from the digestive tract. This possibility will require future pharmacokinetic studies. Furthermore, the drug is probably rapidly hydrolysed at the acidic pH of gastric juice. The unsubstituted ribosylchloroethyl nitrosourea[8] is thus set free.

ACKNOWLEDGMENT

This work has been conducted at the Fondation Simone et Cino del Duca, and in the framework of the French–American Agreement INSERM-NCI.

REFERENCES

1. Carter, S.K.: *Cancer Chemother Rep 4(3): 35, 1973.*
2. Clarysse, A., Kenis, Y., and Mathé, G.: *Cancer Chemotherapy: Its Role in the Treatment Strategy of Hematologic Malignancies and Solid Tumors.* Springer-Verlag, Heidelberg, New York, 1976.
3. Florentin, I., Hayat, P., Kiger, N., Maral, J., Imbach, J.L., and Mathé, G.: *Internat J Immunopharmacol (in press).*
4. Hayat, M., Bourut, C., Chenu, E., Montero, J.L., Imbach, J.L., MacDonald, J.S., and Mathé G.: *Cancer Chemother Pharmacol 3: 217, 1979.*
5. Imbach, J.L., Montero, J.L., Moruzzi, A., Serrou, B., Chenu, E., Hayat, M., and Mathé, G.: *Biomedicine 23: 410, 1975.*
6. Jasmin, C., Mori, K.J., Hayat, M., MacDonald, J.S., and Mathé, G.: *Nitrosoureas in Cancer Treatment.* B. Serrou, P.S. Schein, and J.L. Imbach, Eds., Elsevier-North Holland, Amsterdam, 1981, p. 193.
7. Johnston, T.P., MacCaleb, G.S., and Montgomery, J.A.: *J Med Chem 18: 104, 1975.*
8. Lemoine, R. and Gouyette, A.: *Cancer Treat Rep 63: 1335, 1979.*
9. Marzin, D., Jasmin, C., Imbach, J.L., and Mathé, G.: In *Nitrosoureas in Cancer Treatment.* B. Serrou, P.S. Schein, and J.L. Imbach, Eds., Elsevier-North Holland, Amsterdam, 1981, p. 165.
10. Mathé, G.: *Cancer Chemother Pharmacol (submitted for publication).*
11. Mathé, G. and Jasmin, C.: *Cancer Chemother Pharmacol 3: 203, 1973.*
12. Mathé, G., Serrou, B., Hayat, M., De Vassal, F., Misset, J.L., Schwarzenberg, L., Machover, D., Ribaud, P., Belpomme, D., Jasmin, C., Musset, M., Montero, J.L., and Imbach, J.L.: *Biomedecine 27: 294, 1977.*
13. Moertel, C.H.: *Cancer Chemother Rep 4(3): 27, 1973.*

14. Montero, J.L. and Imbach, J.L.: CR *Acad Sci 279: 809, 1974.*

15. Montero, J.L., Moruzzi, A., Oiry, J., and Imbach, J.L.: *Eur J Med Chem 12: 397, 1977.*

16. Mori, K.J., Jasmin, C., Hayat, M., MacDonald, J.S., and Mathé, G.: *Cancer Res 40: 4282, 1980.*

17. Ribaud, P., Garcia-Giralt, E., Razafimahaleo, E., Vu Choang, C., MacDonald, J.S., Schein, P., and Mathé, G.: *Biomed Pharmacother (in press).*

18. Schein, P.: Personal communication.

19. Schein, P.S., McMenamin, M.G., and Anderson, T.: *Cancer Res 23: 2005, 1978.*

20. Serrou, B., Imbach, J.L., Hayat, M., Mathé, G., and Macieira-Coelho, A.: *Proc Am Assoc Cancer Res 18: 223, 1977.* (Abstract 892).

21. Vlaeminck, M.N., Collyn, M., D'Hooghe, M., Cappelaere, P., Biserte, G., Oiry, J., Montero, J.L., and Imbach, J.L.: *Biomedicine 35: 27, 1981.*

22. Wasserman, T.H., Slavik, M., and Carter, S.K.: *Cancer Treat Rev 1: 131, 1974.*

23. Wasserman, T.H., Slavik, M., and Carter, S.K.: *Cancer Treat Rev 1: 251, 1974.*

24. WHO/EORTC/NCI *Cancer 1982 (in press).*

CHAPTER 3

Phase II Study of Chlorozotocin

G. Mathé,[a] P. Schein,[b] J.S. MacDonald,[c] T. Hercend,[a] J.L. Misset,[a]
P. Ribaud,[a] J. Gouveia,[a] F. De Vassal,[a] D. Machover,[a]
M. Musset,[a] J. Gastiaburu,[a] H. Tapiero,[a] and R. Maral[a]

Introduction

Three nitrosourea (NU) analogs, BCNU, CCNU, and methyl-CCNU[2] are used in clinical cancer chemotherapy. While therapeutic activity has been recorded for digestive tract and brain tumors,[2] the responses are often not clinically meaningful. Moreover, these agents produced serious and accumulative delayed bone marrow toxicity, which limits their usefulness.[13] Based upon the structure–activity analysis of Schein and colleagues,[18] Johnson et al.[10] synthesized a glycosyl analog, chlorozotocin (CZT), 3-(2-chloroethyl) 3-nitroso 1-(D$_2$-glucopyranosyl) urea, which appeared experimentally remarkable for its relatively low bone marrow toxicity.[18]

Two other sugar analogs, RFCNU and RPCNU, were synthesized by Montero et al.,[14] and we compared them to CZT. CZT was less active against specific murine solid tumors.[4] However, it was less toxic for bone marrow CFU-s. It was found to have the same toxicity as RFCNU for CFU-c — which action is stronger than that of RPCNU in acute hematotoxicity tests.[15] In a study of chronic hematotoxicity, CZT and RFCNU appeared less toxic than RPCNU.[9] As far as the effect on immunological reactions, RPCNU only exerted a slight immunodepressive effect, while CZT potentiated delayed type hypersensitivity when administered before the antigen, and increased K-cell activity when injected simultaneously.[3] Finally, CZT is as mutagenic as RFCNU and RPCNU.[12]

Patients and Methods

We report in this paper the results of an oriented phase II trial concerning patients with colorectal carcinomas (25 cases), melanomas (18), sarcomas of soft tissues (14) and bones (3).

A second group of patients received the same protocol for other solid tumors (six of the bronchus, five of the breast, four of the ovary, two of the cavum, and 11 of various origin — 1 per site).

All were in an advanced metastatic stage of their disease, presented with metastasis (Table 1), and had been previously submitted to chemotherapy, to which they were resistant.

All these patients received CZT at a dose of 120–150 mg/m^2 I.V. each month, accord-

[a]Institut de Cancérologie et d'Immunogénétique (INSERM U-50, CNRS LA-149), Hôpital Paul-Brousse; Unité de Pharmacologie Humaine Simone et Cino Del Duca, Villejuif, France
[b]Vincent T. Lombardi Cancer Research Center, Georgetown University, Washington, D.C., in the framework of the French–American Agreement INSERM-NCI
[c]Cancer Treatment Evaluation, Division of Cancer Treatment, National Institutes of Health, Bethesda, Maryland.

TABLE 1.   Chlorozotocin — Results in Advanced Solid Tumors

Diagnosis	Sites of Targets (Metastases)	Number of Patients	Remissions Complete	Partial ≥50%	Local-ization	Responses <50%	Failure (Progressive Disease and Stabili-zation)
Colo-rectum	Liver–Lung	25		1	Lung	4	20
Melanoma	Skin–Lung	18			—	6	12
Soft tissue sarcoma	Lung–Liver	14/17			Lung–Pleural	4	9
Total		57	0	<2%		14/57	41

Age: range 4–75 years (mean 47 years); sex: F, 38 — M, 50.

ing to Hoth's and Schein's phase I study.[7] Monthly administrations, the number of which varied from two to six, were repeated until toxicity appeared. The evaluation of the results was done according to WHO-EORTC-NCI Panel recommendation[21] for lesion evaluation and treatment toxicities.

Our classification of the results considers the three following types: 1) apparently complete remission (CR); 2) partial regression (PR) superior to 50% of the target volumes; 3) minor regression less than 50% (MR), and stabilization (ST), which is not considered as failure when the perceptible doubling time (DT), studied before the trial, is short enough to be evaluated; if not, it is included in 3) or failure, either expressed by progressive disease or by stabilization of a DT which is so long that it could not be measured before the trial.

Results

ANTITUMOR ACTION

The results are presented in Table 1: of 25 colorectal adenocarcinoma patients, one subject with pulmonary metastasis achieve a PR; three patients had a stabilization of disease, and one a response <50%; of 18 patients with melanoma, there were only six cases with MR; none of the 17 patients with sarcomas responded, but four had a MR.

TOLERANCE

Clinical toxicity was evaluated in 75 treatments (Table 2). Digestive intolerance (nausea and vomiting) was noted in 8%. Hematological toxicity was observed in three treatments. The main manifestation was thrombocytopenia. Except in one case in which it was due to long administration, the thrombocytopenia was reversible. It should be emphasized that no renal toxicity was observed.

Discussion

The results of this phase II study do not differ from those of other trials of the literature involving patients with colorectal cancers,[1,11] sarcomas,[16,19] and melanomas.[8]

With regard to melanoma, our results (five stabilizations out of 18 patients and one PR) are identical to those of Houghton et al.,[8] but differ from those of Hoth et al.[5] who, with a dose of 120 mg/m²/6w, obtained one CR and four PR out of 35 patients, and from those of Van Amburg

TABLE 2.   Toxicity of Chlorozotocin — N = 85

Hematologic	75
Anemia (≤10 g)	6
Neutropenia (≤1500/mm³)	4
Thrombocytopenia	21
51–100.000/mm³	16
≤50.000/mm³	5
Digestive (nausea, vomiting)	7
Mucosal ulceration	1

et al.[20] who, with the dose of 150 mg/m^2/ 6w, registered three CR in 10 previously untreated patients, and one PR in 28 previously untreated subjects. The poorer results we have obtained may be due to the fact that our subjects had been previously submitted to chemotherapy.

We were first tempted to explain these results by the relatively small dose of 120–150 mg/m^2/m indicated for phase II studies by the Hoth, Schein, et al. phase I trial.[6-7] Our clinical and biological study in baboons showed that 120 mg/m^2/m were perfectly tolerated. We tried to give 380 mg/m^2/m; it was also tolerated for three cycles.[17] We administered this dose weekly in the case of neoplasias spontaneously complicated by bone marrow insufficiency (such as acute leukemia) and we have already registered three CRs out of four patients. This study, the results of which are promising, is in progress.

ACKNOWLEDGMENT

This work was conducted at the Foundation Simone et Cino del Duca, and in the framework of the French–American Agreement INSERM-NCI.

REFERENCES

1. Bleiberg, H., Rozencweig, M., Michel, J., Clavel, M., Longeval, E., Feremans, W., Bondue, H., Lardinois, J., Crespeigne, N., and Kenis, Y.: In UICC Conference on Clinical Oncology and 7th Annual Meeting of the European Society for Medical Oncology, Lausanne, October 1981 (Abstract 05-0079).
2. Carter, S.K.: Cancer Chemother Rep 4(3): 35, 1973.
3. Florentin, I., Hayat, M., Kiger, N., Maral, J., Imbach, J.L., and Mathé, G.: Internat J Immunopharmacol (in press).
4. Hayat, M., Bourut, C., Chenu, E., Montero, J.L., Imbach, J.L., MacDonald, J.S., and Mathé, G.: Cancer Chemother Pharmacol 3: 217, 1979.
5. Hoth, D.F., Schein, P.S., Winokur, S., Wooley, P.V., Robichaud, K., Binder, R.G., and Smith, F.P.: Cancer 46: 1544, 1980.
6. Hoth, D.F., Schein, P., MacDonald, J., Buscaglia, D., and Hallen, D.: Proc Amer Assoc Cancer Res 18: 302 (Abstract C-169), 1977.
7. Hoth, D., Woolley, P.V., Green, D., MacDonald, J., and Schein, P.S.: Clin Pharmacol Ther 23: 712, 1978.
8. Houghton, A.N., Camacho, J., Gralla, R.J., and Wittes, R.: Cancer Treat Rep 65: 705, 1981.
9. Jasmin, C., Mori, K.J., Hayat, M., MacDonald, J.S., and Mathé, G.: In Nitrosourea in Cancer Treatment. B. Serrou, P.S. Schein, and J.L. Imbach, Eds., Elsevier-North Holland, Amsterdam, 1981, p. 193.
10. Johnston, T.P., MacCalbe, G.S., and Montgomery, J.A.: J Med Chem 18: 104, 1975.
11. Lawton, J.O., Gilles, G.R., Hall, J., MacAdam, A., Hall, R., Matheson, T., and Bird, G.: Cancer Treat Rep 65: 13, 1981.
12. Marzin, D., Jasmin, C., Imbach, J.L., and Mathé, G.: In Nitrosoureas in Cancer Treatment. B. Serrou, P.S. Schein, and J.L. Imbach, Eds., Elsevier-North Holland, Amsterdam, 1981, 165.
13. Moertel, C.H.: Cancer Chemother Rep 4(3): 27, 1973.
14. Montero, J.L., Moruzzi, A., Oiry, J., and Imbach, J.L.: Europ J Med Chem 12: 397, 1977.
15. Mori, K.J., Jasmin, C., Hayat, M., MacDonald, J.S., and Mathé, G.: Cancer Res 40: 4282, 1980.
16. Mouridsen, H.T., Bramwell, V.H.C., Lacave, J., Metz, R., Vendrick, C., Hild, J., McCreanney, J., and Sylvester, R.: Cancer Treat Rep 65: 509, 1981.
17. Ribaud, P., Garcia-Giralt, E., Razafimahaleo, E., Vu Hoang, C., MacDonald, J.S., Schein, P.S., and Mathé, G.: Biomed Pharmacother (in press) 1983.
18. Schein, P.S., McMenamin, M.G., and Anderson, T.: Cancer Res 33: 2005, 1978.
19. Sordillo, P.P., Magill, G.B., and Gralla, R.J.: Cancer Treat Rep 65: 513, 1981.
20. Van Amburg, A., Ratkin, G., and Washington, U.: Proc Am Soc Clin Oncol 21: 354, 1980. (Abstract C-137)
21. WHO/EORTC/N.C.I.: Cancer 1982 (in press).

CHAPTER 4

Cellular Uptake and Metabolism of a New Chloroethyl Nitrosourea Compound (CNCC): Relationship with the Cytotoxic Effect on Human Lymphoid Cells

J.J. Farhi, M. Bennoun, G. Willoquet, and H. Tapiero

Introduction

Nitrosoureas are decomposed under physiological conditions in alkylating and carbamoylating moieties.[5,7,11] Although alkylation of nucleic acids and protein[3,10,11] and carbamoylation of protein[1,4,13] have been demonstrated, the relationship between these two activities and cytotoxicity is still unclear.[2,9,12] In the present study, we assumed that the cytotoxic effect of nitrosoureas is related to their cellular uptake and their affinity for intracellular targets. Those parameters were analyzed with a new chloroethyl nitrosourea compound, di (chloro-2-ethyl)-2 N-nitroso N carbamoyl N,N-cystamine (CNCC) and with its related isomers.[6,8]

Materials and Methods

CELL CULTURE

Namalva cells (a human lymphoblastoid B cell line) were grown in RPMI 1640 medium supplemented with 10% fetal calf serum, 10 mM glutamin, and 20 μg gentamycin per ml. Cell viability was determined by counting on a hemacytometer the cells excluding 0.1% trypan blue.

DRUGS

CNCC and its related isomers were provided by Pr. J.L. Imbach and by Roger Bellon Laboratories (Paris, France). The purity, as well as the concentration of drug used in experimental procedures, was controlled by HPLC.

CELL LABELING

Cells ($0.4.10^6$ per ml) treated or not with drug for different times were 20 minutes pulse-labeled with 2 μCi/ml of tritiated thymidine (Sp. Act.: 50 Ci/mmol), 2 μCi/ml of tritiated uridine (Sp. Act.: 50 mCi/mmol) and 0.5 μCi/ml of (14_C) protein hydrolysate (Sp. Act.: 50 mCi/milliatom carbon). The amount of incorporated radioactive compound was determined by TCA precipitation and by counting in a liquid scintillation counter.

High Pressure Liquid Chromatography (HPLC)

CNCC and related isomers were diluted in the mobile phase: isooctane, dichloro-

Département de Pharmacologie Cellulaire et Moléculaire et de Pharmacocinétique, Unité Simone et Cino Del Duca de Pharmacologie Humaine des Cancers, Institut de Cancérologie et d'Immunogénétique (INSERM U-50), Hôpital Paul-Brousse, Villejuif, France

methane, methanol (79.8, 18.7, 1.5, v/v); eluted on a radial pak silica column using a Waters HPLC model and detected by U.V. absorption at a wavelength of 245 nm. In those conditions, the retention time of M, S, and C were respectively 6.23, 6.80, and 7.26 minutes.

Results and Discussion

CNCC is a mixture of three isomers which differ in the position of the two nitroso groups, and have a different retention time in an HPLC column. CNCC is composed of 51% of the isomer S (the two nitroso groups located on the cystamine side), 1% of the isomer C (nitroso groups on the chloroethyl end), and 48% of the isomer M (one nitroso group on each side of the molecule).

To study the cytotoxic activity and the inhibiting effect of these compounds on DNA, RNA, and protein synthesis, cells were exposed to different concentrations of CNCC at 37°C for various time periods. They were then washed, resuspended in a growth medium without drug and allowed to grow 3 and 6 days in order to determine the cytostatic and the cytotoxic effect. The relative cytostatic effect was related to the time of incubation and to the drug concentration. When cells were exposed to 20 and 40 μg CNCC per ml, this effect was respectively obtained in 15 and 5 minutes. The cytotoxic effect was obtained after 120 and 15 minutes with these respective concentrations (Table 1).

In presence of 20 μg CNCC per ml, only 40% of RNA synthesis was inhibited, whereas about 80% of DNA synthesis and 90% of protein synthesis was inhibited after 20 minutes of incubation. Moreover, the inhibition of RNA synthesis was reversed after the first 20 minutes. We therefore conclude that CNCC mainly inhibits DNA and protein synthesis. Its effect on RNA synthesis can be attributed to the differential inhibiting activity of the isomers and/or to the related metabolites

TABLE 1.   Relationship between Uptake and the Cytotoxic Effect of the Di(chloro-2-ethyl)-2N nitroso-N-carbamoyl N,N-cystamine (CNCC)

CNCC (μg/ml)	Time of Incubation (Minutes)	Number of Viable Cells ($\times 10^6$)	
		3 Days	6 Days
20	0	2.6	4.1
	5	1.6	3.4
	10	0.8	2.8
	15	0.6	2.2
	30	0.2	1.3
	120	0.2	0.2
40	0	2.6	4.1
	5	0.5	2.0
	10	0.4	1.3
	15	0.2	0
	30	0.1	0
	120	0.1	0

Exponentially growing Namalva cells were exposed to 20 and 40 μg CNCC per ml at 37°C. After different times of incubation, cells were centrifuged, washed, and the last pellet was resuspended in growth medium and incubated in a CO_2 incubator for 3 and 6 days. Viable cells were counted as described in Materials and Methods.

(unpublished data). These metabolites were obtained by incubating CNCC at 37°C in medium containing 10% fetal calf serum.

After different times of incubation, cells were seeded and grown for 4 days. The level of CNCC degradation was followed by U.V. absorption after HPLC elution. The amount of drug in the growth medium decreased progressively according to the time of incubation. This decrease was also related to a loss of the cytotoxicity. In presence of 20 μg CNCC per ml, the cytotoxic effect could not be observed after 45 minutes (Fig. 1). We suggest, therefore, that CNCC is decomposed in inactive metabolites. Uptake of intact drug is probably the first limiting step for cytotoxicity.

The effect of the isomers on DNA, RNA and protein synthesis was different, S being the most active. The isomers S, C, and M have about the same alkylating and carbamoylating activities (K. Tew, personal communication). The drug activity is probably determined by the position of

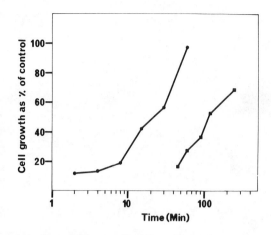

FIGURE 1. The cytotoxic effect of CNCC preincubated in growth medium. CNCC at 20 μg per ml (●———●) and 40 μg per ml (■———■) was incubated in growth medium at 37°C at indicated times. Exponentially growing cells were resuspended in these drug-containing media and allowed to grow for 4 days. Viable cells were counted as described in Materials and Methods.

the nitroso groups and not by the alkylating and carbamoylating properties.

ACKNOWLEDGMENTS

We are indebted to Professor G. Mathé, Nicole Vriz, and Roger Bellon Laboratories for their help. This work was supported by contracts INSERM, CNRS, and ADRC.

REFERENCES

1. Baril, B.E., Baril, E.F., Laszlo, J., and Wheeler, G.P.: Inhibition of rat liver DNA polymerase by nitrosoureas and isocyanates. *Cancer Res 35: 1–5, 1975.*

2. Bray, D.A., De Vita, V.T., Adamson, R.H., and Oliverio, V.T.: Effects of 1-(2-chloroethyl)-3-cyclohexyl-1-nitrosourea (CCNU NSC-79037) and its degradation products on progression of L1210 cells through the cell cycle. *Cancer Chemother Rep 55: 215–220, 1971.*

3. Cheng, C.J., Fujimura, S., Grumberger, D., and Weinstein, I.B.: Interaction of 1-(2-chloroethyl)-3-cyclohexyl-1-nitrosourea (NSC-79037) with nucleic acids and proteins in vivo and in vitro *Cancer Res 32: 22–27, 1972.*

4. Chuang, R.Y., Laszlo, J., and Keller, P.: Effects of nitrosoureas on human DNA polymerase activities from acute and chronic granulocytic leukemia cells. *Biochim Biophys Acta 425: 453–468, 1976.*

5. Colvin, M., Brundhett, R.B., Cowens, W., Jardin, I., and Ludlum, D.B.: A chemical basis for the antitumor activity of chloroethyl-nitrosoureas. *Biochem Pharmacol 25: 695–699, 1976.*

6. Imbach, J.L., Martinez, J., Oiry, J., Bourut, C., Chenu, E., Maral, R., and Mathé, G.: New nitrosourea derivatives and related compounds. In *Nitrosoureas in Cancer Treatment* INSERM Symposium 19, B. Serrou and J.L. Imbach, Eds., Elsevier/North Holland Biomedical Press, Amsterdam, 1981, pp. 123–137.

7. Montgomery, J.A., James R., McCaleb, G.S., Kirk, M.C., and Johnston, T.P.: Decomposition of N-(2-chloroethyl)-N-nitrosourea in aqueous media. *J. Med Chem 18: 568–571, 1975.*

8. Oiry, J. and Imbach, J.L.: CNCC: *bis* (2-chloroethyl)-N-nitroso-N carbamoyl cystamine *(in preparation).*

9. Panasci, L.C., Green, D.C., Nagourney, R., Fox, P., and Schein, P.S.: A structure activity analysis of chemical and biological parameters of chloroethyl nitrosoureas in mice. *Cancer Res 37: 2615–2618, 1977.*

10. Schmall, B., Cheng, C.J., Fujimura, S., Gersten, N., Grunberger, D., and Weinstein, I.B.: Modification of proteins by 1-(2-chloroethyl)-3-cyclohexyl-1-nitrosourea (NSC 79037) in vitro. *Cancer Res 33: 1921–1924, 1973.*

11. Wheeler, G.P. and Chumley, S.: Alkylating activity of 1,3-bis (2-chloroethyl-1-nitrosourea and related compounds. *J Med Chem 10: 259–261, 1967.*

12. Wheeler, G.P., Bowdon, B.J., Grimsley, J., and Lloyd, H.H.: Interrelationships of some chemical, physicochemical and biological activities of several 1-(2-haloethyl)-1-nitrosoureas. *Cancer Res 34: 194–200, 1974.*

13. Woolley, P.V., Dion, R.L., Kohn, K.W., and Bono, V.H.: Binding of 1-(2-chloroethyl)-3-cyclohexyl-1-nitrosourea to L1210 cell nuclear proteins. *Cancer Res 36: 1470–1474, 1976.*

CHAPTER 5

Studies on *Cis*-dichloro-*trans*-dihydroxy-*bis*-isopropylamine Platinum IV (CHIP): A Second Generation Platinum-Containing Complex

J.W. Cowens,[a] L. Pendyala,[b] and P.J. Creaven[b]

Introduction

Pt-containing complexes are an important class of antineoplastic compounds because cisplatin, the prototype compound of this class, is active against several solid tumors (bladder, prostate, and ovarian carcinoma) which are not responsive to other agents, and is curative when used in combination with vinblastine and bleomycin in the treatment of nonseminomatous tumors of the testis. However, the clinical usefulness of cisplatin is limited by its acute and chronic nephrotoxicity. Therefore, it is important to identify second-generation Pt-containing complexes that retain the antitumor activity of cisplatin but do not cause impairment of renal function.

Cis-dichloro-*trans*-dihydroxy-*bis*-isopropylamine Pt (CHIP), synthesized by Tobe of Johnson Matthey Co., is a quadrivalent Pt complex, five times more water soluble than cisplatin. In the preliminary antitumor and toxicological screening carried out by Connors[3] and Cleare et al.,[2] it showed antitumor activity with no nephrotoxicity. Because of these findings, CHIP underwent extensive preclinical toxicological and pharmacological evaluation in the Department of Experimental Therapeutics (Grace Cancer Drug Center, GCDC) at Roswell Park Memorial Institute, and has been entered into phase I clinical trial. This paper will give a brief overview of the preclinical and the initial clinical studies of CHIP.

Preclinical Antitumor Activity Studies

In its initial screening, CHIP showed activity against ADJ/PC6 plasmacytoma in BALB/C mice with a therapeutic index of 12.0.[3] Subsequent studies reported by Cleare et al.[2] demonstrated that CHIP was active against leukemia L1210, Lewis lung carcinoma (LL), and B16 melanoma in BDF$_1$ mice. Their findings were confirmed by Prestayko et al.[13] and Bradner et al.[1] who showed that CHIP had activity against L1210 and LL comparable to that of cisplatin when administered on a single dose or multiple dose (daily ×9) schedule; CHIP was less active than cisplatin against B16 melanoma, however. At the GCDC, the antitumor activity of CHIP and cisplatin were compared by administering equitoxic doses to tumor bearing animals; CHIP was shown to give a greater increase in life-span than cisplatin when administered to DBA/2HADD mice bearing L1210

The Departments of Experimental Therapeutics[a] and Clinical Pharmacology and Therapeutics[b], Roswell Park Memorial Institute, New York State Department of Health, Buffalo, New York

and to be more effective than cisplatin in inhibiting the growth of Walker carcinosarcoma.[6] At equitoxic doses both drugs inhibited Murphy-Sturm Lymphosarcoma to the same extent.[6]

Preclinical Toxicology Studies

The LD_{50} for CHIP when administered as a single intravenous (I.V.) dose in the rat and the dog is 250 mg/m², which is five times the LD_{50} of cisplatin.[7] When 50% of the LD_{50} dose was administered intraperitoneally to rats, CHIP produced bone marrow and GI toxicity with no renal toxicity. When a daily ×5 regimen was used, the results were similar.[7] When an LD_{50} dose was administered intravenously to dogs as a single dose, CHIP produced leukopenia and thrombocytopenia with no change in renal function; renal and hepatic function changes were noted only when twice the LD_{50} dose was administered.[6] In monkeys, both toxicological and histopathological studies indicated that renal and hepatic functional alterations occurred in addition to bone marrow aplasia at lethal doses (40 mg/kg).[6]

Preclinical Pharmacokinetic Studies

STUDIES IN THE RAT

Comparative studies of the pharmacokinetics of total Pt after CHIP and cisplatin administration were performed using flameless atomic absorption spectrophotometry (FAAS). The plasma decay was biphasic for both compounds; however, the elimination phase $t_{\frac{1}{2}}$ was 69 hours for cisplatin and 14 hours for CHIP.[4] The excretion of both compounds in the urine reached a plateau at 24 hours; the percent of total dose excreted at 24 hours was 43% for cisplatin and 53% for CHIP. The concentration of Pt in the kidney also showed biexponential decay; however, the elimination phase $t_{\frac{1}{2}}$ was similar for both compounds.

STUDIES IN THE DOG

Pharmacokinetic studies of total Pt and unchanged CHIP were carried out in the dog after an I.V. bolus of 10 mg/kg.[8] Total Pt studies were performed FAAS; the unchanged drug studies were carried out on urine samples by thin layer chromatography and high-performance liquid chromatography (HPLC) in conjunction with FAAS. The plasma half-life of Pt in the dog was calculated based on the urinary excretion rates.

Both chromatographic procedures indicated a monoexponential decay for unchanged CHIP in the dog with a $t_{\frac{1}{2}}$ of 0.3–0.5 hours. Total Pt, however, conformed to a biexponential decay with a $t_{\frac{1}{2}}\alpha$ of 0.6 hours and a $t_{\frac{1}{2}}\beta$ of 39.4 hours; the β-phase of the plasma decay thus appears to be due to the retention of metabolites. The excretion of Pt containing complexes reached a plateau at 24 hours; the percent of the total dose excreted was variable and ranged from 45–72%. The Pt-containing complexes in urine were separated by HPLC, and it could be shown that the urine contained two metabolites more polar than CHIP.

Phase I Study

Thirty patients with a microscopic diagnosis of cancer who had failed conventional treatment and who had given informed consent were entered into the phase I study.[5] CHIP was administered by a 2-hour infusion preceded by hydration with two L of 0.5 N saline in 12 hours but without diuresis or posttreatment hydration. The initial dose was 20 mg/m² (1/12th of the LD_{50} in the rat and dog). Nausea and vomiting lasting 24 hours was seen in all patients. At the maximum tolerated dose (350 mg/m²), leukopenia and thrombocytopenia were seen in 6/7 patients; the dose-limiting toxicity was thrombocytopenia, which was prolonged. Creatinine clearance measured before and after each course of CHIP showed no evidence of renal impairment (Table 1). Five of the seven patients at this dose received no pretreatment hydration. In order to determine whether the patients suffered subclinical renal toxicity, two urinary enzymes β-glucuronidase (BGA) and leucine aminopeptidase (LAP), were monitored. From a concurrent study with cisplatin, LAP proved to be the more sensitive indicator of renal damage. In this study, a clinically nontoxic dose of cisplatin (40 mg/m²) produced significantly greater increases in urinary LAP than toxic dose of CHIP (350 mg/m²).[9] No tumor responses were seen in this group of patients, most of whom had tumor types which are not responsive to cisplatin.

Clinical Pharmacokinetic Studies

Pharmacokinetic studies of total Pt, filterable Pt (FP) (nonprotein bound Pt) and unchanged CHIP were carried out in the plasma of patients treated during the phase I trial.[10] Pharmacokinetic studies were done at all dose levels; total Pt measurements were done by FAAS, filterable Pt by FAAS after centrifugal ultrafiltration, and CHIP by FAAS after HPLC separation. At all doses studied, the plasma decay of total Pt was biphasic ($t_{\frac{1}{2}}\alpha$ 0.4–2.2 hours; $t_{\frac{1}{2}}\beta$ 47–103 hours). However, the plasma decay of filterable Pt was monoexponential at doses less than 120 mg/m² ($t_{\frac{1}{2}}$ 0.8–1.7 hours) and biphasic at doses greater than 120 mg/m² ($t_{\frac{1}{2}}\alpha$ 0.4–2 hours; $t_{\frac{1}{2}}\beta$ >24 hours). CHIP at all doses showed a monoexponential decay with $t_{\frac{1}{2}}$ ranging from 0.7–1.3 hours. Urinary excretion of Pt was variable and ranged from 15–61% at 24 hours and 16.5–63% at 48 hours. HPLC separation of CHIP and metabolites in plasma and urine indicated the presence of at least two metabolites in plasma and five in urine (Fig. 1). One of the less polar metabolites, present both in plasma and urine, had similar chromatographic properties to cis-dichloro-bis-isopropylamine Pt (II) and co-chromatographs with it.[11]

Conclusion

CHIP is a quadrivalent second generation platinum complex presently undergoing clinical evaluation. In the phase I study, the dose-limiting toxicity was myelosuppression, especially prolonged thrombocytopenia. Pharmacokinetic studies showed that the decay of unchanged CHIP in plasma was monoexponential while that of total Pt was biexponential with a long β-phase half-life; this indicates that CHIP metabolites are retained. Because of its low potential for producing renal impairment at toxic doses in man, CHIP warrants further clinical study.

ACKNOWLEDGMENT

This work was supported in part by grants from the United States Public Health Service (CA-21071 and CA-13038) and from Bristol Laboratories, Syracuse, New York.

TABLE 1. Toxicity of CHIP — 350 mg/m²

Pt. No.[a]	WBC Nadir	Platelet Nadir	Serum Creatinine, mg/dl		Creatinine Clearance, ml/min	
			Pretreatment	Post-treatment[b]	Pretreatment	Post-treatment[b]
1	2,300	74,000	0.7	0.6	100	117
2	3,200	62,000	0.6	0.6	142	155
3	2,500	8,000	0.8	0.8	105	113
4	2,300	27,000	0.9	0.8	110	110
5	2,500	34,000	0.8	0.7	120	154
6	3,200	18,000	1.3	1.3	—	—

[a] Seven patients were entered at this dose. One who received one dose only and developed no toxicity except nausea and vomiting is not included in the table.
[b] At the time of the second treatment.

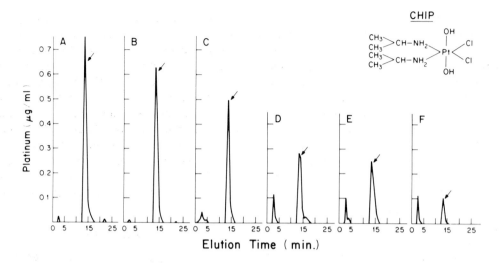

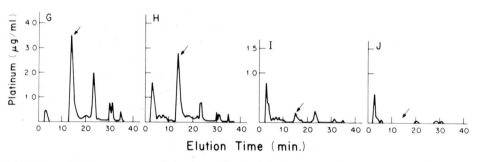

FIGURE 1. Platinum compounds in plasma (A–F) and urine (G–J) of a patient, at different times after administration of CHIP (120 mg/m^2). Plasma: A, mid infusion; B, end infusion; C, 5 minutes after infusion; D, 30 minutes after infusion; E, 60 minutes after infusion; F, 90 minutes after infusion. Urine: G, 0–4 hours after infusion; H, 4–8 hours after infusion; I, 8–16 hours after infusion; J, 16–24 hours after infusion (arrows indicate CHIP).

REFERENCES

1. Bradner, W.T., Rose, W.C., and Huftalen, J.B.: Prestayko, A.W., Crooke, S.T., and Carter, S.K., Eds., Academic Press, Inc., New York, 1980, pp. 171–182.
2. Cleare, M.J., Hydes, P.C., Malerbi, B.W., and Watkins, D.M.: *Biochimie 60: 835–850, 1978.*
3. Connors, T.A., Cleare, M.J., and Harrap, K.R.: *Cancer Treat Rep 63: 1499–1502, 1979.*
4. Creaven, P.J., and Mihich, E.: Mihich, E., Ed., *New Leads in Cancer Therapeutics.* G.K. Hall Medical Publishers, Boston, 1981, p. 1.
5. Creaven, P.J., Mittelman, A., Pendyala, L., Tseng, M., Pontes, E., Spaulding, M., Moyaeri, H., Madajewicz, S., Cowens, J.W., and Solomon, J.: *Proc Am Soc Clin Oncol 1: 22, 1982.*
6. Mihich, E., Bullard, G., Pavelic, Z., and Creaven, P.: *Proc Am Assoc Cancer Res Am Soc. Clin. Oncol. 20: 426, 1979.*

7. Mihich, E., and Bullard, G.A. Unpublished data.
8. Pendyala, L., Cowens, J.W., and Creaven, P.J.: *Cancer Treat Rep 66: 509–516, 1982.*
9. Pendyala, L., Cowens, J.W., Lele, S., Greco, W., and Creaven, P.J.: *Am Coll Clin Pharmacol 1982.*
10. Pendyala, L., Cowens, J.W., Mittelman, A., and Creaven, P.J.: *Proc Am Assoc Cancer Res 23: 127, 1982.*
11. Pendyala, L., Cowens, J.W., and Creaven, P.J.: *Thirteenth International Cancer Congress, 1982, (in press).*
12. Pfister, M., Pavelic, Z.P., Bullard, G.A., Mihich, E., and Creaven, P.J.: *Biochimie 60: 1057, 1978.*
13. Prestayko, A.W., Bradner, W.T., Huftalen, J.B., Rose, W.C., Schurig, J.E., Cleare, M.J., Hydes, P.C., and Crooke, S.T.: *Cancer Treat Rep 63: 1503–1508, 1979.*

CHAPTER 6

Cardiac and Skin Toxicity of Mitoxantrone in Comparison with Anthracyclines

D. Dantchev, M. Paintrand, C. Bourut, I. Pignot, R. Maral, and G. Mathé

Introduction

Mitoxantrone hydrochloride (MTX) is an anthracenedione compound with a potential antineoplastic effect as has been already demonstrated in experimental and also in clinical trials.[12,23,25,26] Using our golden hamster model, we submitted this new drug to the same electron microscopic (EM) study of cardiotoxicity and the same light microscopic (LM) study of skin toxicity that we employ for evaluation of these toxicities of different anthracyclines.[6-8] As previously reported, in a first trial we studied eight anthracyclines: adriamycin (ADM), detorubicin (DTR), daunorubicin (DNR), 4'-epi-adriamycin (e-ADM), rubidazone (RBZ), aclacinomycin (ACM), N-trifluoroacetyl-adriamycin-14-valerate (AD-32), and tetra-hydropyranyl-adriamycin (THP-ADM). In a second trial, MTX was studied as well as four other anthracyclines: N-L-leucyl-daunorubicin (l-DNR), carminomycin (CAM), rubicyclamin (RBC), and N-trifluoroacetyl-adriamycin-14-9-hemiadipate (AD-143). In this paper we report the results of this comparative study of the cardiotoxicity and skin toxicity of all studied drugs, according to our grading system and classification.

Institut de Cancérologie et d'Immunogénétique, Hôpital Paul-Brousse, 14 et 16, Villejuif, France

Materials and Methods

Twenty-four adult female golden hamsters were used for each drug, 12 of which served for evaluation of mortality. They received an i.p. administration three times a week during four weeks. The dose was equivalent to ¾ of the optimally oncostatic dose on murine L1210 leukemia, when injected at days 1, 5, and 9 after tumor cell inoculation.[6,7,11] These doses are shown in Table 1.

Each week three hamsters for each drug and three controls were sacrificed and relevant tissues were quickly removed; the ventricular cross (apex) was immediately fixed for EM study in 5% cacodylate-buffered glutaraldehyde adjusted to pH 7.25, and the apex of the myocardium was minced under fixative into 1–2 mm³ blocks. The remainder of the heart and some other tissues including the skin, were collected for LM examination and fixed in 10% neutral-buffered formalin.

The blocks for the E.M. study were postfixed in 2% osmium tetroxyde, dehydrated in graded ethanols, transferred to propylene oxide, and embedded in Epon. Thin sections cut at 400–500 Å with a Porter-Bloom ultramicrotome were mounted on Formvar-coated 300-mesh copper grids, stained with uranyl acetate and lead citrate, and examined with a Jeol 100 C ASSID electron microscope at 100

TABLE 1. Drugs Used and Doses Employed

Drug	Dose Used in Hamster
First Trial	
Adriamycin (ADM)	3 mg/kg
Daunorubicin (DNR)	3 mg/kg
Detorubicin (DTR)	3 mg/kg
4' Epi-adriamycin (e-ADM)	3 mg/kg
Rubidazone (RBZ)	9 mg/kg
Aclacinomycin (ACM)	6 mg/kg
N-Trifluoroacetyladriamycin-14-valerate (AD-32)	30 mg/kg
Tetrahydropyranyladriamycin (THP-ADM)	3 mg/kg
Second Trial	
Adriamycin (ADM)	3 mg/kg
N-L-leucyl-daunorubicin (1-DNR)	6 mg/kg
Carminomycin (CAM)	0.15 mg/kg
Mitoxantrone (MTX)	1 mg/kg
Rubicyclamin (RBC)	7.5 mg/kg
N-Trifluoroacetyladriamycin-14-0-hemiadipate (AD-143)	60 mg/kg

KV. For histopathological study the tissues were embedded in paraffin, sectioned at 6 μm and stained with hematoxylin end eosin.

Results

MORTALITY AND GENERAL TOXIC OBSERVATIONS

Table 2 summarizes the number of surviving hamsters at the end of each week, and Figures 1 and 2 the curves of mortality by toxicity in our two trials. It is evident that mortality was very high for the animals treated with ADM, DTR, DNR, e-ADM, RBZ, 1-DNR, CAM, and MTX; the majority of treated hamsters were dead between the first and third week and all animals were dead before the end of the fourth week, with a loss of 20–40% of their weight and severe digestive troubles, particularly abundant diarrhea and hair loss. Mortality was a little lower for the group of RBC-treated hamsters, in which some animals survived until the

seventh week. On the contrary, mortality was very low for the animals receiving ACM, AD-32, THP-ADM, and AD-143: only one out of 12 ACM- and AD-32-treated hamsters died during 4 weeks of treatment, and there were no deaths in the groups of THP-ADM- and AD-143-treated animals; all these animals preserved their good general status, without loss of body weight, without digestive trouble, and without loss of hair. According to these data, it is evident that MTX is in the group of studied drugs with very high general toxicity or mortality.

EM ALTERATIONS OF THE MYOCARDIUM

To establish a possible comparative appreciation of the degree of EM myocardial alterations, we used a grading system which derived from that proposed by Billingham et al.[2] *Grade 0* was used for a normal cardiac morphology and *grade 1* for the cases which contained some cells with moderate alterations. *Grade 2* was assigned when more than 50% of myocardial cells showed severe alterations. In *grade 3,* the myocardium was diffusely affected by very severe cell alterations. We also used the intermediate grades of 0–1, 1–2, and 2–3, which indicate that about half the myocardial cells showed the morphologic structure or changes of each of the two grades. For instance grade 0–1 signifies that half of the observed cells were normal (grade 0) and that half had grade 1 lesions.

In the preceding paper we showed examples of EM structures and alterations classified as grades 0, 1, 2, and 3.[8] In this paper we show examples of myocardial alterations observed at the end of each week after treatment, especially with MTX.

Most frequently, at the end of the first week of treatment with MTX, mitochondria, sarcomeres, myofilaments and nucleus are well preserved, but some cells show swelling of mitochondria with clear-

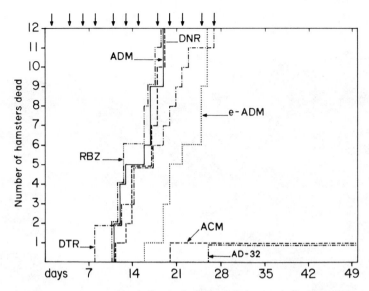

FIGURE 1. Curves of mortality in the first trial. Arrows indicate the I.P. administration of the drugs. There were no deaths with THP-ADM.

ing of their matrices, lysis of the crests, and formation of myelinic figures (Figs. 3*a* and 3*b*); these structure and lesions are classified as grade 0–1. At the end of the second week of treatment with MTX, the myocardium shows some cells well preserved, but also some other cells with more important alterations of the mito-

chondria, separation and lysis of myofilaments, dilatation of sarcoplasmic reticulum and vacuolization (Figs. 4*a* and 4*b*); these alterations are classified as grade 1–2. At the end of the third week of treatment, the myocardial alterations are still more severe and more frequent, with swelling and clearing of mitochondria,

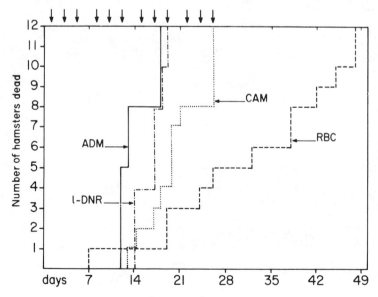

FIGURE 2. Curves of mortality in the second trial. The arrows indicate the I.P. administration of the drugs. There were no deaths with AD-143.

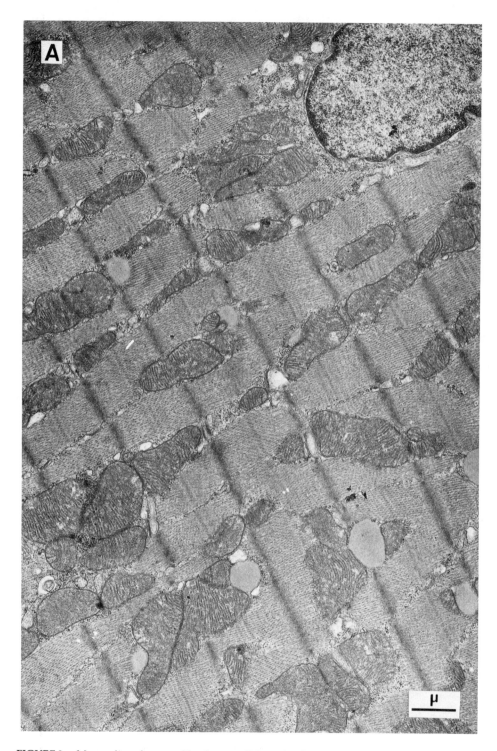

FIGURE 3. Myocardium from a golden hamster 7 days after treatment with MTX. Most frequently, mitochondria, sarcomeres, myofilaments, and nucleus are well preserved (A), but some cells show swelling of mitochondria with clearing of their matrices, lysis of the crests, and formation of myelinic figures (B), Grade 0–1.

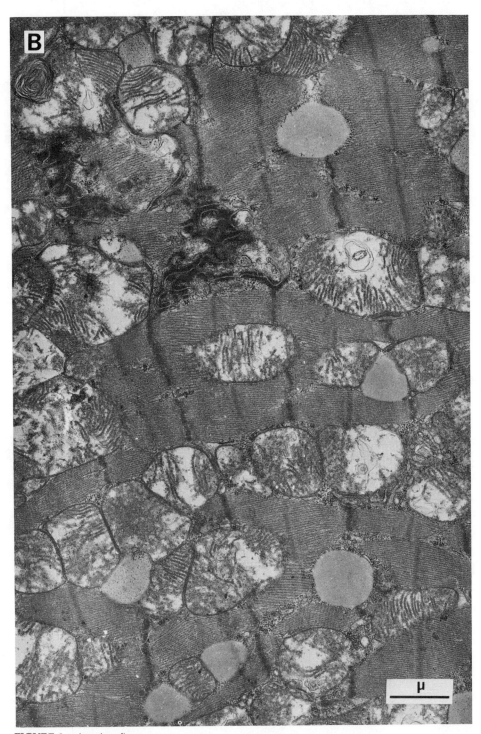

FIGURE 3. *(continued).*

lysis of their crests, condensation of the chromatin into electron-dense masses adjacent to the irregular nuclear membrane, dilatation of sarcoplasmic reticulum, separation of fascia adherens of intercalated disks and formation of myelinic figures

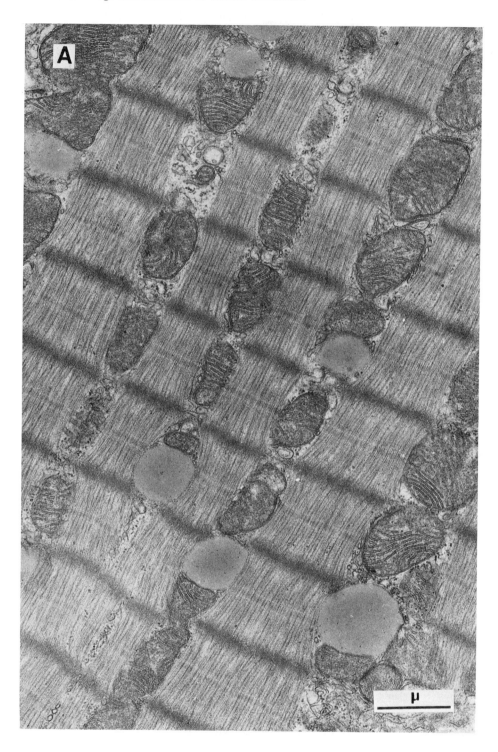

FIGURE 4.   Myocardium from a golden hamster 14 days after treatment with MTX: some cells are well-preserved (A), but some other cells show alterations of the mitochondria, separation and lysis of myofilaments, dilatation of sarcoplasmic reticulum, and vacuolization (B), Grade 1–2.

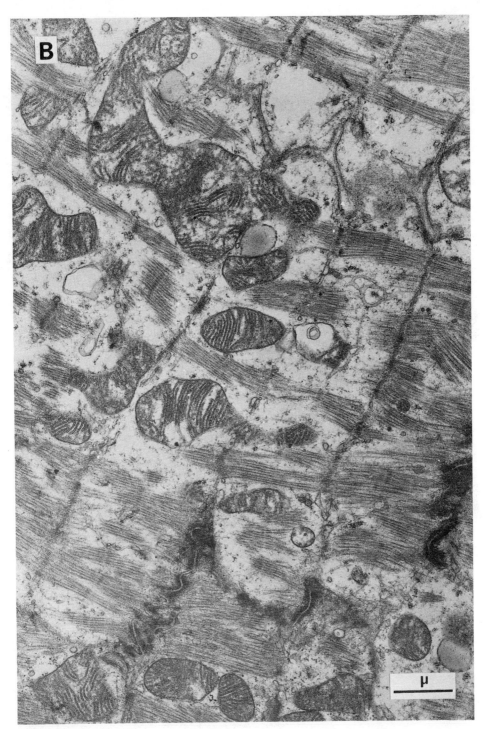

FIGURE 4. (continued).

(Figs. 5a and 5b); these alterations are classified as grade 2. At this time — the end of the third week — seven out of 12 animals were dead and the remaining five animals died before the end of the fourth week. Thus, under our experimental con-

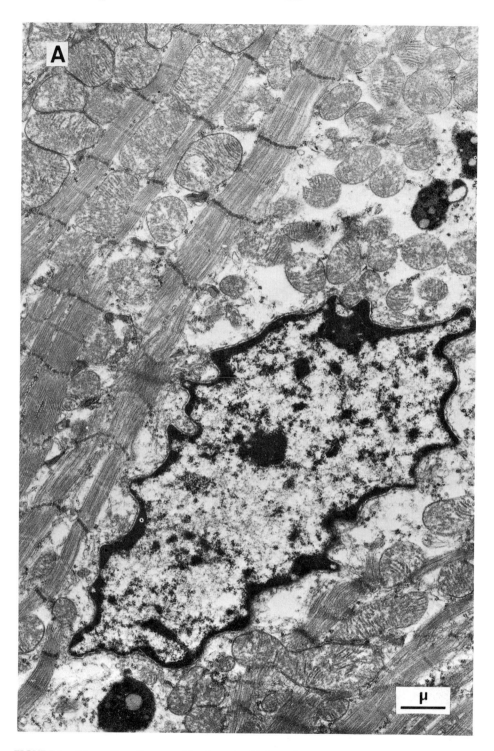

FIGURE 5. Myocardium from a golden hamster 21 days after treatment with MTX: swelling and clearing of mitochondria, lysis of their crests, condensation of the chromatin into electron-dense masses adjacent to the irregular nuclear membrane, dilatation of sarcoplasmic reticulum, separation of fascia adherens of intercalated disks, and formation of myelinic figures (A and B), Grade 2.

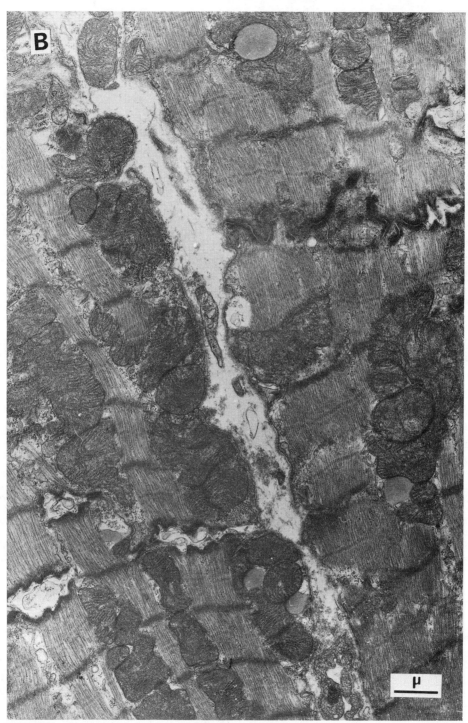

FIGURE 5. (*continued*).

ditions, MTX must be considered as not very cardiotoxic, especially during the first 2 weeks of treatment, but as possessing severe general toxicity that kills the animals before the end of our experiment.

According to the degree of their car-

TABLE 2. Mortality Due to Toxicity (12 Animals per Group)

	Number of Animals Surviving at End of			
	1st Week	2nd Week	3rd Week	4th Week
First Trial				
ADM	12	7	0	0
DNR	12	7	0	0
DTR	12	7	4	0
E-ADM	12	12	7	0
RBZ	12	6	0	0
ACM	12	12	11	11
AD-32	12	12	12	11
THP-ADM	12	12	12	12
Second Trial				
ADM	12	4	0	0
L-DNR	12	8	0	0
CAM	12	11	4	0
MTX	12	11	5	0
RBC	11	11	9	7
AD-143	12	12	12	12

diotoxicity and their general toxicity or mortality, it is possible to classify all studied drugs in three groups: *the first group* causes severe myocardial alterations (grade 2–3) and high mortality and in- cludes ADM, DNR, 1-DNR, and RBZ; *the second group* causes less myocardial alter- ations (grade 1–2), but high mortality or general toxicity, and includes e-ADM, DTR, CAM, RBC, and MTX; and *the third*

TABLE 3. Degree of Myocardial Electron Microscopic Alterations at End of Each Week according to a Semiquantitative Grading System[a]

Classification of the Drugs according to Their Degree of Cardiotoxicity and General Toxicity or Mortality		Degree of Myocardial Alterations at End of:			
		1st Week	2nd Week	3rd Week	4th Week
1st Group					
With very severe myocardial	ADM	1–2	2–3	2–3	
alterations (grade 2–3) and very	DNR	1–2	2–3		
high mortality	1-DNR	1	1–2	2–3	
	RBZ	1–2	2–3		
2nd Group					
With less severe myocardial	e-ADM	0–1	1–2	2	
alterations (grade 1–2) and high	DTR	0–1	1–2	2	
mortality	CAM	0–1	1–2	2	1–2
	RBC	0–1	1	1–2	
	MTX	0–1	1–2	2	
3rd Group	ACM				
With less severe myocardial	THP-ADM	0–1	1	1–2	1–2
alterations (grade 1–2) and very	AD-32	0–1	1	1–2	1–2
low mortality	AD-143	0–1	1–2	2	2
		0–1	1	1–2	2

[a]Grade 0 = no pathologic alterations; Grade 1 = moderate cell alterations; Grade 2 = severe cell alterations; Grade 3 = very severe cell alterations. Intermediate grades of 0–1, 1–2, and 2–3 indicate that about half of myocardial cells showed the morphologic structure or alterations of each of the two grades.

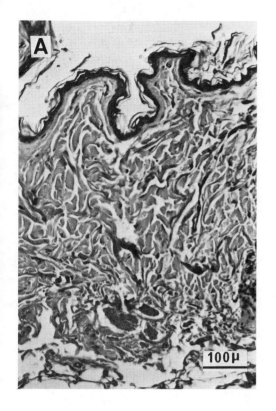

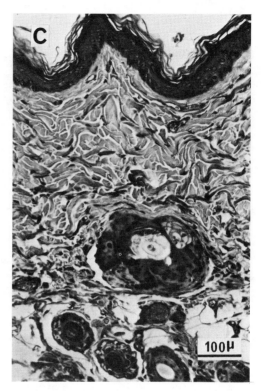

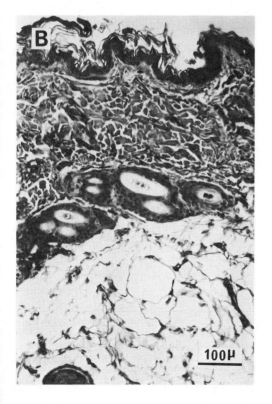

FIGURE 6. (*A*) Examples of very severe degenerative lesions of the skin of a golden hamster at the end of the third week of treatment with ADM: atrophy of all epidermic layers and disappearance of hair.

(*B*) Example of moderate degenerative alterations of the skin of a golden hamster at the end of the third week of treatment with MTX: moderate lesions of epidermic cells and morphologic structure of the hair still like that in controls.

(*C*) Example of normal histological structure of the skin, without loss of hair, of a golden hamster at the end of 4 weeks of treatment with ACM.

group also causes less myocardial alterations (grade 1–2), and low mortality and general toxicity, and includes ACM, THP-ADM, AD-32, and AD-143. Almost all animals treated with the last four drugs survived after 4 weeks of treatment, with well-preserved general status, and 2 months after the treatment had been stopped, the EM study of their myocardium revealed a recovery of myocardial alterations. Table 3 summarizes this classification and the degree of cardiotoxicity at the end of each week and for each drug.

LM LESIONS OF THE SKIN

As EM study of the myocardium permits us to detect and specify the degree of cardiotoxicity of different drugs, the histopathologic study of the skin can detect degenerative lesions of the skin with alopecia caused by these drugs. Using the same grading system and classification of the drugs, a comparative study enabled us to establish correlations between the cardiac and skin toxic effects in the three groups of drugs. All very cardiotoxic drugs, in the first group (ADM, DNR, 1-DNR, and RBZ), were also very skin-toxic and caused severe atrophy of all epidermic layers and loss of hair or alopecia. Figure 4*a* shows an example of this histopathological structure of the skin at the end of the third week of treatment with ADM, with atrophy of epidermic layers and disappearance of hair. The five drugs included in the second group of our classification (e-ADM, DTR, CAM, RBC, and MTX), which are less cardiotoxic, also showed less skin toxicity and only slight alopecia. Figure 4*b* shows an example of moderate degenerative alterations of epidermic cells and a morphologic structure of the hair, still like that in controls, at the end of the third week of treatment with MTX. The four anthracyclines included in the third group (ACM, THP-ADM, AD-32, and AD-143), which are also less cardiotoxic but with, in addition, a very low

general toxicity and mortality, are almost completely nonskin-toxic and do not provoke alopecia. Figure 6*c* shows an example of normal histological structure of the skin without alopecia, at the end of four weeks of treatment with ACM.

Discussion

In clinical and experimental studies, many authors already showed several biochemical changes and tissue alterations after treatment with different anthracyclines.[1,2,4,5,9,10,13–16,18–20,22,24,27,28] The ultrastructural and histopathological myocardial alterations reported here were similar to those in our published golden hamster model.[6–8] Using our method and grading system, the comparative study of general toxicity or mortality, EM alterations of the myocardium and LM lesions of the skin permit us to classify studied drugs and to show the advantages or disadvantages of each one.

According to our data, all studied drugs, including MTX, were cardiotoxic, but with different degrees of cardiotoxicity. The comparative study of their cardiotoxicity and general toxicity or mortality permit us to establish our classification. The MTX was classified in the second group, with less severe cardiotoxicity, moderate skin toxicity, but very high general toxicity or mortality. The present findings about MTX are not in agreement with others.[23,26] Further clinical and experimental studies are required to elucidate the cause of the divergent results. Concerning some other drugs, our experimental findings and classification seem to be consistent with clinical data already published.[3,17,21]

REFERENCES

1. Benjamin, R.S., Mason, Y.W., and Billingham, M.E.: *Cancer Treat Rep 62: 935–939, 1978.*
2. Billingham, M.E., Mason, J.W., Bristow, M.R., and Daniels, J.R.: *Cancer Treat Rep 62: 865–872, 1978.*
3. Blum, R.H., Garnick, M.B., Israel, M., Canellos,

G.P., Henderson, I.G., and Frei, III, E.: *Cancer Treat Rep 63: 919–923, 1979.*

4. Buja, L.M., Ferrans, V.J., Mayer, R.J., Roberts, W.C., and Henderson, E.S.: *Cancer, 32: 771–788, 1973.*

5. Clarysse, A., Kenis, Y., and Mathé, G.: Springer-Verlag, Heidelberg, New York, 1976.

6. Dantchev, D., Slioussartchouk, V., Paintrand, M., Bourut, C., Hayat, M., and Mathé, G.: *Cancer Treat Rep 63: 375–388, 1979.*

7. Dantchev, D., Slioussartchouk, V., Paintrand, M., Bourut, C., Hayat, M., and Mathé, G.: In *Recent Results in Cancer Research, Vol. 74,* G. Mathé, and F.M. Muggia, Eds., Springer-Verlag, Berlin–Heidelberg, 1980, pp. 221–249.

8. Dantchev, D., Paintrand, M., Bourut, C., Pignot, I., Maral, R., and Mathé, G.: In *Anthracyclines: Current Status and Future Developments,* G. Mathé, R. Maral, R. DeJager, Eds., Masson, New York, 1983, pp. 25–35.

9. EORTC Clinical Screening Group: *Cancer Clin Trials 3: 115–120, 1980.*

10. Ferrans, V.J.: *Cancer Treat Rep 62: 955–961, 1978.*

11. Freireich, E.J., Gehan, E.A., Rall, D.P., Schmidt, L.M., and Skipper, H.E.: *Cancer Chemother Rep 50: 219–245, 1966.*

12. Henderson, B.M., Dougherty, W.J., James, V.C., Tilley, L.P., and Noble, J.F.: I. Clinical observations. *Cancer Treat Rep 66: 1139–1143, 1982.*

13. Jacquillat, Cl., Auclerc, M.F., Weil, M., et al.: *Cancer Treat Rep 63: 889–893, 1979.*

14. Jaenke, R.S.: *Lab Investigation 30: 292–304, 1974.*

15. Jaenke, R.S., Deprez-de Campeneere, D., and Trouet, A.: *Cancer Res 40: 3530–3536, 1980.*

16. Lampidis, T.J., Henderson, I.C., Mervyn, Israel, and Canellos, George P.: *Cancer Res 40: 3901–3909, 1980.*

17. Mathé, G., Bayssas, M., Gouveia, J., Dantchev, D., Ribaud, P., Machover, D., Misset, J.L., Schwarzenberg, L., Jasmin, C., and Hayat, M.: *Cancer Chemother Pharmacol 1: 259–262, 1978.*

18. Mettler, F.P., Young, D.M., and Ward, J.M.: *Cancer Res 37: 2705–2713, 1977.*

19. Olson, H.M., and Capen Ch. C.: *Lab Investigation 37: 386–394, 1977.*

20. Olson, H.M., Young, D.M., Prieur, D.J., Le Roy, A.F., and Reagan, R.L.: *Am J Pathol 77: 439–450, 1974.*

21. Ogawa, M., Inagaki, J., Horikoshi, N., et al.: *Cancer Treat Rep 63: 931–938, 1979.*

22. Rosenoff, S.H., Olson, H.M., Young, D.M., Bostick, F., and Young, R.C.: *Natl Cancer Inst 55: 191–194, 1975.*

23. Sprano, B.M., Gordon, G., Hall, C., Iatropoulos, M.J., and Noble, J.F.: *Cancer Treat Rep 66: 1145–1158, 1982.*

24. Trouet, A. and Sokal, G.: *Cancer Treat Rep 63: 895–898, 1979.*

25. Von Hoff, D.D., Coltman, C.A., and Forseth, B.: *Cancer Res 41: 1853–1855, 1981.*

26. Von Hoff, D.D., Pollard, E., Kuhn, J., Murray, E., and Coltman, C.A., Jr.: *Cancer Res 40: 1516–1518, 1980.*

27. Wakabayashi, Takashi, Oki, Toshikazu, Tone, Hiroshi, Hirano, Shinichi, and Omori, K.: *Electron Microsc 29(2): 106–118, 1980.*

28. Young, D.M.: *Cancer Chemother Rep 6(3): 159–175, 1975.*

CHAPTER 7

Phase II Studies of Aclacinomycin A in Patients with Hematologic Malignancies

D. Machover, J. Gastiaburu, M. Delgado, F. De Vassal,
P. Ribaud, M. Bayssas, J.L. Misset, T. Dorval, H. Tapiero,
J. Gouveia, C. Jasmin, L. Schwarzenberg, and G. Mathé

Introduction

Aclacinomycin A (ACM) is a cytostatic anthracycline antibiotic produced by fermentation of *Streptomyces galileus*.[7] It presents major chemical differences from daunorubicin (DNR) and doxorubicin (adriamycin, ADM). The molecule comprises an aglycone moiety called aklavinone and a triglycosidic chain in C_7, formed of L-Rhodosamine, 2-Deoxy-L-Fucose and L-cinerulose (Fig. 1).

ACM was selected for clinical trials on the basis of its wide spectrum of activity against experimental tumors[3,8] and low myocardiotoxicity in animal models.[3,1,11] Also, using the Ames' test, ACM was found nonmutagenic, whereas ADM and DNR are highly potent in this respect.[10]

Preliminary clinical studies with ACM were reported by Japanese authors.[2,6,9] We report here the results of two consecutive phase II studies with ACM in patients with hematologic malignancies, conducted since 1977 in the Service des Maladies Sanguines et Tumorales, Hôpital Universitaire Paul-Brousse.[4,5]

Service des Maladies Sanguines et Tumorales, and Institut de Cancérologie et d'Immunogénétique (INSERM U-50), Hôpital Paul-Brousse, Villejuif, France

Patients

Fifty-one patients entered the first phase II study (Table 1); forty-five were considered evaluable for antitumor response. Of these, 17 had AML, 19 had ALL, eight had leukemic lymphosarcoma (LLS) and one had CML blastic crisis. Four patients in the AML group, four in the LLS group, and one with CML blastic crisis were initially resistant to standard chemotherapy before initiation of ACM. The remaining patients were in relapse; some of these patients were submitted to ACM after an unsuccessful attempt to obtain a new CR with standard chemotherapy and others were submitted to the drug immediately after the diagnosis of relapse.

Twenty-five patients entered the second phase II trial (Table 2). Twenty-two patients with overt AML were evaluated; all patients were in relapse or initially refractory to standard chemotherapy. Seven patients were resistant to a prior treatment with DNR or ADM administered as single agents or in combination regimens.

Treatment

In the first trial, ACM was administered daily by I.V. bolus injection at a dose ranging from 10 to 30mg/m²/day for 10–30

41

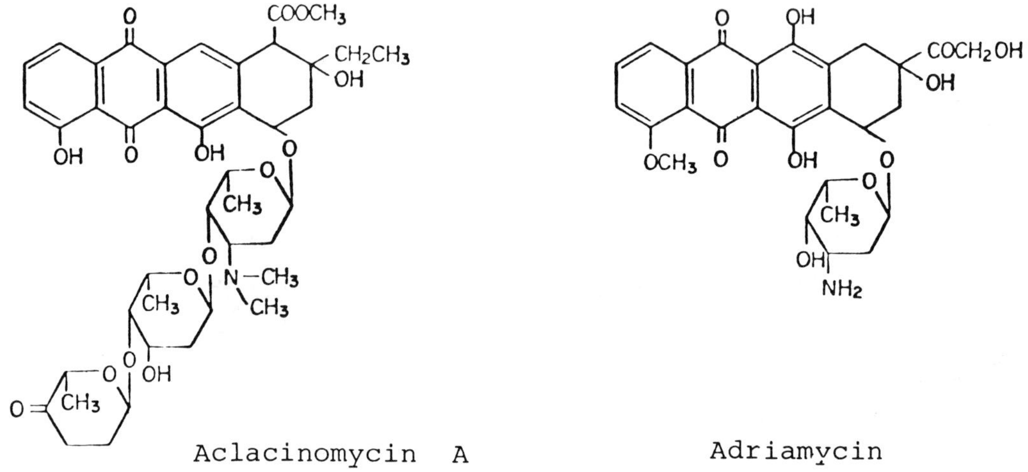

Aclacinomycin A   Adriamycin

FIGURE 1. Structural formulae.

consecutive days. The majority of the patients received a dose of 15mg/m^2/day for 20 consecutive days. In this study, the aim was to continue drug administration to the point of the maximum tolerable amount; the maximum dose administered per course did not exceed 300mg/m^2, however. If antitumor response was observed after one course, a second course was recommended after a drug-free interval of variable duration, depending on the clinical condition of the patient.

In the second trial, based mainly upon the toxic effects observed in the former study, we decided to modify the ACM administration schedule. In this regimen, ACM was administered in courses of 10 consecutive days at a daily dose of 15mg/m^2 as a rapid I.V. injection with a 10-day, drug-free interval. Courses were repeated until CR, or until failure of treatment became evident.

TABLE 1. Aclacinomycin A in Acute Leukemia and Leukemic Lymphosarcoma — Patients' Characteristics (First Trial)[a]

Leukemia Type	Patients' Number	Number of Evaluable Patients	Age Median (Range)	Sex M/F	Prior Treatment: No. of Prior CRs Obtained	Prior Treatment: No. of Patients
AML	20	17	25	12/5	0	4
			(14–56)		1	7
					2	5
					3	1
ALL	19	19	12	13/6	1	4
			(3–47)		2	9
					3	4
					4	1
					7	1
LLS	11	8	19	7/1	0	4
			(7–49)		1	3
					3	1
Blastic CML	1	1	29	0/1	0	1

[a]Treatment schedule 10–30 mg/m^2/day, 10–30 days.

TABLE 2.   ACM-A in AML — Patients' Characteristics (Second Trial)[a]

Number of Patients Entered	Patients Evaluable	Mean Age (Range)	Sex (M/F)	Previous Resistance to Anthracyclines		Cytologic Type	
				Yes	Unknown	AML	AMMoL
25	22	40.5 (8–79)	11/11	7	15	19	3

[a]15 mg/m²/day × 10 days per course; drug-free interval: 10 Days.

Results

FIRST CLINICAL TRIAL

The response rate is shown in Table 3. The number of CRs was analyzed according to the total dose of ACM. Of the patients with AML, four (23%) achieved CR; the four complete responders received total doses of ACM ranging from 300 to 390mg/m². Of those with ALL, two patients (10%) attained CR. Of those with LLS, two patients (25%) reached CR with total doses ranging between 200–300mg/m².

We have particularly focused our attention on AML patients; in fact, 11 of the 17 evaluable patients received an inefficient chemotherapy combining ADM (50mg/m² day 1), VCR (1mg/m² day 2) and ARA-C (160mg/m²/day from days 2 to 8) immediately before receiving ACM. This enabled us to consider these patients resistant to this combination regimen. Four out of 11 resistant patients achieved CR with ACM (Table 4).

SECOND CLINICAL TRIAL

The response rate is shown in Table 5. CR was obtained in 12 patients (55%); CRs were observed as often in AML as in AMMoL patients. Forty-two percent of the complete responders achieved CR after one course (150mg/m²), 42% after two courses (300mg/m²), and 16% after three courses (450mg/m²). As shown in Table 6, five of seven previously anthracycline-resistant patients achieved CR with ACM. In none of the two studies was disease-free survival studied, because all complete responders were submitted, when in CR, to different types of maintenance regimens.

Toxicity

FIRST CLINICAL TRIAL

Forty-three patients were evaluable for toxic effects (Table 7). Severe myeloid toxicity occurred in all patients, requiring supportive treatments. The most promi-

TABLE 3.   Aclacinomycin A in Acute Leukemia and Leukemic Lymphosarcoma — Response Rate according to Total Dose Administered (First Trial)[a]

Leukemia Type	Total Dose (mg/m²)	Number of Evaluable Patients	Type of Response		
			Complete	Partial	Failure
AML	300–390	7	4 ⎫	2	1
	200–299	4	0 ⎬ 23%	2	2
	130–199	6	0 ⎭	1	5
ALL	321–412	2	0 ⎫	1	1
	200–299	8	1 ⎬ 10%	1	6
	60–199	9	1 ⎭	0	8
LLS	200–299	5	2 ⎫ 25%	1	2
	90–199	3	0 ⎭	0	3

[a]Treatment schedule, 10–30 mg/m²/day, 10–30 days.

TABLE 4. Aclacinomycin A in Acute Myelocytic Leukemia Response Rate According to Previous Clinical Resistance to Anthracyclines (N = 17) (First Trial)[a]

	ADM-Resistant[b] (N = 11)	ADM Resistance Unknown (N = 6)
CR	4	—
PR	2	3
Failure	5	3

[a] Treatment schedule 10–30 mg/m²/day, 10–30 days.
[b] Clinical resistance to previous induction chemotherapy combining ADM (50 mg/m²) d 1 + VCR (1 mg/m²) d 2 and ARA-C (160 mg/m²/d) days 2–8.

TABLE 6. ACM-A in AML — Response Rate According to Prior Resistance to Anthracyclines (Second Trial)[a]

	Number of Patients with	
	Previous Resistance to Anthracyclines (N = 7)	Unknown Resistance (N = 15)
CR	5	7
PR	0	2
Failure	2	6

[a] 15 mg/m²/day × 10 days; drug-free interval: 10 days.

nent toxicity effects were severe diarrhea, which was observed in 34 patients (79%), and severe erosive stomatitis which developed in 16 patients (37%). This toxicity usually appeared when the total dose of ACM by course went over 200mg/m². Abnormalities of the ST-T segment on EKG were observed in six patients (13%), and congestive heart failure (CHF) with contributing factors of prior high-dose anthracycline treatment, pneumonia, and fluid overload occurred in two patients. Alopecia was not observed in the 12 patients evaluable for this type of toxicity.

SECOND CLINICAL TRIAL

The overall toxicity is shown in Table 8. The 22 evaluable patients received a mean total dose of 350mg/m², with a range from 120 to 600mg/m². Severe myeloid toxicity related both to the disease and the treatment was observed in all patients; in most instances, it required hematologic supportive treatments. Four patients died of uncontrolled sepsis and one of visceral hemorrhage. Intestinal toxicity and oral mucositis was much less prevalent during this study. In fact, diarrhea, usually moderate, was observed in four patients (18%), and oral mucositis in one patient (5%). Only minor and transient abnormalities of the ST-T segment on EKG were observed in two patients; CHF was not recorded during the follow-up time. There was no evidence of cumulative toxicity when courses were repeated according to this schedule of administration of ACM.

TABLE 5. ACM in AML — Response Rate (Second Trial)[a]

Type of response (N = 22)

CR	PR	Failure
12(55%)	2(9%)	8(36%)

CR rate according to cytologic type (N = 22)

AML	AMMoL
10/18	2/3

Number of courses necessary to attain CR (N = 12)

Number of Courses	Number of patients in CR
1	5 (42%)
2	5 (42%)
3	2 (16%)

[a] 15 mg/m²/ × 10 days per course; drug-free interval: 10 days.

TABLE 7. Aclacinomycin A in Acute Leukemia and Leukemic Lymphosarcoma 8 Toxicity (First Trial)[a] (N = 43)

Type of Toxicity	Number of Patients	Percent
Severe myeloid toxicity	All patients	
Diarrhea (hemorrhagic)	34 (3)	79 (7)
Nausea and vomiting	17	40
Stomatitis	16	37
Abnormal EKG	6	13
Congestive heart failure	2	4
Hemorrhagic cystitis	1	—
Hepatic	—	—
Renal	—	—
Alopecia	0/12 Evaluable patients	

[a] Treatment schedule 10–30 mg/m²/day, 10–30 days.

TABLE 8.   Aclacinomycin in AML — Toxicity (N = 22) (Second Trial)

Toxic Effects	Number of Patients Experiencing Toxicity	Percent
All patients had severe granulo-cytopenia and thrombocytopenia complicated with:		
Severe infectious syndromes	17	(77)
Severe hemorrhage	2	(9)
Diarrhea	4	(18)
Oral mucositis	1	(5)
Transient abnormalities of hepatic functions tests	3	(14)
Transient ST–T wave abnormalities	2	(9)
Alopecia	0/7 Evaluable patients	

15 mg/m²/day I.V. × 10 days; 10-day rest period. Twenty-two patients received a mean total dose of 350 mg/m² ranging from 120 to 600 mg/m².

Alopecia was not observed in the seven evaluable patients for this type of toxicity.

Discussion

The results obtained in our preliminary study enable us to consider that ACM administered at total doses greater than 200mg/m² is an active drug in AML and in leukemic lymphosarcoma; furthermore, it appears that ACM is effective in some AML patients previously resistant to combination therapy including ADM. However, intestinal toxicity and oral mucositis are unacceptable in daily dose schedules at total doses per course greater than 200mg/m².

The second phase II trial confirms the antitumor efficacy of ACM in AML. In fact, we observed CRs in 55% of the patients. Furthermore, five out of seven previously anthracycline-resistant patients achieved CR with ACM. The toxicity observed during this study is within acceptable limits; particularly, severe intestinal and oral toxicities are much less prevalent. ACM definitely causes no alopecia.

Our data suggest that ACM is not necessarily cross-resistant with either DNR or ADM in AML; this contrasts with experiments using DNR-resistant L1210 and ADM-resistant P388 leukemias which showed that ACM had cross-resistance to both agents.[8] The results obtained in our studies together with the clinical experience of Japanese authors[12] lead to the conclusion that ACM is a first-line drug for induction treatment in AML.

REFERENCES

1. Dantchev, D., Slioussartchouk, V., Paintrand, M., Hayat, M., Bourut, C., and Mathé, G.: Electron microscopy studies of the heart and light microscopic studies of the skin after treatment of golden hamsters with adriamycin, detorubicin, AD-32, and aclacinomycin. Cancer Treat Rep 63: 875–888, 1979.
2. Furue, H., Komita, T., Nakao, I., Furukawa, I., Kanko, T., and Yokohama, T.: Clinical experiences with aclacinomycin-A. In Antitumor Antibiotics, S.K. Carter, H. Umezawa, J. Douros, and Y. Sakurai, Eds. RRCR, 63, Springer-Verlag, Heidelberg, 1978, pp. 241–246.
3. Hori, S., Hurano, S., Oki, T., Inui, T., Tsukagoshi, S., Ishizura, M., Takeuchi, T., and Umezawa, H.: Antitumor activity of new antracycline antibiotics, aclacinomycin-A and its analogs, and their toxicity. Gann 68: 685–690, 1977.
4. Mathé, G., Bayssas, M., Gouveia, J., Dantchev, D., Ribaud, P., Machover, D., Misset, J.L., Schwarzenberg, L., Jasmin, C., and Hayat, M.: Preliminary results of a phase-II trial of aclacinomycin in acute leukemia and lymphosarcoma. An oncostatic that is rarely cardiotoxic and induces no alopecia. Cancer Chemother Pharmacol 1: 259–262, 1978.
5. Mathé, G., Gil, M.A., Gescher, F., Delgado, M., Bayssas, M., Ribaud, P., Misset, J.L., Hayat, M., and Machover, D.: Aclacinomycin in acute leukemias and lymphomas. Lancet 2: 310–311, 1979.
6. Ogawa, M., Inagaki, J., Horikoshi, N., Inoue, K., Chinen, T., Ueoka, H., and Nagura, E.: Clinical study of aclacinomycin-A. Cancer Treat Rep 63: 931–934, 1979.
7. Oki, T., Matsuzawa, Y., Yoshimoto, A., Numata, K., Kimatura, I., Ori, S., Takamatsu, A., Umezawa, H., Ishizuka, M., Nagawa, H., Suda, H., Hamada, M., and Takeuchi, T.: New antitumor antibiotics, aclacinomycins A and B. Jpn J Antibiot 28: 830–834, 1975.
8. Oki, T.: New anthracycline antibiotics. Jpn J Antibiot (Suppl) 30: 570–584, 1977.
9. Sakano, T., Okasaki, N., Ise, T., Kitaoka, K., and Kimura, K.: Phase I study of aclacinomycin A. Jpn J Clin Oncol 8: 49–53, 1978.
10. Umezawa, H., Sawamura, M., Matsushima, T., and Sugimura, T.: Mutagenicity of aclacinomy-

cin A and Daunomycin derivatives. *Cancer Res* *38: 1782–1874, 1980.*

11. Wakabayashi, T., Oki, T., Tone, H., Hirano, S., and Omori, K.: A comparative electron microscopic study of aclacinomycin and adriamycin cardiotoxicities in rabbit and hamsters. *J Electron Microsc (Tokyo) 29: 106–118, 1980.*

12. Yamada, K., Nakamura, T., Tsuruo, T., Kitahara, T., Maekawa, T., Uzaka, Y., Kurita, S., Masaoka, T., Takaku, F., Hirota Y., Amaki, I., Osamura, S., Ito, M., Nakano, N., Oguro, M., Inagaki, J., and Onozawa, K.: A phase II study of aclacinomycin A in acute leukemia in adults. *Cancer Treat Rev 7: 177–182, 1980.*

CHAPTER 8

Present State of BHAC Clinical Studies in Japan

Masanori Fukushima and Kazuo Ota

Introduction

BHAC is a prodrug of Ara-C which was developed by Aoshima et al. in 1976.[1] The phase II study of its effect on acute leukemia was completed in 1980 by the Japanese Cooperative Clinical Study Group for Acyl Ara-C[4] and this Ara-C derivative is now widely used in Japan. We present here a brief review of: 1) the characteristics and pharmacokinetics of BHAC; 2) a phase II study of the effect of BHAC on acute leukemia; 3) the BHAC–DMP regimen (BHAC, daunorubicin, 6MP, and prednisone) for ANLL; 4) the BHAC–AMP regimen (BHAC, aclacinomycin A, 6MP, and prednisone) for previously treated ANLL; 5) a phase II study on malignant lymphoma; and 6) PLAC, an orally administrable Ara-C derivative.*

Patients and Methods

PATIENTS

The subjects of these studies were adults with acute leukemia or malignant lymphoma who had been admitted to hospitals belonging to the Clinical Study Group.

DRUG

BHAC and PLAC were supplied by Asahi Chemical Industry Co., Ltd. (Tokyo).

DRUG ADMINISTRATION

BHAC dissolved in 5% glucose was administered by intravenous infusion with 2–3 hour duration. Details of the administration schedule in the BHAC–DMP and the BHAC–AMP regimen were described in cited references 2 and 9.

EVALUATION

Through all the studies, the effectiveness of the drug was evaluated according to the criteria proposed by Kimura.[3]

Results and Discussion

CHARACTERISTICS OF BHAC AND ITS PHARMACOKINETICS

As shown in Table 1, a series of N^4-acyl-Ara-C derivatives exhibited a marked antitumor activity against mouse L1210 leukemia cells comparing with the effect of Ara-C. From studies of the toxicity of acyl-Ara-Cs, the C_{22}-analog BHAC was found to have the most promising therapeutic index.[1] BHAC seems to undergo β-oxidation, with ultimate liberation of Ara-C through deacylation.[5] After clinical administration of the drug, megaloblasts were observed in the bone marrow, suggesting the typical Ara-C effect. BHAC is

Aichi Cancer Center, Department of Internal Medicine, Chikusa-ku, Nagoya, Japan
*Abbreviations: BHAC = N^4behenoyl-1-β-D-arabinofuranosylcytosine; PLAC = N^4-palmitoyl-1-β-D-arabinofuranosylcytosine; and AL = acute leukemia.

47

TABLE 1. Antitumor Activity and Toxicity of N^4-acyl-Ara-C Analogs

		T/C (Percent)			Dead/3 Mice
N^4-acyl Group	$n + 1$	100	200	400 (mg/kg)	1000
Butyryl	4	131	131	139	—
Caproyl	6	125	133	150	—
Caprylyl	8	123	127	163	—
Capryl	10	159	188	284	0
Lauroyl	12	177	272	296	2
Myristoyl	14	211	191	90	3
Pentadecanoyl	15	246	309	91	3
Palmitoyl	16	361	242	78	3
Margaroyl	17	405	152	99	3
Stearoyl	18	329	123	111	3
Nonadecanoyl	19	298	260	134	3
Arachidoyl	20	313	363	329	0
Behenoyl	22	241	298	342	0
Oleoyl		218	214	109	—
Ara-C		127	144	159	—
Cyclocytidine		163	188	191	—

L1210 mouse leukemia cells (1×10^5 cells) were inoculated intraperitoneally and drugs were given on day 2 and day 6 I.P. (Courtesy of Dr. M. Aoshima.)

remarkably resistant to cytidinedeaminase and a relatively long presence of Ara-C in blood has been demonstrated after administration of BHAC.[8] A further advantage of this drug is its accumulation in marrow. Since BHAC is highly lipophilic, it is provided in 50 mg BHAC vials containing 350 mg of hydrogenated castor oil polythylene glycol ether as solvent, and prior to use, incubation in a boiling bath is required.

PHASE II STUDY OF BHAC ON ACUTE LEUKEMIA

As shown in Table 2, 44% complete remissions were obtained in adult AML patients under 60 years old. During the ad-

ministration of this drug, the patients' complaints were chiefly gastrointestinal. They occurred in approximately 10% of the patients and were easily tolerated. Allergy-like manifestations such as fever, itching, and rashes occurred in a few cases, but were generally not serious.

BHAC is thus a remarkably effective agent against acute leukemia. In the group achieving complete remission, patients received 5–8 mg/kg of BHAC daily for over 10 days. Two to 3 weeks after the start of administration of BHAC, the level of platelets and leukocytes dropped and recovery was made in approximately 2 weeks. As shown in Table 3, administra-

TABLE 2. Therapeutic Effect of BHAC on Adult Acute Leukemia

Diagnosis	Cases	CR	PR	NR	CR Rate Percent
AML	35	15	7	12	44.1
AMoL	8	1	3	4	12.5
ALL	3	1	2	0	33.0
SAL[a]	3	0	0	3	0
APL[b]	2	0	1	1	0
Total	51	17	13	20	(34.0)

[a] Smoulder AL.
[b] Promyelocytic AL.

TABLE 3. Total Dosage of BHAC and Response in Adult Acute Leukemia

Dose (mg)	Cases	CR	PR	NR	CR Rate Percent
1080–1999	12	0	4	8	0
2000–2999	6	0	2	4	0
3000–3999	11	7	2	2	63.6
4000–4999	9	4	2	3	44.4
5000–10350	12	6	3	3	50.0
Total	50	17	13	20	(34.0)[a]

[a]53.1% for cases treated with more than 3000 mg.

TABLE 4. Effect of BHAC-DMP Therapy on Adult ANLL

Age	Cases	CR	PR	NR	CR Rate Percent
15–59	111	91	5	15	82.0
60–	30	12	3	15	40.0
Total	141	103	8	30	73.1

TABLE 5. Effect of BHAC-AMP Therapy on Adult ANLL

Diagnosis	Cases	CR	PR	NR	CR Rate Percent
Without prior treatment					
AML	18	15	2	1	83.3
AMoL	11	8	2	1	72.7
APL[a]	1	0	0	1	0
EL[b]	2	2	0	0	100
Total	32	25	4	3	(78.1)
With prior treatment					
AML	19	13	1	5	68.4
AMoL	2	1	0	1	50.0
APL	2	2	0	0	100
Total	23	16	1	6	(69.6)

[a]Promyelocytic AL.
[b]Erythroleukemia.

tion of more than 3000 mg (total dose) was required for complete remission. CR rate for these cases was 53.1%.

BHAC–DMP REGIMEN (BHAC, DAUNORUBICIN, 6MP, AND PREDNISONE) FOR ANLL

For treatment of adult ANLL, the DCMP regimens (daunorubicin, Ara-C, 6MP, and prednisone) are the most common in Japan. In the BHAC–DMP regimen 170 mg/m^2 of BHAC is administered daily for 2 weeks. As shown in Table 4, complete remission was obtained in approximately 80% of the 111 patients under 60 years old. Over 50% of patients who achieved complete remission survived over 2 years. These results suggest that this regimen is superior to the DCMP regimen, and that BHAC is a safe, effective drug against ANLL.

BHAC–AMP REGIMEN (BHAC, ACLACINOMYCIN A, 6MP, AND PREDNISONE) FOR ANLL PREVIOUSLY TREATED

Aclacinomycin A has been used instead of daunorubicin in the above regimen in some recent studies, and the preliminary results are shown in Table 5. The rate of complete remissions was 83% in AML and 72% in AMoL. Even in the cases having received prior treatment, this regimen was found to induce 68% complete remission in AML and 50% in AMoL.

PHASE II STUDY OF BHAC ON MALIGNANT LYMPHOMA

BHAC was also found to have some effect on malignant lymphoma.[6] In a phase II study for malignant lymphoma, the overall response rate was 30%. The response was mostly only partial remission even where the total dose was over 2000 mg, suggesting that the agent remains a supplemental one for lymphoma. Again, the most frequent side effect was gastrointestinal, and rashes also appeared in a few cases. Myelosuppression was a dose-limiting factor.

PALMITOYL-ARA-C, AN ORALLY ADMINISTRABLE ARA-C DERIVATIVE

Among the acyl-Ara-Cs, palmitoyl-Ara-C has been found to be promising for development as an orally administrable drug.[7] When 400 mg of this drug was administered orally, a considerable amount of Ara-C was found in blood (3 ng/ml). The absorption profile was markedly modified by simultaneous administration of bile acid or by a fatty diet (unpublished observations). For this drug, phase I–II studies are now in progress.

ACKNOWLEDGMENT

We thank Drs. Kimura, K. and Yamada, K. (Nagoya) for their generous support in relation to this presentation. This study was carried out by the Japanese Cooperative Clinical Study Group for Acyl Ara-C.

REFERENCES

1. Aoshima, M., Tsukagoshi, S., Sakurai, Y., Ohishi, J., Ishida, T., and Kobayashi, H.: *Cancer Res* 37: 2481–2486, 1977.
2. Hirano, M., Morishita, Y., Ino, T., Matsui, T., Shimizu, S., Shigemura, H., Nakamura, K., Ono, Y., and Saito, M.: *Jpn J Clin Oncol* 11: 87–92, 1981.
3. Kimura, K.: *A Seminar on Chemotherapy of Acute Leukemia under the US–Japan Cooperative Science Program*, September 27–28, Bethesda, Maryland, pp. 21–23. Published by the Editorial Committee for the Symposium on Recent Advances in Acute Leukemia, Nagoya, 1965.
4. Kimura, K., Yamada, K., Uzuka, Y., Maekawa, T., Takaku, F., Shimoyama, M., Ogawa, M., Amaki, I., Osamura, S., Ito, M., Sakai, T., Oguro, M., Kimura, I., and Ichimaru, M.: In *Recent Results in Cancer Research*, vol. 71, S.K. Carter, Y. Sakurai, and H. Umezawa, Eds., Berlin, Heidelberg, and New York, Springer-Verlag, 1981, pp. 232–240.
5. Oh-ishi, J., Kataoka, T., Tsukagoshi, S., Sakurai, T., Shibukawa, M., and Kobayashi, H.: *Cancer Res* 41: 2501–2506, 1981.
6. Takagi, T., Sueyama, H., and Oguro, M.: Abstract of Joint Meeting of the 18th Congress of the International Society of Hematology and 16th Congress of the International Society of Blood Transfusion, Montreal, 1980. No. 910, p. 179, 1980.
7. Tsuruo, T., Iida, H., Hori, K., Tsukagoshi, S., and Sakurai, Y.: *Cancer Res* 41: 4484–4488, 1981.
8. Yamada, K., Kawashima, K., Kato, Y., Morishima, Y., Tanimoto, M., and Ohno, R.: In *Recent Results in Cancer Research* vol. 70, S.K. Carter and Y. Sakorai, Eds., pp. 219–229, 1980.
9. Yamada, K., Suzuki, H., and Kato, Y.: *Acta Haematol Jpn* 43: 1080–1085, 1980.

CHAPTER 9

A Phase II Trial of Pepleomycin:
A Preliminary Report

EORTC Clinical Screening Group[a]

Introduction

Pepleomycin (PPM) or 3-[(s)-1-phenyl-ethylamino]-propylaminobleomycin is an analog of bleomycin (BLM) obtained from a strain of *Streptomyces verticillus*. It can be obtained either by fermentation and semisynthesis or prepared from bleomycin A2 by bleomycinic acid reaction with diaminopropane phenyl ethyl.[7]

PPM was selected among BLM analogs because it causes less pulmonary fibrosis than other BLM analogs.[2] Other toxicities were moderate and it is not mutagenic.[1]

The experimental activity of PPM on murine tumors was identical to that of BLM (i.e., in Ehrlich's ascites carcinoma) or even greater (i.e., in solid Ehrlich tumor or in chemically induced gastric tumors in rats).[2] PPM absorption, clearance, and pyrogenicity after subcutaneous injection are similar to those of BLM.[5]

Japanese colleagues have conducted phase I and II clinical trials of PPM showing its efficacy, mainly in head and neck epidermoid tumors, cervix carcinoma, prostate cancer, and lymphomas.[6]

Methods and Patients

Two protocols have been applied during two successive periods: 1) 10mg/m²/d × 5 consecutive days (5mg twice a day, I.M.)

with a 9-day interval between the cycles, and 2) 5mg/m²/day × 5 consecutive days (2.5mg/m² twice a day I.M.) with a 9-day interval between the cycles.

Two hundred and four patients entered the first protocol. One hundred ninety-two are evaluable. The age range is 13–80 years and the median 55.5. There are 96 females and 108 males. The number of cycles varied from one to seven, and the median was 2.73. The total dose range was 75–560 mg/m².

Fifty-six patients were included in the second protocol; 51 are evaluable. The age ranged from 24–81 years with a median of 56.6. There were 33 females and 19 males. They received between one and eight cycles; the mean dose was 137 mg/m². Eleven patients (21%) had been previously treated with BLM.

Results and Discussion

The results of the first protocol are summarized in Table 1. Only four diseases have been the object of a study in which one can quantify the incidence of apparently complete (CR) and partial remissions (PR) — more than to 50% of the volume evaluated according to the WHO-EORTC-NCI rules.[8]

The results concerning these diseases indicate a response (CR + PR) in 5/11 lymphomas, 4/35 breast carcinomas, 6/63 head and neck tumors, and 1/22 cervix car-

[a]J.P. Armand (Chairman), G. Mathe (Secretary), and F. De Vassal (Study Coordinator)

TABLE 1. Complete and Partial Remissions in a Phase II Trial of Pepleomycin and Bleomycin EORTC Clinical Screening Group

	Pepleomycin				Bleomycin (3)
	10mg/m²/D × 5D CR + PR		5mg/m²/D × 5D CR + PR		
Tumor	Nᵃ	Percent	Nᵃ	Percent	Percent
Head and neck	6/63	10	0/3	—	—
Breast	4/35	11	2/18	0.11	20
Cervix	1/22	04	—	—	30
NHL	5/11	45	2/10	0.20	—
Melanoma	1/8	—	—	—	60
Esophageal	1/7	—	—	—	50
Hodgkin's	1/4	—	2/6	—	20
Vulvar	2/4	—	—	—	50
Skin	2/3	—	1/3	—	50
Mycosis Fungoïdes	1/2	—	—	—	—

ᵃ N = Number responding.

cinomas. Localizations of responding lesions suggest that node, skin, and pleuropulmonary metastasis are the most sensitive to PPM.

The results of second protocol are shown in Table 1. Sufficient patient numbers were found only for non-Hodgkin's lymphoma (NHL) and breast carcinomas.

Two out of 10 NHL patients had remissions, complete in one and partial in another. Two out of 18 breast tumor patients had a PR, as had 2/6 Hodgkin patients and 1/3 skin carcinomas.

Toxicities are shown in Table 2. They consist of fever, nausea, vomiting, asthenia, dyspnea, pulmonary fibrosis, alopecia, skin pigmentation, fibrosis, swelling of hands, rash, stomatitis in 5% of the patients, and hematopoietic depression. Only three secondary effects were more frequent with the first protocol than with the second: fever (46–15%), nausea and vomiting (30–14%), and alopecia (14–6%).

The results previously obtained by our Group with BLM and the toxicity collected

TABLE 2. EORTC Clinical Screening Group Phase II Trial Toxicities of Pepleomycin and Bleomycin

	Pepleomycin			Bleomycin
	10mg/m²	5mg/m²	Total	JMHᵃ
	Percent			Percent
No. of Patients	201	52	253	1.613
Fever	46	15	40	40
Nausea–vomiting	30	14	27	15
Asthenia	31	24	30	16
Pulmonary (Dyspnea)	20	4	9	10
Pulmonary (Fibrosis-pneumonia)	5	5	5	
Alopecia	14	6	12	30
Skin	16	16	16	22
Stomatitis	6	8	6	13
Hematologic	5	2	5	0.2
Swelling of hands	3	—	2	3
Shock	1	2	0.02	0.1
Others	1	—	0.01	—

ᵃ Japanese Ministry of Health, 1973.⁴

by the Japanese Ministry of Health[4] can be compared in Tables 1 and 2 to the present PPM results.

NOTES

Members who have introduced more than five patients: Villejuif: G. Mathé; Strasbourg: R. Keiling; Bordeaux: J. Chauvergne; Lyon: E. Pommateau; Lille: P. Cappelaere; Montpellier: B. Serrou; Nice: M. Schneider; Toulouse: J.P. Armand; Dijon: J. Guerrin; Coimbra (Portugal): C. De Oliveira; Reims: A. Cattan; Rouen: C. Jeanne; Paris: C. Jacquillat; Saint-Cloud: B. Clavel; Besançon: S. Schraub; Saint-Etienne: P. Serpantié; Nantes: B. Le Mevel.

REFERENCES

1. Abe, F., Koyu, A., Inoue, H., Yamashita, I., Ezura, H., Yoshizawa, K., and Matsuda, A.: *Jpn J Antibiotics 31: 859, 1978.*
2. Ebihara, K., Ekimoto, H., Itchoda, H., Abe, F., Inoue, H., Aoyagi, S., Yamashita, T., Kohu, A., Takahashi, K., Yoshioka, O., and Matsuda, A.: *Jpn J Antibiotics 31: 872, 1978.*
3. EORTC Clinical Screening Co-operative Group. *Br Med J 2: 643, 1970.*
4. Extracted from the Summary of Adverse Reactions to BLM submitted to the Japanese Ministry of Health and Welfare in October 1973.
5. Matsuda, A., Yoshioda, O., Yamashita, T., Ebihara, K., Umezawa, H., Miura, T., Katayama, K., Yokoyama, M., and Nagais, S.: In *Antitumor Antibiotics*, S.K. Carter, H. Umezawa, J. Douros, and Y. Sakurai, Eds., Springer Verlag, Heidelberg, New York, 1978, p. 191.
6. Oka, S.: In *Cancer Chemo- and Immunopharmacology. 1. Chemopharmacology*, G. Mathé and F. M. Muggia, Eds., Springer Verlag, Heidelberg, New York, 1979, p. 163.
7. Umezawa, H.: *Adv Pharmacol Chemother 10: 127, 1979.*
8. WHO-EORTC-NCI. *Cancer, 1983, (in press).*

CHAPTER 10

Studies on 2,4-Diamino-5-Adamantyl-6-Methyl Pyrimidine (DAMP), A New Lipid Soluble Antifolate

Sigmund F. Zakrzewski and Patrick J. Creaven

Introduction

In this paper we present the background, preclinical data and an outline of the initial clinical studies of 2,4-diamino-5-adamantyl-6-methyl pyrimidine (DAMP). DAMP was developed as part of an investigation of the structure–activity relationships of substituted pyrimidines as inhibitors of dihydrofolate reductase (DHFR). In the course of this investigation it was shown that the requirements for optimal inhibition of the enzyme DHFR were the 2,4-diamino-pyrimidine structure, a bulky lipophilic group in the 5 position, and an alkyl group in the 6 position. These investigations led to the development of DAMP.[3]

Synthesis

Ethylaceto (1-adamantyl) acetate is condensed with guanidine hydrochloride in absolute ethanol to form 2-amino-4-hydroxy-5-(1-adamantyl)-6-methylpyrimidine. Refluxing of this material with a mixture of PCl_5 and $POCl_3$ leads to the formation of the 4-chloro-analog. The chloro-analog is converted to the final product (DAMP) by heating it with

ethanolic ammonia in a bomb at 160°. The crude product is purified by chromatography on a silica gel column followed by chromatography on an alumina column and crystallization from absolute ethanol. The final product has m.p. 274–275°, and its elemental analysis corresponds to $C_{15}H_{22}N_4 \cdot 0.5H_2O$. M.W. = 267.[3]

Experimental Antitumor Activity

DAMP is a strong inhibitor *in vitro* of DHFR isolated from sarcoma 180, though not as strong as methotrexate (Table 1).[2] However, its activity against the TA3 mouse mammary carcinoma cell line is essentially identical with that of methotrexate (Table 1).[2] *In vivo*, it shows activity against a methotrexate-resistant tumor, the Walker 256 carcinosarcoma, but is inactive against the methotrexate-sensitive Murphy-Sturm lymphosarcoma (Table 1).[4] Because of its powerful inhibition of DHFR and its spectrum of activity which is different from that of methotrexate, the compound was advanced to toxicology in preparation for clinical trial.

Animal Toxicity Studies

Toxicity has been evaluated in rodents and dogs.[5] When given to dogs by rapid I.V. injection, the compound caused vom-

Department of Clinical Pharmacology and Therapeutics, Roswell Park Memorial Institute, Buffalo, New York

TABLE 1. Preclinical and Clinical Data for DAMP-ES

		Reference
In Vitro activity		
Ki for DHFR	6×10^{-9} m $(10^{-10}$ m)[a]	2
ID_{50} for TA3 cells	6×10^{-9} m $(8 \times 10^{-9}$ m)[a]	2
ID_{50} for S180 cells	4×10^{-7} m $(1.2 \times 10^{-5}$ m)[a]	2
In Vivo antitumor activity		
Maximum tumor shrinkage:		
Walker 256 carcinosarcoma	92%	3
Murphy-Sturm lymphosarcoma	19%	3
Toxicity and pharmacokinetics in the dog		
LD_{50}	120 mg/m^2/day $\times$ 5 days	4
$t_{\frac{1}{2}}\alpha$	0.38 minute	4
$t_{\frac{1}{2}}\beta$	177.60 minutes	4
Clinical Studies		
Maximum tolerated dose	75–90 mg/m^2/day $\times$ 5 days	6
$t_{\frac{1}{2}}\alpha$	25 minutes	7
$t_{\frac{1}{2}}\beta$	1242 minutes	7

[a]Numbers in parenthesis are the corresponding values for methotrexate.

iting, convulsions, and a minor drop in temperature. These effects were seen within 30 minutes of drug administration with complete recovery 24 hours after drug administration. When given in divided doses (every 12 hours) the acute toxicity was largely circumvented and toxicity consisted of diarrhea, anorexia, and loss of weight, noted in most dogs at doses of 125, 250, and 500 mg/m^2/day $\times$ 5 with leukopenia also being observed. Biochemical changes were slight and of doubtful significance. Pathological findings in dogs treated with nonlethal doses of DAMP were minor; in dogs receiving lethal doses, pulmonary edema and signs of gastrointestinal toxicity were most frequently observed. Lymphoid atrophy, pancreatic necrosis, and bone marrow atrophy were also seen, as were degenerative changes in the bladder and one case of ovarian necrosis. Testicular atrophy or hypoplasia was noted in male animals.

Folinic acid (100 mg/m^2/day) did not prevent the acute CNS toxicity of DAMP but prevented the antiproliferative effect of doses up to 125 mg/m^2/day $\times$ 10 days. In studies with dogs, both oral and intravenous administration were used. For intravenous administration, because of the low water solubility of DAMP, the ethane sulfonate salt of DAMP, DAMP-ES, was used. The data indicate that the two compounds are biologically equivalent. The approximate LD_{50} when the drug was given on a daily $\times$ 5 schedule was 150–200 mg/m^2/day in rats, and somewhat less — in the order of 125 mg/m^2/day — in beagle dogs. The rhesus monkey tolerated up to 200 mg/m^2/day for 10 days.

Preclinical Pharmacokinetic Studies

STUDIES IN THE RAT

These studies were carried out using 2-[^{14}C]-DAMP or 2-[^{14}C]-DAMP-ES in CD male rats weighing about 200 g.[6] Radioactivity in the liver, spleen, kidney, and pancreas was at higher levels than that of plasma at 1 hour after intraperitoneal drug

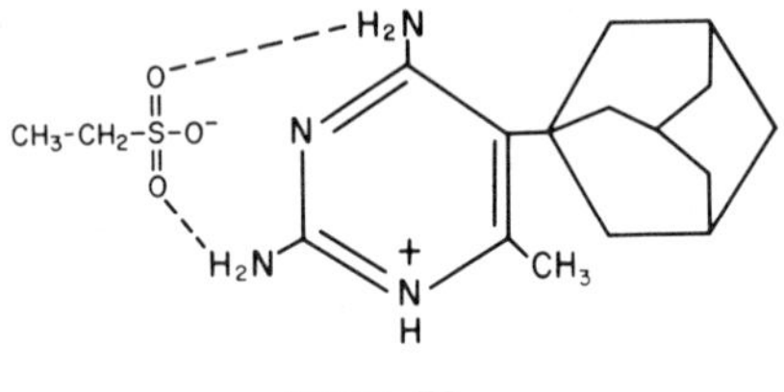

FIGURE 1. Structure of DAMP-ES.

administration. Levels in these tissues, as well as in plasma, fell rapidly except for the level in the pancreas, which remained relatively high (about 40% of the level at 1 hour at 24 hours). Over 90% of the drug was excreted in 24 hours. At 4 hours the drug in the urine was 70% unchanged DAMP, but at 24 hours only 5% was unchanged drug.

STUDIES IN THE DOG

In these studies, ^{3}H-DAMP-ES was used.[5] At 48 hours after injection of the drug, 63% of the radioactivity was recovered in the urine and 10% in the feces. Metabolism was rapid; two metabolites, one lipophilic, and the other hydrophilic were found in the plasma and urine, the hydrophilic metabolite being the predominant form. Pharmacokinetic analysis indicated a two-compartment, open model with extremely rapid diffusion of the drug from the central to the peripheral compartment; an alpha-phase half-life of 23 seconds, and an elimination phase half-life of 3 hours were calculated.

Clinical Studies

A PHASE I STUDY

A phase I study was carried out in 30 patients at doses of 10–90 mg/m^2/day for 5 days, given as a 1-hour infusion. Dose-limiting toxicity was myelosuppression and the maximum tolerated dose was 75–90 mg/m^2/day for 5 days. Other toxicities seen were nausea and vomiting that was mild in all patients except one, maculopapular rash in five patients, mucositis in three, and diarrhea in two. A variety of CNS symptoms, many not dose-related and most mild and transient, were observed. Tumor benefit short of a partial response was observed in five patients, two patients with colorectal carcinoma showed tumor shrinkage on scan, one patient with prostate carcinoma had an improvement on bone scan, and another had disappearance of pain. A patient with carcinoma of the breast had improvement in performance status and marked decrease in pain.

HUMAN PHARMACOKINETIC STUDIES

Ten patients received [^{3}H]-DAMP-ES and pharmacokinetics were studied.[7] Biexponential plasma decay was found with an alpha-phase half life of 25 ± 10.4 minutes and a beta-phase half life of 20.7 ± 9.7 hours. These studies are ongoing.

ACKNOWLEDGMENT

This work was supported in part by grants from the United States Public Health Service, grants CA-21071 and CA-13038.

REFERENCES

1. Creaven, P.J., Zakrzewski, S.F., Mittelman, A., Pontes, E., Tseng, M., Wajsman, L.Z., Karakousis, C., Moayeri, H., Madajewicz, S., and Perry, A.: Proceedings of the 13th International Cancer Congress, Seattle, Washington, September 1982 p. 531, 1982.
2. Ho, Y.K., Hakala, M.T., and Zakrzewski, S.F.: Cancer Res 32: 1023–1028, 1972.
3. Jonak, J.P., Zakrzewski, S.F., and Mead, L.H.: J Med Chem 14: 408–411, 1971.
4. Zakrzewski, S.F., Dave, C., and Rosen, F.: J Natl Cancer Inst 60: 1029–1033, 1978.
5. Zakrzewski, S.F., Pavelic, Z., Bullard, G., Creaven, P.J., and Mihich, E.: Cancer Res 42: 2177, 1982.
6. Zakrzewski, S.F., Dave, C., Mead, L.H., and Delluomo, D.S.: J Pharmacol Exper Therap 205: 19–26, 1978.
7. Zakrzewski, S.F. and Creaven, P.J.: Proc Am Assoc Cancer Res 23: 130, 1982.

CHAPTER 11

Phase II Trials of Vindesine in Hematological Malignancies: A Survey

R. Hulhoven

Introduction

Vindesine (VDS), a semisynthetic derivative of vinblastine, has been selected because of a cytostatic activity in murine tumors more related to vincristine (VCR) and a toxicity and pharmacokinetics more related to vinblastine.[1,9] Phase I trials proposed a dosage of 3–4 mg/m² once a week for future phase II trials.[2]

Phase II trials using VDS alone or in combination with prednisolone in hematological malignancies, were conducted in the hematology departments of the ICIG at Villejuif and of the St-Luc hospital at the Catholic University of Louvain. A total of 115 treatments was evaluable for therapeutic response.[5-7] Others also used VDS alone or in combination with prednisone in smaller series.[3,10] The aim of this short survey was to define thoroughly the cytostatic efficacy of VDS in hematological malignant diseases.

Results

The most impressive activity of VDS was shown in childhood acute lymphoblastic leukemia (ALL) (Table 1). Indeed, 40% of patients achieved a complete remission (CR) and 63% a response of more than 50%. VDS appeared also active in

Pharmacotherapy Unit (Professor C. Harvengt), St-Luc Hospital, Catholic University of Louvain, Avenue E., Mounier 53, Brussels, Belgium

adult ALL. Fifteen percent of patients achieved a CR and 30% a response > 50%. Its activity thus seemed lower than in childhood ALL.

In malignant lymphomas, the cytostatic efficacy of VDS was also obvious. Twenty-eight percent of patients achieved a response of > 50%, but CRs were uncommon (5% of patients). As yet, only partial responses (PR) were seen in Hodgkin's disease (17% of the patients treated).

In acute myeloid leukemia (AML), efficacy appeared poor. Indeed, only 7% of the patients responded favorably. In contrast, its efficacy was impressive in the blastic crisis of chronic myeloid leukemia (CML). Twenty-eight percent of the patients achieved a CR and 52% a response of > 50%. Responses appeared better in the undifferentiated or lymphoid-like blastic crises, but occurred also in the classical myeloid-like types. In multiple myeloma, VDS was also effective, at least in combination with prednisone, as shown by Houwen.[4] Forty-two percent favorable responses were observed. In other hematological disorders there were too few patients treated to draw firm conclusions.

When patients failed to respond to VDS, they could respond to a continuous infusion of 2 or 5 days. In Villejuif, out of 12 refractory patients, two CRs and four PRs were observed.[6] In Marseille, out of 18 pa-

TABLE 1. Cytostatic Efficacy of VDS Alone or in Malignancies (Cumulative Data of the Literature) Response

	n	CR	PR	Response > 50%
Childhood ALL	57	22	13	35
Adult ALL	27	4	4	8
Malignant lymphoma	75	4	17	21
Hodgkin's disease	42	—	7	7
AML	29	1	1	2
CML blastic crisis	61	17	15	32
Multiple myeloma	26	—	11	11

tients, seven PRs were achieved.[8] Therefore, this mode of VDS administration should be further investigated. However, it necessitates the use of a central venous catheter because of the caustic properties of VDS, involving a high risk of phlebitis and extravasation.

A particularly exciting point is the apparent lack of clinical cross-resistance between VDS and VCR. In Villejuif and at the St-Luc hospital, out of 38 VCR-resistant patients, a CR or PR was achieved in 17 instances.

Toxicity

The toxicity of VDS was essentially hematological. This toxicity was expected because most patients had poor bone marrow reserves due to massive invasion by leukemic cells and prior chemo- and/or radiotherapy treatments. Leukopenia was observed in nearly all patients; thrombocytopenia occurred in half the patients and was sometimes severe. Neurotoxicity, in such induction treatment, appeared generally moderate; loss of reflexes was very common, sometimes accompanied by paresthesias and constipation or abdominal pain. More severe neurotoxicity occurred occasionally. This was sometimes difficult to evaluate because of previous VCR treatment. Moreover, an induction course is too short to permit evaluation of cumulative neurotoxicity. Another very common toxicity was alopecia.

Conclusion

VDS phase II trials exhibited an impressive cytostatic efficacy in childhood ALL and in the blastic crisis of CML. Efficacy was also evident in adult ALL, malignant lymphoma and multiple myeloma. In contrast, efficacy appeared poor in AML and Hodgkin's disease. The poor results achieved in Hodgkin's disease were probably due to prior therapy with both VCR and vinblastine. Toxicity appeared acceptable, consisting mainly of hematological depression and, to a lesser degree, of neurological side effects. The apparent lack of clinical cross-resistance between VDS and VCR must be emphasized.

REFERENCES

1. Barnett, C.J., Cullinan, G.J., Gerzon, K., Hoying, R.C., Jones, W.E., Nelson, W.M., Poore, G.A., Robinson, R.L., Sweeney, M.J., Todd, G.C., Dyke, W.R., and Nelson R.L.: J Med Chem 21: 88, 1978.
2. Dyke, W.R., and Nelson R.L.: Cancer Treat Rev 4: 135, 1977.
3. Hellriegel, K.P.: In Proceedings of the International Vinca Alkaloid Symposium — Vindesine, Karger, Basel, 1981, pp. 159–170.
4. Houwen, B., Van Dobbenburgh, O.A., Marrink, J., Oekhuizen, T., and Nieweg, H.O.: In Proceedings of the International Vinca Alkaloid Symposium — Vindesine, Karger, Basel, 1981, pp. 239–249.
5. Hulhoven, R., Michaux, J.L., Cornu, G., Ferrant, A., Symann, M., Bosly, A., Delannoy, A., Dutrieux-Fauchet, M.C., and Sokal, G.: In Proceedings of the International Vinca Alkaloids symposium — Vindesine, Karger, Basel, 1981, pp. 143–150.
6. Mathé, G., Hulhoven, R., Sokal, G., Bayssas, M., Belpomme, D., Bosly, A., Cornu, G., Delannoy, A., de Luca, L., de Vassal, F., Ferrant, A., Gouveia, J., Hayat, M., Jasmin, C., Machover D., Michaux, J.L., Misset, J.L., Musset, M., Pico, J.L., Ribaud P., and Schwartzenberg, L.: Anticancer Res 1: 1, 1981.
7. Mathé, G., Misset, J.L., de Vassal, F., Gouveia, J., Hayat, M., Machover, D., Belpomme, D., Pico, J.L., Schwartzenberg, L., Ribaud, P., Musset, M., Jasmin, C., and de Luca, L.: Cancer Treat Rep 62: 805, 1978.
8. Maraninchi, D., Gastaut, J.A., Tubiana, N., and Carcassonne, Y.: Bull Cancer 68: 338, 1981.
9. Todd, G.C., Gubson, W.R., and Morton, D.M.: J Toxicol Environ Health, 1: 843, 1976.
10. Vats, T.S., Mehta, P., Trueworthy, R.C., Smith, S.D., and Klopovich, P.: Cancer 47: 2789, 1981.

CHAPTER 12

Pharmacokinetics and Metabolism of Etoposide (VP 16-213) and Teniposide (VM 26)

P.J. Creaven

Introduction

The epipodophyllotoxins etoposide (4' demethylepipodophyllotoxin-9-[4,6-0-eth-ylidene-β-D-glucopyranoside] VP 16-213 EPEG) and teniposide (4' demethylepi-podophyllotoxin-9-[4,6-0-tenylidene-β-D-glucopyranoside] VM 26 PTG) have been in clinical use for over a decade. Their pharmacokinetics were reported in 1975[1,6,7] in studies using tritium-labeled material. More recently, high-performance liquid chromatographic (HPLC) methods for these two drugs have been developed[2,11,13,16,24,25] and this has led to a substantial increase in our knowledge of the pharmacokinetics and metabolism of these agents these will be briefly reviewed here.

Gastrointestinal Absorption

Both these drugs are normally given intravenously but there have been studies with oral forms of etoposide, a lipophilic capsule,[4,9,12,17] an oral solution,[4,5,9] and a hydrophilic soft gelatin capsule.[15] With the lipophilic capsule, toxicity indicated poor and erratic absorption,[4,17] while results were better with the oral solution and the hydrophilic capsule.[4,5,15,18] Ab-

sorption by measurement of the integral of the plasma concentration × time curve was calculated to be 91% for the oral solution.[9] For the capsule it was calculated to be 57% in one study[9] and 48–78% in another.[16]

Distribution

In the original studies, a biexponential plasma decay was found for etoposide[6] and a triexponential decay for teniposide.[7] Most of the reported studies confirm a biexponential plasma decay for etoposide although Lawrie et al. have reported that in some patients a third exponential phase could be detected.[16] The elimination phase half-life is in the range of 3–11 hours for those studies reporting a biexponential decay. The plasma decay of teniposide has been reported to be biexponential in children.[11] Some of the half-lives reported for these two agents are listed in Table 1. The plasma decay is more rapid for etoposide than for teniposide and for both drugs is probably shorter in children than adults.

A two-compartment open model has been developed for etoposide and a three-compartment model for teniposide.[1] The central compartment in the model for etoposide corresponds to the combined volumes of the central and shallow peripheral compartments for teniposide. The difference in pharmacokinetics of the two drugs may thus be due to a difference in

Department of Clinical Pharmacology and Therapeutics, Roswell Park Memorial Institute, New York State Department of Health, Buffalo, New York

61

TABLE 1. Plasma Kinetics of Etoposide and Teniposide

Dose mg/m²	Kinetics of Plasma Decay	Terminal $t_{\frac{1}{2}}$ (Hour)	Authors (References)
Etoposide			
Adults			
70–290	Biexponential	11.06 ± 6.0 ($n = 20$)	Creaven and Allen[6]
200	Biexponential	6–8	Lawrie et al.[16]
	Triexponential	20–46	Lawrie et al.[16]
100–200	Biexponential	7.05 ± 0.67 ($n = 14$)	D'Incalci et al.[9]
80	Biexponential	5.95 ($n = 6$)	Scalzo et al.[22]
400–800	Biexponential	8.1 ± 4.3 ($n = 12$)	Hande et al.[14]
Children			
200	Biexponential	3–5	Snodgrass et al.[24]
200–250	Biexponential	5.8 ± 3.2 ($n = 9$)	Evans et al.[11]
95–216	Biexponential	3.37 ± 0.5 ($n = 6$)	D'Incalci et al.[9]
Teniposide			
Adults			
67	Triexponential	21.2 ± 9.9 ($n = 6$)	Creaven and Allen[7]
Children			
165	Biexponential	9.6 ± 27 ($n = 6$)	Evans et al.[11]

plasma protein binding (at typical plasma concentrations of the two drugs, the observed affinity constants calculate out to a 94% plasma protein binding for etoposide and 99.4% for teniposide).[1] The turnover of teniposide in the deep peripheral compartment is 10 times slower than that of etoposide in the peripheral compartment, which may account for the slower elimination of the former agent. Another factor governing the differences in pharmacokinetics is that the excretion rate constant is three times and the renal clearance six times larger for etoposide than for teniposide. The estimate of fraction of drug metabolized derived from these models agrees well with the fraction of the dose of each compound not recovered in the urine as unchanged drug, but poorly with the fraction of the dose recovered as metabolite. This observation led to the development of a more comprehensive model for etoposide to include metabolite as well as unchanged drug.[19] This model showed a body clearance of metabolites of 111.7 ml/minute considerably greater than its renal clearance (31 ml/minute), indicating loss or sequestration of metabolite.

The data derived from these pharmacokinetic models indicate a much greater plasma clearance (Cl_P) for etoposide than for teniposide (28.9 and 10.5 ml/minute/m², respectively, with values for body clearance (Cl_B) essentially identical). The plasma clearance for etoposide reported by D'Incalci et al. for adults is in close agreement with this figure (26.8 ml/minute/m²).[9] These authors found a higher clearance in children (39.3 ml/minute/m²). Evans et al. report a lower body clearance for etoposide in children (17.8 ml/minute/m²), but confirm the approximate threefold greater clearance of etoposide than of teniposide (5.2 ml/minute/m² in their studies).[11] Plasma clearances of 19.2 ml/minute/m² after 80 mg/m² and 50.7 ml/minute (approximately 30 ml/minute/m²) after 400–800 mg/m² have recently been reported.[22,14]

Levels of both drugs in the cerebrospinal fluid are low both by radioactive[8] and by HPLC assays.[8,10,14,23] Penetration of etoposide into pleural effusion and of teniposide into ascites fluid have both been reported to be poor.[14,23]

Metabolism and Excretion

In studies with tritiated etoposide, urinary recovery of total radioactivity was variable — a maximum recovery of 87.5% of the dose being found[8]; however, the mean recoveries were considerably lower than this, ranging from 43.3% at a dose of 220 mg/m[2] to 67.3% at 170 mg/m[2]. Recovery of total radioactivity after tritiated teniposide was 44.5%. Maximum recoveries in feces were 16.3% and 10.1% for the two drugs, respectively.[8] This is in contrast to studies in the rat in which biliary excretion was the major route of elimination of the drugs.[20,21] However, in one patient studied with a tube in the bile duct, recovery of etoposide in the bile was less than 2% of the dose.[10]

In the case of etoposide, the majority of the radioactivity (66.8%) is in the form of unchanged drug, whereas with teniposide the reverse is the case (21.3%).[8] In terms of recovery of metabolite as a percent of the dose administered, it is 18% in the case of etoposide and 32% in the case of teniposide. However, as indicated above, calculations based on the pharmacokinetic model indicate a much higher percentage of both drugs metabolized (66% and 86%, respectively), with the majority of the metabolites unrecovered.[1] Urinary recoveries of unchanged etoposide of 20–30% of the dose in 24 hours[10] and 30–46.5% of the dose in 48 hours[22] have been reported. Recovery of unchanged teniposide was 3–15% of the dose in the study by Sessa et al.[23]

Studies of plasma radioactivity indicate that at the end of the infusion radioactivity is 95.5% unchanged drug in the case of etoposide and 94.8% in the case of teniposide. By 12 hours, these percentages have fallen to 70.6% and 63.8%, respectively, and by 48 hours, to 45.3% and 41.6%.[8]

Studies on metabolism thus indicate that the extent of metabolism of both drugs is considerable and relatively greater for teniposide than for etoposide. A recent report that liver failure can increase the plasma half-life and markedly decrease the plasma clearance of etoposide

would seem to confirm the importance of metabolism in the elimination of these drugs.[10]

Studies on the structure of the human metabolites of both drugs were carried out following administration of tritium-labeled material.[3] The major urinary metabolite of etoposide was identified by mass spectroscopy following derivatization with diazomethane as 4'-dimethyl-epipodophyllic acid-9-[4,6-0-ethylidene-β-D-glucopyranoside] (Fig. 1). The corresponding acid derived from teniposide was identified as the probable metabolite of that compound, although in these studies definitive identification could not be made. The probable identification of these acids as the major metabolites of these two drugs have now been confirmed by other groups.[25,11] Characterization of the stereochemical form of the metabolite is made difficult by the fact that the trans-hydroxy acid cannot be produced directly by alkaline hydrolysis of the lactone ring, since epimerization to the cis-lactone with subsequent ring opening to give the acid in the cis-conformation (the hydrolyzed picro-isomer) occurs rapidly. However, Strife et al.[25] have produced indirect evidence that the metabolite of etoposide is the trans-isomer by demonstrating a difference in retention time on paired ion chromatography between the natural metabolite and the cis-hydroxy acid produced from picro-etoposide. This suggested that the metabolite is enzymatically produced, and Van Maanen et al.[26] have recently demonstrated the production of the hydroxy acid by a rat liver microsomal preparation. Strife et al. could not detect the picro-isomer of etoposide in patient plasma,[25] but relatively low concentrations of this isomer have been detected in the plasma of some children treated with these drugs.[11]

Conclusion

The pharmacokinetics and metabolism of both etoposide and teniposide have

renal clearance of etoposide than teniposide. Metabolism of both drugs is extensive, but more so for teniposide than etoposide. The corresponding epipodophyllic acid — probably the *trans*-isomer — is the major metabolite in the case of each drug.

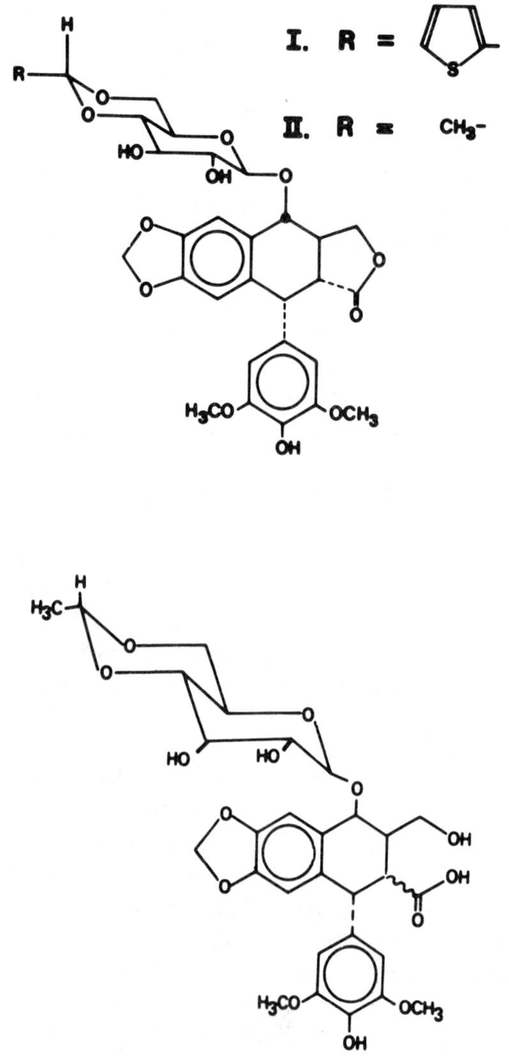

REFERENCES

1. Allen, L.M., and Creaven, P.J.: *Eur J Cancer 11: 697, 1975.*
2. Allen, L.M.: *J Pharm Sci 69: 1440, 1980.*
3. Allen, L.M., Marcks, C., and Creaven, P.J.: *Proc Am Assoc Cancer Res Am Soc Clin Oncol 17: 6, 1976.*
4. Brunner, K.W., Sonntag, R.W., Ryssel, H.J., and Cavalli, F.: *Cancer Treat Rep 60: 1377, 1976.*
5. Cavalli, F., Sonntag, R.W., Jungi, F., Senn, H.J., and Brunner, K.W.: *Cancer Treat Rep 62: 473, 1978.*
6. Creaven, P.J., and Allen, L.M.: *Clin Pharmacol Ther 18: 221, 1975.*
7. Creaven, P.J., and Allen, L.M.: *Clin Pharmacol Ther 18: 227, 1975.*
8. Creaven, P.J.: *Cancer Chemother Pharmacol 7: 133, 1982.*
9. D'Incalci, M., Farina, P., Sessa, C., Mangioni, C., Conter, V., Masera, G., Rocchetti, M., Brambilla Pisoni, M., Piazza, E., Beer, M., and Cavalli, F.: *Cancer Chemother Pharmacol 7: 141, 1982.*
10. D'Incalci, M., Sessa, C., Farina, P., Rossi, C., Beer, M., Cavalli, F., Masera, G., Mangioni, C.: *Proc Am Assoc Cancer Res 23: 131, 1982.*
11. Evans, W.E., Sinkule, J.A., Crom, W.R., Dow, L., Look, A.T., and Rivera, G.: *Cancer Chemother Pharmacol 7: 147, 1982.*
12. Falkson, G., Van Dyk, J.J., Van Eden, E.B., Van Der Merwe, A.M., Van Den Bergh, J.A., and Falkson, H.C.: *Cancer 35: 1141, 1975.*
13. Farina, P., Marzillo, G., and D'Incalci, M.: *J Chromatogr 222: 141, 1981.*
14. Hande, K.R., McKay, C.M., Wedlund, P.J., Noone, R.M., Shea, W.K., Fer, M.F., Greco, F.A., and Wolff, S.N.: *Proc Am Assoc Cancer Res 23: 131, 1982.*
15. Lau, M.E., Hansen, H.H., Nissen, N.I., and Pedersen, H.: *Cancer Treat Rep 63: 485, 1979.*
16. Lawrie, S., Dodson, M., Arnold, A., and Whitehouse, J.M.A.: *Cancer Chemother Pharmacol 7: 236, 1982.*
17. Nissen, N.I., Hansen, H.H., Pedersen, H., Stroyer, I., Dombernowsky, P., and Hessellund, M.: *Cancer Chemother Rep 59: 1027, 1975.*
18. Nissen, N.I., Dombernowsky, P., Hansen, H.H., and Larsen, V.: *Cancer Treat Rep 60: 943, 1976.*
19. Pelsor, F.R., Allen, L.M., and Creaven, P.J.: *J Pharm Sci 67: 1106, 1978.*
20. Sandoz Pharmaceuticals, Preclinical Brochure. VM26. Research Department, Hanover, New Jersey, 1967.

FIGURE 1. Upper panel shows structure of teniposide (I) and etoposide (II). • indicates the position of the radioactive label in the studies by Creaven and Allen.[6,7] Lower panel shows structure of the major metabolite of etoposide 4'-demethylepipodophyllic acid-9-(4,6-0-ethylidene-β-D-glucopyranoside).[3]

now been studied by isotopic and by HPLC techniques. The gastrointestinal absorption of etoposide is adequate if the compound is given in solution. The plasma decay is relatively rapid for etoposide, slower for teniposide. Data on clearance in the literature are variable but indicate a more rapid body clearance and

21. Sandoz Pharmaceuticals, Preclinical Brochure. VP16-213. Research Department, Hanover, New Jersey, 1971.

22. Scalzo, A.J., Comis, R., Fitzpatrick, A., Issell, B.F., Nardella, P.A., Pfeffer, M., Smyth, R.D., and Harken, D.R.: *Proc Am Soc Clin Oncol 1: 129, 1982.*

23. Sessa, C., D'Incalci, M., Farina, P., Rossi, C., Cavalli, F., Mangioni, C., and Garattini, S.: *Proc Am Assoc Cancer Res 23: 128, 1982.*

24. Snodgrass, W., Walker, L., Heideman, R., Odom, L.F., Hays, T., and Tubergen, D.G.: *Proc Am Assoc Cancer Res Am Soc Clin Oncol 21: 333, 1980.*

25. Strife, R.J., Jardine, I., and Colvin, M.: *J Chromatogr 182: 211, 1980.*

26. Van Maanen, J.M.S., Van Oort, W.J., and Pinedo, H.M.: *Cancer Chemother Pharmacol 7: 236, 1982.*

CHAPTER 13

Teniposide (VM 26)

F.R. Macbeth

Introduction

Teniposide (VM 26) is a semisynthetic derivative of podophyllotoxin, which has been in experimental clinical use for over 10 years, but has, in general, been much less studied than its congener etoposide (VP16-213). There have been several reviews of its pharmacology and activity over the past few years.[10,16,20,25,35]

Dosage, Administration, and Toxicity

Teniposide is usually administered by intravenous infusion over at least 30 minutes. As with etoposide, more rapid infusion is associated with collapse and hypotension. It has been administered intravesically with some success and minimal toxicity[17] but at present there is no specific oral formulation or reported experience of oral administration.

The usual dosage schedules are either 70–130 mg/m² weekly or 30–60 mg/m² daily × 5 repeated every 3–4 weeks. These schedules derived from phase I studies in heavily pretreated patients are probably somewhat conservative, and higher dose rates such as 180 mg/m² weekly or 100 mg/m² daily × 5 have been used in previously untreated patients with acceptable levels of toxicity. This may be important in assessing clinical response rates be-

CRC Medical Oncology Unit, Centre Block, Southampton General Hospital, Southampton, England

cause there is a suggestion of a dose–response relationship in small cell carcinoma.

The major toxicity of teniposide is undoubtedly bone marrow suppression, and this is often dose-limiting. Leukopenia seems to be more common than thrombocytopenia, with nadir counts occurring at around 10–14 days with recovery in a further 7–10 days. In other respects, it is a fairly well-tolerated drug. Nausea and vomiting are fairly common but not severe, and alopecia is infrequent. Other less common toxicities are listed in Table 1.

ANTITUMOR ACTIVITY

Over the past 10 years, the activity of teniposide has been adequately studied in 18 tumors (Tables 2 and 3). It is a significantly active agent in Hodgkin's disease — with an overall response rate of 40% in pretreated patients — and it has a similar level of activity in non-Hodgkin's lymphoma of various histological subtypes. It is also an active single agent in childhood neuroblastoma and in combination with cisplatin has been reported as giving six CRs (27%) and nine PRs (33%) in 22 children resistant to adriamycin and cyclophosphamide.[11]

Teniposide is being widely used in the management of primary brain tumors. The initial premise for this was that it is a small lipophilic molecule and therefore likely to cross the blood–brain barrier.

TABLE 1.   Toxicity of Teniposide

Common, dose-limiting	Bone marrow suppression
Fairly common	Nausea and vomiting Alopecia
Rare	Raised serum SGOT Acute hypertension Fever Anaphylaxis Congestive cardiac failure[a] Seizures[a] Raised serum amylase[a] Hypercalcemia[a] Pulmonary hyaline membrane disease Acute intravascular haemolysis

[a] Doubtful relationship to teniposide administration.

However, pharmacokinetic studies indicate that less than 1% of the administered I.V. dose does, in fact, get into the CSF, unless there has been previous surgery or radiotherapy.[25]

At first, a response rate of about 30% for primary brain tumors, mainly gliomas, appears encouraging. But response assessment in brain tumors is very difficult, and, in the three papers quoted, response was defined as any improvement in clinical signs. Few of the responses were confirmed by CT or isotope scan, and, in fact, Gerosa[9] specifically points out that there was no concordance between clinical response and CT scans and that some "responders" had worsening CT scans. If the more rigorous response criteria proposed by Edwards et al.[6] were used (a responder being a patient who shows improvement in two or more tests — clinical examination and/or isotope scan and/or CT scan), then the response rates would be much less impressive. A randomized, prospective study comparing CCNU with teniposide or teniposide plus CCNU in well-documented patients with rigorous response assessment is now needed to settle the question of whether teniposide is a significantly useful drug in primary brain tumors.

The efficacy of teniposide in small-cell bronchial and bladder carcinomas remains controversial. For small-cell carcinoma, Samson et al.[26] reported 0/14 responses at 30 mg/m² daily × 5, whereas Woods et al.[34] using 60–100 mg/m² daily × 5, found 7/25 responses, including two complete responders, which suggests a dose–response relationship. However, even the higher response rate is lower than that usually reported for etoposide. The European experience of teniposide in bladder carcinoma consists of an 18% overall response rate in 65 patients,[17,18] whereas Qazi, of the Eastern Cooperative Oncology Group,[19] found only 2/40 partial re-

TABLE 2.   Tumours Responsive to Teniposide

Tumor	References	Patients				CR + PR Percent
		Total	Evaluable	CR	PR	
Hodgkin's	7,14,28	50	50	3	17	40
Non-Hodgkin's lymphoma	4,7,14,31	128	127	4	40	35
Neuroblastoma	3,22	52	38	1	12	34
Primary brain tumors (adults)	9,13,27	57	52	—	15[a]	29[a]
Small-cell carcinoma of bronchus	26,34	39	36	2	5	19
Breast	7,29	45	42	0	7	17
Acute lymphoblastic leukemia (children)	3,24	43	27	1	3	15
Colorectal	28	20	17	0	2	12
Bladder	7,17–19	105	105	4	10	10

[a] Special response criteria.

TABLE 3. Tumours Not Responsive to Teniposide

Tumor	References	Total	Evaluable	CR	PR	CR + PR Percent
Acute non-lymphoblastic leukemia (children)	3	28	19	1	0	5
Bladder (Bilharzia-induced)	8	24	24	0	1	4
Non-small-cell carcinoma of bronchus	2,26	59	56	0	1	2
Ovary	26	16	16	0	0	0
Kidney	12	13	12	0	0	0
Esophagus	7	12	12	0	0	0
Head and neck	7	16	16	0	0	0
Malignant melanoma	1	22	21	0	0	0
Sarcoma (miscellaneous)	32	12	12	0	0	0
Primary brain tumors (children)	3,30	34	25	0	0	0

sponses (5%), and Gad-el-Mawla of Egypt only one partial response in 24 patients with bilharzia-induced tumors.[8] All studies used a similar dose rate of 30 mg/m² daily × 5.

Teniposide is an active agent in childhood ALL and Rivera has recently reported the St. Jude's experience of using it in combination with cytosine arabinoside in consolidation and induction failures.[23] Teniposide also has limited activity in breast and colon carcinomas, and Table 3 lists the tumors in which it has been adequately assessed and shown to be inactive. There has not yet been any assessment in germinal tumors, adult leukemias, and childhood tumors other than neuroblastoma.

REFERENCES

1. Bellet, R.E., Catalano, R.B., Mastrangelo, M.J., Berd, D., and Koons, L.S.: Cancer Treat Rep 62: 445, 1978.
2. Bhuchar, K., Boyle, L.E., and Lanzotti, V.J.: Proc Am Soc Clin Oncol 19: 407, 1978.
3. Bleyer, W.A., Krivit, W., Chard, R.L., and Hammond, D.: Cancer Treat Rep 63: 977, 1979.
4. Chiuten, D.F., Bennet, J.M., Creech, R.H., Glick, J., Falkson, G., and Brodovsky, H.S.: Cancer Treat Rep 63: 7, 1979.
5. Dombernowsky, P., Nissen, N.I., and Larsen, V.: Cancer Chemo Rep 56: 71, 1972.
6. Edwards, M.S., Levin, V.A., and Wilson, C.B.: Cancer Treat Rep 64: 1179, 1980.
7. EORTC: Br Med J 2: 744, 1972.
8. Gad-el-Mawla, N.M., Muggia, F.M., Hamza,

M.R., El-Morsi, B., and Sherif, M.: Cancer Treat Rep 62: 993, 1978.
9. Gerosa, M.A., DiStefano, E., and Olivi, A.: Surg Neurol 15: 128–134, 1981.
10. Gutierrez, M.L. and Crooke, S.T.: Cancer Treat Rev 6: 153, 1979.
11. Hayes, A., Green, A.A., Casper, J., Cornet, J., and Evans, W.E.: Cancer 48: 1715–1718, 1981.
12. Hire, E.A., Samson, M.K., Fraile, R.J., and Baker, L.H.: Cancer Clin Trials 2: 293, 1979.
13. Kessinger, A., Lemon, H.M., and Foley, J.F.: Cancer Treat Rep 63: 511, 1979.
14. Mathé, G., Schwarzenberg, L., Pouillart, P., Oldham, R., Weiner, R., Jasmin, C., Rosenfeld, C., Hayat, M., Misset, J.L., Musset, M., Schneider, M., Amiel, J.L., and De Vassal, F.: Cancer 34: 985, 1974.
15. Muggia, F.M., Selawry, O.S., and Hansen, H.H.: Cancer Chemother Rep 55: 575, 1971.
16. Nissen, N.I., Dombernowsky, P., Hansen, H.H., and Pedersen, A.G.: Rec Res Cancer Res 69: 98, 1980.
17. Pavone-Macaluso, M., Caramia, G., Rizzo, F.P., and Messana, V.: Eur Urol 1: 53, 1975.
18. Pavone-Macaluso, M.: Eur Urol 2: 138, 1976.
19. Qazi, R., Elson, P., and Khandekar, J.D.: Cancer Treat Rep 66(2): 405–406, 1982.
20. Radice, P.A., Bunn, P.A., and Ihde, D.C.: Cancer Treat Rep 63: 1231, 1979.
21. Rivera, G., Avery, T., and Pratt, C.: Cancer Chemo Rep 59: 743, 1975.
22. Rivera, G., Green, A., Hayes, A., Avery, T., and Pratt, C.: Cancer Treat Rep 61: 1243, 1977.
23. Rivera, G., Dahl, G.V., Murphy, S.B., Bowman, W.P., Aur, R.J., Avery, T.L., and Simone, J.V.: Cancer Chemother Pharmacol 7: 169–172, 1982.
24. Rosenstock, J.G. and Donaldson, M.H.: Cancer Treat Rep 60: 265, 1976.
25. Rozencweig, M., Von Hoff, D.D., Henney, J.E., and Muggia, F.M.: Cancer 40: 334, 1977.
26. Samson, M.K., Baker, L.H., Talley, R.W., and Fraile, R.J.: Eur J Cancer 14: 1395, 1978.
27. Sklansky, B.D., Mann-Kaplan, R.S., Reynolds,

A.F., Rosenblum, M.L., and Walker, M.D.: *Cancer 33: 460, 1974.*

28. Sonntag, R.W., Senn, H.J., Nagel, G., Giger, K., and Alberto, P.: *Eur J Cancer 10: 93, 1974.*

29. Spremulli, E., Schulz, J.J., Speckhart, V.J., and Wampler, G.L.: *Cancer Treat Rep 64: 147, 1980.*

30. Sullivan, M.P., van Eys, J., Herson, J., Starling, K.A., Ragab, A., and Sexhauer, C.: *Cancer Treat Rep 63: 155, 1979.*

31. Terelli, U., Carbone, A., Tumulo, S., Galligori, E., Veronesi, A., Trovo, M.G., Frustaci, S., Ron-cadin, M., Zaganel, V., Figoli, F., Longlus, S., Grigoletto, E., and Cannale, V.C.: *Proc Am Soc Clin Oncol 1: 163, 1982.*

32. Trempe, G., Sykes, M., Young, C., and Krakoff, I.: *Proc Am Soc Clin Oncol 11: 79, 1970.*

33. Wilson, W.W., Bull, F., and Solomon, J.: *Proc Am Soc Clin Oncol 17: 250, 1976.*

34. Woods, R.L., Fox, R.M., and Tattersall, M.H.N.: *Cancer Treat Rep 63: 2011, 1979.*

35. Macbeth, F.R.: *Cancer Chemother Pharmacol 7: 87–91, 1982.*

CHAPTER 14

Recent Clinical and Experimental Developments with Methylglyoxal-*bis*(guanylhydrazone)

C.W. Porter, D.L. Kramer, and E. Mihich

Clinical History

Since being introduced as an anticancer agent in the late 1950s,[16,34] methylglyoxal-*bis*(guanylhydrazone) (MGBG, also known as methyl-G or methyl-GAG) has experienced continual but limited clinical use. The early clinical trials using the drug on a daily dose schedule[8,17,27,49,50] revealed very impressive activity, particularly against acute myelocytic leukemia, where at optimal dose levels (150 mg/m² daily), MGBG produced up to 45% complete remissions as a single agent.[27] In combination with 6-mercaptopurine and/or other anticancer agents, remission rates of 35–45% have been reported among leukemia patients.[4,58] Unfortunately, the potent activity of the drug was achieved at the cost of severe host toxicities and the drug was gradually withdrawn from clinical use as new alternative agents became available.

Clinical Developments

A resurgence in clinical interest occurred when minimal toxicity and good response rates (36%) were reported by the Southwest Oncology Group[26] in phase I and II trials employing MGBG on a weekly, rather than daily, infusion sched-

ule. Among 47 patients studied, 74% were virtually without significant toxicity. It has since been determined from pharmacokinetic studies[50] that MGBG has a very low urinary excretion rate and a relatively rapid plasma clearance suggesting that MGBG may be sequestered in the body. Moreover, MGBG is not broken down or metabolized in biological systems.[1,33]

Although initial indications suggested that weekly MGBG would be very useful in treating certain solid tumors, this has not been confirmed in subsequent studies. Recently, Warrell et al.[57] found that weekly MGBG resulted in partial responses in 46% of Hodgkin's disease and in 37% of nonHodgkin's lymphomas refractory to conventional therapy. Finally, recent findings in Finland[22,56] indicate that the antitumor activity of MGBG can be selectively enhanced by pretreatment (priming) patients with α-difluoromethylornithine (DFMO), a specific inhibitor of polyamine biosynthesis. The basis for this effect will be discussed later. DFMO is particularly well suited for drug combination studies since, by comparison to other anticancer agents, it is virtually atoxic to humans. Rapid and distinct therapeutic responses were obtained in a number of children with advanced lymphoblastic and myeloblastic leukemia by sequential treatment with DFMO and MGBG. Thus, MGBG continues to demonstrate clinical

Department of Experimental Therapeutics, Grace Cancer Drug Center, Roswell Park Memorial Institute, New York State Department of Health, Buffalo, New York

usefulness, particularly in the treatment of lymphomas and leukemias.

Mechanism of Action; Polyamine Effects

Until recently, the mechanism of action of MGBG was thought to be related to its various interactions with the biological polyamines (Table 1). It resembles spermidine structurally,[18] competes with spermidine and spermine for uptake,[11,46,47] strongly inhibits the polyamine biosynthetic enzyme, S-adenosylmethionine decarboxylase,[19,61] and inhibits the polyamine degradative enzyme, diamine oxidase.[19] It was the inhibition of S-adenosylmethionine decarboxylase by MGBG that was thought to be responsible for the antiproliferative activity of the drug. In cells treated with MGBG, putrescine pools increase while those of spermidine and spermine decrease slowly as a consequence of pathway blockade. However, a number of laboratories[20,21,37,43,53] have been unable to correlate these decreases in pool sizes with inhibition of cell growth. The ability of spermidine to prevent the antiproliferative effects of MGBG,[32] which was a key observation in linking MGBG to polyamines, is now attributed to competition for cellular uptake rather than replenishment of MGBG-depleted spermidine pools.[47] Moreover the effect of DFMO — a highly specific inhibitor of polyamine biosynthesis — on cell growth is cytostatic,[28] while that for MGBG is definitely cytotoxic, suggesting different mechanisms of action.

Mitochondrial Effects

On the basis of considerable biochemical and ultrastructural evidence (Table 1), there is now sufficient cause to believe that another site of drug action, the mitochondrion, may, in fact, be responsible for the antiproliferative activity of the drug. Much of the impetus for this belief

TABLE 1. Biological Consequences of MGBG Treatment

Relating to Polyamines
  Competition with spermidine for uptake [11,47]
  AdoMet decarboxylase inhibited [10,61]
  AdoMet decarboxylase increased due to enzyme stabilization [15,19,40]
  Ornithine decarboxylase increased [15,25,39]
  Putrescine pools increased [15,25,39]
  Spermidine and spermine pools decreased [15,25,39]
  Methylthioadenosine levels decreased [60]
  Diamine oxidase inhibited [19,40]

Relating to Mitochondria
  Drug present in mitochondrial fraction [1]
  ATP pools decreased; ADP pools increased [42,49]
  Acetate incorporation into lipids decreased [42]
  Selective ultrastructural damage to organelle [36,38,43,49]
  Pyruvate oxidation inhibited [43,48]
  Lactate production increased [48]
  Inhibition of respiration in isolated mitochondria [6]
  Synthesis of mtDNA inhibited [13]
  Kinetoplast damaged in trypanosomes [9]
  Ultrastructural damage to mitochondria of yeast [12]
  Mitochondrial damage to intestinal crypt cells [44]
  Hypoglycemic response in animals [32]

came from ultrastructural studies which showed that, in a variety of cell types treated *in vitro*[36,38,62,63] or *in vivo*[43,49] with MGBG, the mitochondria are selectively and significantly damaged. Confirmation of these findings has recently been made in yeast by Diala et al.[12]

The ultrastructural effects are now supported by a number of findings which demonstrate that, in addition to being structurally damaged, the mitochondria are functionally impaired. These include decreased ATP pools with increased ADP pools,[42,50] decreased acetate incorporation into lipids,[42] decreased pyruvate oxidation,[43] increased lactate production,[48] and selective inhibition of mitochondrial DNA biosynthesis.[13] Of these various parameters, we have found pyruvate oxidation to be particularly reliable for detecting and assessing mitochondrial integrity. The assay relies on the measurement of radiolabeled carbon dioxide released from cells incubated in the presence of ^{14}C-pyruvate labeled in the 2-position. It requires that the substrate cycles at least twice through an intact tricarboxcylic acid cycle before the $^{14}CO_2$ is released and trapped. In studies with ascites L1210 leukemia cells,[48] pyruvate oxidation is significantly decreased by 4 hours after exposure to MGBG, while growth inhibition does not occur until after 10–12 hours and depletion of spermidine pools to levels comparable to those attained during DFMO-induced cytostasis does not occur even after 24 hours.

A study of the effects of MGBG on isolated rat liver mitochondria[6] has been used to characterize the interaction of MGBG with mitochondria in general. At drug concentrations comparable to those attained intracellularly, MGBG significantly inhibited state 4 respiration, but had less of an effect on state 3, or uncoupled, respiration. This may be due to the fact that in the absence of ADP (state 4) mitochondria generate a significant electrochemical gradient across their inner membrane. MGBG, being a cation under physiological conditions, might be electrophoretically attracted to the membrane by the negative potential at its interior. Similar selective binding characteristics have been noted for other cationic compounds. Rhodamine dyes, which are positively charged, stain mitochondria specifically, whereas uncharged rhodamines and the negatively charged dye, fluoroscein, do not.[24]

The inhibition of mitochondrial respiration was prevented by potassium cations and enhanced by valinomycin, suggesting drug competition for potassium-binding sites, possibly membrane phospholipids. Pretreatment of mitochondria with MGBG protected against the nonspecific swelling effects of Triton X-100, as might be expected with membrane binding. Finally, the electrophoretic mobility of mitochondria was markedly slowed by MGBG. Overall, the data suggest that MGBG neutralizes the net negative surface potential of isolated mitochondria by binding to sites (possibly phospholipids) at the inner mitochondrial membrane. Subsequent interference with cation binding and/or transport results in inhibition of bioenergetic functions.

Antiproliferative Action

While the numerous effects of MGBG on mitochondria (Table 1) seems to be a compelling reason to believe that they are responsible for the antiproliferative activity of the drug, this relationship has not yet been definitively established. Some of the arguments in favor of this mechanism of action for MGBG are as follows. First, for reasons given above, there seems little cause to believe that the effects of MGBG on polyamine biosynthesis can account for its antiproliferative activity. This is supported by studies with 4,4'-diacetyl-diphenylurea-*bis*(guanylhydrazone), an aromatic *bis*-(guanylhydrazone) having potent antiproliferative activity. The drug causes profound ultrastructural damage to mitochondria[35] and has no effect on polyamine biosynthesis.[10]

More direct evidence is the early appearance of mitochondrial effects, particularly those involving pyruvate oxidation. These appear as early as 4 hours in *in vitro*[48] and *in vivo* systems,[43] whereas inhibition of cell growth does not occur until several hours later. Similarly, ultrastructural damage also precedes detectable inhibition of cell growth.[38] Damage to mitochondrial ultrastructure is selective for proliferating cells and this is consistent with the action of MGBG. This has been observed among cultured cells[36] and more recently in the intestinal epithelium,[44] a site of MGBG toxicity, where damage only occurs to mitochondria of the dividing crypt cells but not to the nondividing villous cells. Although the appropriate uptake studies were not performed, Diala et al.[12] made the interesting observation that wild-type yeast is growth-inhibited by MGBG while petite mutants, lacking mitochondria, are not. Recently, mutants of human fibroblast VA_2 cells have been developed which are 20- to 30-fold more resistant to the growth inhibitory effects of MGBG than the parent line.[62,63] Although mitochondrial function is definitely resistant to MGBG, the cells take up about 40% less MGBG than the parent cells. This uptake difference is considered very minor among transport mutants,[29] but it is sufficient to make definitive experiments regarding the basis for resistance difficult to achieve. As indirect evidence for the significance of the mitochondrial effects, we have recently shown[7] that the hypoglycemic agent, phenethylbiguanide, potentiated the inhibitory effects of MGBG on the respiration of isolated mitochondria and, likewise, potentiated the antileukemic effects as well. Overall, the absolute contribution of the mitochondrial effects to the antiproliferative action of MGBG has yet to be defined, but the accumulation of these effects provides compelling reason to believe that such a relationship does indeed exist.

MGBG Uptake

That MGBG may have the mitochondrion as its primary site of action would certainly make it unusual among existing anticancer agents. Although a large number of mitochondrial poisons exists, and their use as anticancer agents has been proposed,[59] their development into clinically useful drugs has generally been limited by lack of selectivity for tumor tissue. In the case of MGBG, the tissue selectivity might be afforded by its rather unique uptake characteristics. It is a structural analog of spermidine[18] and is capable of utilizing the facilitated carrier mechanism for spermidine to gain entry into cells.[11,47] Proliferating tissues are particularly rich in polyamines (see review by Janne et al.[23]) and, as a consequence, an increased exchange of polyamines across the plasma membrane is expected. In fact, increased

quantities of polyamines are present in the urine and serum of humans and animals bearing tumors.[52] Pohjanpelto[45] reported that uptake of putrescine, the precursor of spermidine, increased 18- to 100-fold in cells stimulated to proliferate with serum, and that it was greater in sparsely populated (rapidly growing) than in densely populated (slowly growing) cultures of fibroblasts.

By sharing transport with spermidine, MGBG is probably taken up to the greatest extent by proliferating tissues and this may account for its selectivity. In fact, Seppanen et al.[54] found that MGBG uptake is critically dependent on the growth rate of tumor cells (i.e., slowly dividing cells transport less MGBG than rapidly dividing cells) and Mikles-Robertson et al.[36] found that MGBG cytotoxicity also correlates with growth rate. Since the mechanism of MGBG uptake involves a saturable carrier that is energy-dependent[14,46] cells can actually concentrate the drug. Concentration gradients across the plasma membrane as high as 1000-fold have been reported,[29,55] so that millimolar quantities of MGBG can accumulate intracellularly.

Thus, the spermidine carrier mechanism offers a unique and effective means for concentrating MGBG intracellularly. In fact, derivatives of the spermidine molecule can also be delivered and concentrated in a similar manner and serve as vector molecules for biologically active moieties.[46] This assumes, of course, that the uptake characteristics of the molecule are not lost during derivatization. We have recently shown[46] that the determinants of uptake for spermidine are the terminal amines primarily and the aliphatic chain length separating the amines secondarily. Accordingly, the optimal site on the spermidine molecule for derivatization is the central amine and we have demonstrated that moieties as large as a benzyl group at this position are well-tolerated by the spermidine carrier mechanism.[46] Using this rationale, we are presently developing a new family of N^4-spermidine derivatives as potential anticancer agents.

DFMO/MGBG Combination

One of the major developments in the use of MGBG is its sequential administration with DFMO. As mentioned earlier, DFMO is a highly specific inhibitor of ornithine decarboxylase,[28] the initial enzyme in polyamine biosynthesis. Its specificity resides in the fact that it does not irreversibly alkylate the enzyme until first being decarboxylated by it.[30] In cells treated with DFMO, putrescine and spermidine pools are completely depleted after two cell cycles while spermine pools remain the same or increase slightly.[28] By contrast, the putrescine pools of cells treated with MGBG increase while those of spermidine and spermine decrease. The original reason for using DFMO in combination with MGBG was to achieve a more effective and complete blockade of the polyamine pathway since the two drugs inhibit different enzymes leading to the formation of spermidine.[20] Although synergistic effects were obtained using the drugs concomitantly in the treatment of murine L1210 leukemia,[5] it soon became apparent that the basis for the synergism was different than first expected.

Alhonen-Hongisto et al.[2] found that during putrescine and spermidine depletion induced by DFMO, the transport of spermidine into cells is increased several-fold as a compensatory mechanism to conserve cellular polyamines stores. Because MGBG shares the transport mechanism with spermidine,[11] the uptake of MGBG is also enhanced. It then became apparent that the most effective means to utilize the DFMO/MGBG combination was by sequential administration of the drugs. Prior treatment with DFMO decreases putrescine and spermidine pools and enhances the accumulation of subsequently added MGBG. We suggest that increased uptake

of MGBG leads to increased interference with mitochondrial function and studies. Examining pyruvate oxidation in cells treated *in vitro* with DFMO and MGBG or MGBG alone support this notion (Fig. 1). This leads in turn to increased cytotoxicity by the drug.[54] There is also some indication that DFMO pretreatment actually enhances the selectivity of MGBG for tumor tissues, by increasing MGBG uptake much more into tumor tissues than into normal host tissues.[2,3] The effect is relative, however, so that uptake into normal tissues is also increased, but to a smaller extent. The latter requires, therefore, that clinical doses of MGBG in combination with DFMO be less than those given with MGBG alone. The sequential DFMO/MGBG combination has been used with success in Europe[22,56] in the treatment of leukemia patients and will soon undergo testing in the United States.

Conclusions

Despite being introduced into clinical use as an anticancer agent some 20 years ago, MGBG remains an experimental drug. It is apparent from the recent clinical advances with MGBG, particularly its administration on a weekly rather than daily basis, that the drug is deserving of further investigation in the treatment of lymphoma and leukemia. Further, the possibility that its clinical usefulness might be significantly improved by DFMO pretreatment is an exciting one. It represents one of those infrequent instances in combination chemotherapy where the basis for the drug interactions is well understood and highly rational.

The success of the clinical studies will determine the future of the laboratory investigations with MGBG. However, if MGBG is to achieve maximum usefulness as an anticancer agent, it is essential that the basis for its antiproliferative activity be defined. Not only will such information be relevant to clinical issues such as dose

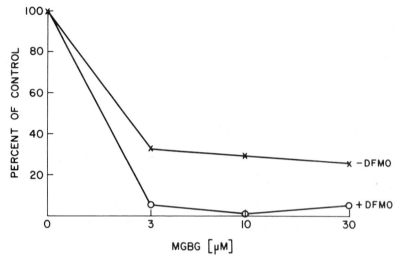

FIGURE 1.   Pyruvate oxidation by intact cultured L1210 leukemia cells treated for 6 hours with 10 μM MGBG. Certain of the cells (O——O) were pretreated with 100 mM DFMO for 24 hours and the others (x——x) were not. The assay was performed as described elsewhere.[43]

scheduling or the selection of agents for combination chemotherapy but it will also provide an indication of the potential of the target site, be it the mitochondrion or otherwise, in anticancer strategies. In any case, the fact remains that MGBG is a potent anticancer agent which, when compared to other anticancer agents, has very unique and interesting biological properties.

Note added in proof: Since the writing of this chapter, an excellent review of the clinical aspects of MGBG has been published by Warrell and Burchenal in the Journal of Clinical Oncology 1:52–65, 1983.

ACKNOWLEDGMENTS

Studies originating from this laboratory were supported in part from research grants CA-22153 and CA-24538 from the National Cancer Institute, U.S.P.H.S.

REFERENCES

1. Adamson, R.H., Denhum, C., and Oliverio, V.T.: *Arch Int Pharmacodyn 161: 364–374, 1966.*
2. Alhonen-Hongisto, L., Seppanen, P., and Janne, J.: *Biochem J 192: 941–945, 1980.*
3. Barrett, M., Porter, C.W., and Cowens, W.: *Cancer Res (Submitted).*
4. Boiron, M., Jacquillat, Cl., Weil, M., and Bernard, J.: *Cancer Chemother Rep 45: 69–75, 1965.*
5. Burchenal, J.H., Lokys, L., Smith, R., Cartmell, S., and Warrell, R.: *Proc Am Assoc Cancer Res 23: 230, 1981.*
6. Byczkowski, J., Salamon, W., Harlos, J., and Porter, C.: *Biochem Pharmacol 30: 2851–2860, 1981.*
7. Byczkowski, J., Zychlinski, L., and Porter, C.: *Cancer Res 42: 3592–3595, 1982.*
8. Carbone, P.P., Freireich, E.J., Frei, E., III, Rall, D.P., Karon, M., and Brindley, C.O.: *Acta Unio Int Can 20: 340–343, 1964.*
9. Chang, K.P., and Steiger, R.F.: *J Parasitol 62 (Suppl): 32, 1976.*
10. Corti, A., Dave, C., Williams-Ashman, H.G., Mihich, E., and Schenone, A.: *Biochem J 139: 351–357, 1974.*
11. Dave, C., and Caballes, L.: *Fed Proc 32: 736, 1973.*
12. Diala, E.S., Evans, I.H., and Wilkie, D.: *J Gen Microbiol 119: 35–40, 1980.*
13. Feuerstein, B., Porter, C.W., and Dave, C.: *Cancer Res 39: 4130–4137, 1979.*
14. Field, M., Block, J.B., Oliverio, V.T., and Rall, D.P.: *Cancer Res 24: 1939–1946, 1964.*
15. Fillingame, R.H. and Morris, D.R.: *Biochem Biophys Res Commun 52: 1020–1025, 1973.*
16. Freelander, B.L. and French, F.A.: *Cancer Res 18: 360–363, 1958.*
17. Freireich, E.J., Frei, E., III, and Karon, M.: *Cancer Chemother Rep 16: 183–186, 1962.*
18. Hamilton, W.C. and LaPlaca, S.J.: *Acta Crystl B24: 1147–1156, 1968.*
19. Holtta, E., Hannonen, P., Pipsa, J., and Janne, J.: *Biochem J 136: 669–676, 1973.*
20. Holtta, E., Pohjanpelto, P., and Janne, J.: *FEBS Lett 97: 9–14, 1979.*

21. Holtta, E., Korpela, H., and Hovi, T.: *Biochim Biophys Acta 677: 9–102, 1981.*
22. Janne, J., Alhonen-Hongisto, L., Seppanen, P., and Siimes, M.: *Med Biol 59: 448–457, 1981.*
23. Janne, J., Poso, H., and Raina, A.: *Biochim Biophys Acta 473: 241–293, 1978.*
24. Johnson, L.V., Walsh, M.L., and Chen, L.B.: *Proc Natl Acad Sci USA, 77: 990–994, 1980.*
25. Kay, J. and Pegg, A.E.: *FEBS Lett 29: 301–304, 1973.*
26. Knight, W.A., III, Livingston, R.B., Fabian, C., and Costanzi, J.: *Cancer Treat Rep 63: 1933–1937, 1979.*
27. Levin, R.H., Henderson, E., Karon, M., and Freireich, E.J.: *Clin Pharmacol Ther 6: 31–42, 1965.*
28. Mamont, P.S., Duchesne, M-C., Grove, J., and Bey, P.: *Biochem Biophys Res Commun 81: 58–66, 1978.*
29. Mandel, J.L. and Flintoff, W.F.: *J Cell Physiol 97: 335–344, 1978.*
30. Metcalf, B.W., Bey, P., Danzin, C., Jung, M.J., Casara, P., and Vevert, J.P.: *J Am Chem Soc 100: 2551–2553, 1978.*
31. Mihich, E.: *Pharmacologist 5: 270, 1963.*
32. Mihich, E.: *Arch Ital Pathol Clin Tumori 8: 153–206, 1965.*
33. Mihich, E.: In *Handbook of Experimental Pharmacology, New Series, Vol. 38/2,* A.C. Sartorelli and D.G. Johns, Eds., Springer Verlag, New York, pp. 766–788.
34. Mihich, E., Simpson, C.L., and Mulhern, A.I.: *Proc Am Assoc Cancer Res 3: 43, 1959.*
35. Mikles-Robertson, F., Dave, C., and Porter, C.W.: *Cancer Res 40: 1054–1061, 1980.*
36. Mikles-Robertson, F., Feuerstein, B.F., Dave, C., and Porter, C.W.: *Cancer Res 39: 1919–1926, 1979.*
37. Newton, N.E. and Abdel-Monem, M.M.: *J Med Chem 20: 249–252, 1977.*
38. Pathak, S.N., Porter, C.W., and Dave, C.: *Cancer Res 37: 2246–2250, 1977.*
39. Pegg, A.E.: *Biochem J 132: 537–540, 1973.*
40. Pegg, A.E., Corti, A., and Williams-Ashman, H.G.: *Biochem Biophys Res Commun 52: 696–701, 1973.*
41. Pegg, A.E. and McGill, S.M.: *Biochem Pharmacol 27: 1625–1629, 1978.*
42. Pine, M.J. and DiPaolo, J.: *Cancer Res 26: 18–25, 1966.*
43. Pleshkewych, A., Kramer, D.L., Kelly, E., and Porter, C.W.: *Cancer Res 40: 4533–4540, 1980.*
44. Pleshkewych, A. and Porter, C.W., *Cancer Res 43: 646–652, 1983.*
45. Pohjanpelto, P.: *J Cell Biol 68: 512–520, 1976.*
46. Porter, C.W., Bergeron, R.J., and Stolowich, N.J.: *Cancer Res (in press), 1982.*
47. Porter, C., Dave, C., and Mihich, E.: In *Polyamines in Biology and Medicine,* D. Morris and L. Marton, Eds., Marcel Dekker, Inc., New York, 1981, pp. 407–436.
48. Porter, C.W., Kramer, D.L., and Luthringer, O.: Manuscript in preparation, 1982.
49. Porter, C.W., Mikles-Robertson, F., Kramer, D., and Dave, C.: *Cancer Res 39: 2414–2421, 1979.*
50. Regelson, W. and Holland, J.F.: *Cancer Chemother Rep 27: 15–26, 1963.*
51. Rosenblum, M., Keating, M., Yap, B., and Loo, T.: *Cancer Res 41: 1748–1750, 1981.*
52. Russell, D.H. and Durie, B.G.M.: *Prog Cancer Res Ther 8: 1–178, 1978.*
53. Seppanen, P., Alhonen-Hongisto, L., and Janne, J.: *Eur J Biochem 110: 7–12, 1980.*
54. Seppanen, P., Alhonen-Hongisto, L., and Janne, J.: *Biochim Biophys Acta 674: 169–177, 1981.*
55. Seppanen, P., Alhonen-Hongisto, L., Poso, H., and Janne, J.: *FEBS Letts 111: 99–103, 1980.*
56. Siimes, M., Seppanen, P., Alhonen-Hongisto, L., and Janne, J.: *Int J Cancer 28: 567–570, 1981.*
57. Warrell, R.P., Lee, B.J., Kempin, S.J., Lacher, M.J., Strauss, D.J., and Young, C.W.: *Blood 57: 1011–1014, 1981.*
58. Weil, M., Jacquillat, Cl., Boiron, M., and Bernard, J.: *Eur J Cancer 5: 271–275, 1969.*
59. Wilkie, D.: *J R Soc Med 27: 599–601, 1979.*
60. Williams-Ashman, H.G. and Canellakis, Z.: *Persp Biol Med 22: 421–453, 1979.*
61. Williams-Ashman, H.G. and Schenone, A.: *Biochem Biophys Res Commun 46: 288–295, 1972.*
62. Wiseman, A., Kramer, D.L., and Porter, C.W.: *J Cell Biol 87: 186a, 1980.*
63. Wiseman, A., Kramer, D., and Porter, C.W.: *Cancer Res (in press), 1982.*

PART II

New Modalities of Tumor Treatment

A Review of the Combination of Radiotherapy and Chemotherapy in the Treatment of Cancer

M. Tubiana

Radiotherapy (RT) is, together with surgery, one of the two oldest methods for the treatment of cancer. Currently, as occurred two decades ago, about half of the patients with solid tumors are treated with RT in France, the United Kingdom, and Canada. Likewise, approximately half of the patients who are cured have received RT.

During these two decades the technique and theory of RT, as well as the knowledge of oncology, did not stand still. RT and surgery are increasingly used in combination, and the advances of chemotherapy have led — for several cancer sites — to an integration of RT, surgery, and chemotherapy in combined protocols.

The simplistic view of a competition, or even an antagonism, between RT and CT has fortunately disappeared. A decision to choose between the two treatments is unusual. Instead, the two main problems are to identify the subsets of patients who can benefit from an association of the two modalities, and to find the optimal way to combine them.

Cell Survival

Before illustrating these two points with a few examples, I would like to remind you that, following a fractionated scheme of irradiation or the administration of

cytostatic drug, the proportion of surviving tumor cells is approximately exponential. Therefore, it takes the same amount of irradiation to deplete the same percentage of surviving cells. For example, if after a dose, D_{50}, the proportion of surviving tumor cells is 50%, after a dose $2 \times D_{50}$ this proportion is 25%, and after $10 \, D_{50}$ it is 0.1%. A partial tumor regression is generally defined as a 50% reduction in tumor size; this corresponds to the death of approximately 50% of the cells. Total clinical disappearance (complete regression) of a tumor of 100 g, that is 10^{11} cells, requires that the tumor mass become smaller than 100 mg. Clinically, 100 mg are no longer detectable. This effect is obtained when at least 999 cells out of 1,000 are killed. If D_{50} kills half the cells, complete remission requires a dose 10 times larger: $10 \, D_{50}$.

If all the tumor cells were clonogenic, the total cure of a tumor of 100 g would require a dose equal to $36 \, D_{50}$. If only 1% of the tumor cells are clonogenic, which appears more likely, then a dose $30 \, D_{50}$ would be sufficient. Whatever the precise proportion of clonogenic cells, the important point is that the dose needed for the cure of a tumor is approximately 30 times larger than the dose which achieves a significant partial regression and at least three times larger than the dose which achieves a complete clinical remission. As the survival of one clonogenic cell is sufficient to cause a recurrence, it is easy

Director, Institute Gustave-Roussy, Rue Camille Desmoulins, Villejuif, France

to understand why, although it may have some relationship with cure, complete remission cannot reliably predict for it.

Combination RT + CT

What are the implications of these data for the combination of RT and CT? Let us assume that a radiation dose equal to approximately 30 D_{50} is required to control a tumor treated by RT solely. If previous CT decreases the tumor volume by half, the necessary RT dose is reduced to 29 D_{50}. If the CT has decreased the tumor diameter by half, the necessary RT dose becomes 26 D_{50}.

It is only when CT has produced a complete disappearance of the tumor that RT given to treat the areas of the original gross mass to eradicate the remaining subclinical disease can be reduced to 20 D_{50}. Even when this is the case, a combination of RT + CT is useful only if the sum of the effects is less for the normal tissues than for the tumor.

Identification of Patient Subgroups for Whom RT + CT is Beneficial

The combination of RT and CT has two purposes:[11,12]

1) Spatial cooperation — The two target volumes are different. CT is used to control disseminated disease while RT is either directed against the localized tumors or used for sanctuaries in which the drug concentration is low, i.e., brain in acute leukemia. In these situations, the chance for cure is equal to that of the less effective of the two treatments.

2) Eradication — The modalities both aim at eradication of the primary tumor. This method deserves to be considered both when the tumor is sensitive to both CT and RT — which unfortunately is not always the case — and when the therapeutic ratio is improved by com-

bination therapy. This means that by adding the two modalities a greater effect could be obtained on the tumor by the doses which are tolerated by the critical normal tissues. Finally, combination therapy is considered when one of the two modalities alone, at doses tolerated by normal tissues, is insufficient to control the disease. Combination therapy is useful either when it increases the proportion of cures or when it enables one to reduce the incidence of side effects or late sequelae.

A Subgroup of Hodgkin's Needing Only RT

For example, let us consider Hodgkin's disease. In clinical stages I and II, association of MOPP + RT results in long-term survival of the order of 90% or higher. This combination causes severe late effects, however, such as gonadal damage and a nonnegligible incidence of second malignancies. During the past decade it has become increasingly clear that for many patients the combination of MOPP + RT is an unnecessarily aggressive treatment. An important question is the delineation of the subgroup of patients which can be treated by RT alone.

Since 1969, the EORTC radiotherapy–chemotherapy group has conducted three clinical trials.[10,13] The first trial (1963–1971) compared regional radiotherapy (RT) with regional RT plus monochemotherapy.[10] The second trial (1972–1976) compared splenic irradiation with splenectomy and assessed the prognostic significance of laparotomy.[13] In the third (1976–1982), laparotomy was intended to select a good prognosis group for which RT alone might be sufficient. Laparotomy was not performed for patients with poor prognostic factors.

Multivariate analysis showed that for patients treated by RT alone (mantle field + paraaortic irradiation + splenectomy or spleen irradiation), the two most important prognostic indicators were the number of involved lymphatic areas and the erythrocyte sedimentation rate (ESR). Patients with stages I or II$_2$ (two lymphatic areas involved) and with ESR below 50 mm can be treated by RT alone with excellent results when staging laparotomy is negative. Staging laparotomy is of limited benefit for patients with poor prognostic indicators, since they require combination of RT and CT even when the laparotomy is negative.

A Subgroup of Ovarian Cancer Sensitive to Abdominal–Pelvic RT

The treatment of ovarian cancers may illustrate how surgery, RT, and CT can be combined. At the Princess Margaret Hospital in Toronto, patients with localized disease were randomized following surgery between pelvic irradiation and observation only.[3,4] The frequency of tumor relapses did not differ significantly between the two groups. This was not due to the inefficacy of RT, but to the fact that only the pelvis had been irradiated. The sites of relapse extended throughout the whole peritoneal cavity. This demonstrated that the irradiation of the entire peritoneal cavity was needed. The first attempts of this technique were not satisfactory because liver and kidney were shielded in order to avoid severe late effects. When it was recognized that the drainage of fluid and cells from the peritoneal cavity was via the diaphragmatic lymphatics, the Stanford group[5] and the Toronto group[3] decided to encompass the entire diaphragm in the treatment portal without liver shielding. Therefore, a radiation dose within liver tolerance was required. This new strategy was successful, and with this relatively small dose (22.5 Gy), excellent results were obtained, but only for tumors with no gross residue. For patients with a macroscopic residue that cannot be controlled by these doses, the results are much less satisfactory. In

this case at IGR we[2] surgically debulk the tumor and/or remove the peritoneal implants. CT is then started to decrease the size of the remaining implants. A second-look operation is carried out after the sixth course of CT. When the residual peritoneal disease is either subclinical or small ($\leq$ 2 cm), RT which aims to deliver 25 Gy to the whole of the peritoneal cavity is given. The preliminary results show the feasibility of this approach.

On the other hand, for several other cancer sites, trials with combination treatment have failed to improve the results. This is the case in particular for head and neck tumors. All the trials which have been carried out in Europe or the United States have affected normal tissues as much as the tumor.[1,7,11,12]

Schedule for the Combination of RT and CT

SIMULTANEOUS OR SEQUENTIAL

Simultaneous administration of drugs and radiation mainly adds to the complications. Analysis of the published data show that the therapeutic gain of such simultaneous administration appears to be very small, if any; often it is more detrimental than beneficial.[11,12] In particular, the hopes of enhancing the effect on the tumor by a so-called synchronisation of the neoplastic cells have not been fulfilled in clinical practice.[11,12]

On the other hand, a short gap between the two treatment modalities generally reduces the cumulative toxic effects on normal tissues. For most drugs, a time interval of 1 week between their administration and radiation therapy is sufficient.

In sequential regimens, the schedule is of great importance. Early administration of both radiotherapy and chemotherapy is advisable for many reasons. First, delaying the start of chemotherapy until after the completion of radiation therapy allows occult metastases to grow and to become less sensitive to chemotherapy. For example, if the tumor doubling time is equal to 1 month, a delay of 2 months allows the metastases to become four times bigger. Since the size is a very critical parameter, such delay could significantly reduce the effectiveness of adjuvant therapy. Similarly, delaying radiotherapy for a long period is also risky, as chemotherapy is not effective on bulky tumors while the effectiveness of radiation decreases with the size of the tumor.

Early irradiation is also advantageous in that it prevents the proliferation of drug-resistant cells. Spontaneous mutation to single drug resistance is relatively frequent. In addition to selection of drug-resistant cells which were initially present, mutation to drug resistance may occur during treatment. Whatever the mechanism, it is commonly observed, both in man and rodent, that initially drug-sensitive tumors become progressively less responsive and ultimately fail to respond during continuous treatment.[9]

One of the aims of polychemotherapy was to avoid the consequences of the presence of drug-resistant cells. However, resistance to as many as six separate drugs has been shown to occur in the treatment of human or experimental tumors. Moreover, when many drugs are used in combination, the individual drug doses must be reduced in order to avoid cumulative toxicity, and some of the drugs are only toxic to vital normal cells without contributing to tumor cell kill. This underlines the usefulness of irradiation, an agent without cross resistance with drugs and for which the cross toxicity is minimal.

The mathematical model constructed by Goldie and Coldman[6] shows that when two agents are used, scheduling is critical, because a delay in the administration of one of them increases the probability of development of a resistant tumor cell line.

COMBINED RT AND CT IN OAT CELL CANCER AND LYMPHOMA

In order to reconcile the needs for early administration of both RT and CT and for sequential administration, we have proposed a new treatment schedule which alternates radiotherapy and chemotherapy.[11,12,14] Chemotherapy is initiated without delay and the interval between the successive courses is, as usual, about 1 month. Radiotherapy starts 1 week after completion of the first cycle of chemotherapy and is continued for about 2 weeks. It is then interrupted 1 week prior to the second cycle of chemotherapy and is resumed 1 week after its completion.

Since it is impossible to deliver more than 25 Gy in 2 weeks, the radiotherapy course should be carried out as a split course, for example twice 25 Gy in 2 weeks separated by a time interval of about 2 weeks. The efficacy of such a treatment is about equal to that of a continuous irradiation delivering 50 Gy in 5 weeks. Such an alternating protocol avoids simultaneous administration of drugs and radiation and does not alter the rhythm of chemotherapy. It has been used at Villejuif in two feasibility trials in order to assess both the tolerance of normal tissues and the effects on the tumor.[14]

For anaplastic oat-cell carcinoma of the lung, each chemotherapy cycle includes: adriamycin, 40 mg/m^2; VP 16, 10 mg/m^2; methotrexate, 10 mg/kg; and cyclophosphamide, 300 mg/m$^2 \times 4$. The duration of this cycle is 4 days. One week after completion of the first cycle, the irradiation of the brain starts and 15 Gy are delivered in 10 days. The second cycle of chemotherapy begins 10 days after the last session of irradiation. One week after its completion, a second series of radiotherapy is given to two target volumes: the brain and the tumor mass and mediastinum. Fifteen Gy in 10 days are given to each volume. Between the second and the third cycle of chemotherapy, and between the third and the fourth, the irradiation of the mediastinum and of the tumor mass is continued. Thereafter, no irradiation is performed between the chemotherapy cycles. Therefore, the total dose of radiotherapy is 30 Gy to the brain in two series and 45 Gy to the tumor mass in three series of irradiation. Twenty-eight patients have been treated with this protocol during the past 2 years. The actuarial relapse-free survival at 1 year is 45%, the incidence of local recurrence 17%, and of distant metastasis 21%. Ten percent of the patients died from complications due to treatment (Arriagada et al., unpublished data). The follow-up is still too short to allow any conclusion, but these preliminary results are promising.

In non-Hodgkin's lymphoma of unfavorable histological types, we have undertaken, under the auspices of the Radiotherapy–Chemotherapy group of the EORTC, a feasibility trial comparing a conventional radiotherapy–chemotherapy combination with this new alternated chemotherapy–radiotherapy regimen for stage II patients. Treatment is started with chemotherapy (adriamycin, vincristine, cyclophosphamide, and prednisone). No irradiation is performed between the first and the second cycle in order to allow an assessment of the effect of this polychemotherapy on neoplastic tissues.

Ten days after the end of the second cycle an irradiation of the areas which were initially involved is carried out, and 15 Gy are delivered in 12 days. Ten days after completion of this first series of radiotherapy, a third cycle is administered. Radiotherapy is performed again between the third and the fourth chemotherapy cycles in order to deliver 30 Gy to all irradiated volumes. A booster irradiation of 15 Gy might be given to bulky masses after the fourth cycle. Chemotherapy is continued up to eight cycles. The immediate tolerance to treatment has been excellent and complete remission was obtained in all of the patients who have so far completed this alternating regimen. The relapse-free survival at one year is higher than 85%.

These promising clinical data have been recently supported by an interesting series of experiments reported by Looney et al.[8] These authors studied a rat hepatoma for which no cure was achieved with either radiotherapy or chemotherapy given alone. They obtained a tumor cure rate of 60% when three series of combined radiation (15 Gy) and cyclophosphamide (150 mg/kg) were given sequentially and the time between modalities held constant at 7 days. The time interval between the two modalities and between successive sequences was relatively critical. For example, a time interval of 7 days between radiation and cyclophosphamide was the most effective in controlling tumor growth with least host toxicity. The cure rate was reduced to 10% when the time between the first sequence of cyclophosphamide and radiation and the following one was increased from 7 to 25 days. This reduction in cure rate was probably due to greater tumor repopulation.

It is difficult to extrapolate from rodent tumors to human tumors. This is why critical investigation of the optimal tumor interval should continue. The reactions may vary from tumor to tumor; therefore, it is probably preferable to base scheduling on the study of the effects on normal tissues. Further clinical research will show whether the time interval chosen in this first series of patients is the optimum. It at least has the advantage of not altering the usual chemotherapy schedule and of allowing only a short period for possible tumor repopulation.

REFERENCES

1. Cachin, Y., Jortay, A., Sancho, H., Eschwege, F., Madelain, M., Desaulty, A., and Gerard, P.: Eur J Cancer 13: 1389, 1977.
2. Chassagne, D.: In Therapeutic Progress in Ovarian Cancer, Testicular Cancer and the Sarcomas, A.T. Van Oosterom, et al., Eds., Martinus Nijhoff, Boston, 1980, pp. 27–40.
3. Dembo, A.J. and Bush, R.S.: In Cancer Research

and Treatment — *Gynecological Malignancy I*, C.T. Griffiths, Ed., Martinus Nijhoff, Boston, 1982.

4. Dembo, A.J., Bush, R.S., and Brown, T.C.: *Bull Cancer* (Paris) *69: 292, 1982.*

5. Glatstein, E., Fuks, Z., and Bagshaw, M.A.: *Int J Radiat Oncol Biol Phys 2: 357, 1977.*

6. Goldie, J.H. and Coldman, A.J.: *Cancer Treat Rep 63: 1727, 1979.*

7. Kramer, S.: *Can J Otolaryngol 4: 213, 1975.*

8. Looney, W.B., Ritenour, E.R., and Hopkins, H.A.: *Cancer 47:860, 1981.*

9. Schabel, F.M., Skipper, H.E., Trader, M.W., Laster, W.R., Corbett, T.H., and Griswold, D.P.: In *Breast Cancer, Experimental and Clinical Aspects,* H.G. Mouridsen and T. Palshof, Eds., Pergamon Press, London 1980, p. 199.

10. Tubiana, M., Henry-Amar, M., Hayat, M., Breur, K., Van Der Werf Messing, B., and Burgers, M.: *Eur J Cancer 15: 645, 1979.*

11. Tubiana, M.: *J Eur Radiother 1: 107, 1980.*

12. Tubiana, M.: *Bull Cancer 68: 109, 1981.*

13. Tubiana, M., Hayat, M. Henry-Amar, M., Breur, K., Van Der Werf-Messing, B., and Burgers, M.: *Eur J Cancer 17: 355, 1981.*

14. Tubiana, M., Arriagada, R., and Cosset, J.M.: In *Progress in Radio-Oncology II,* K.H. Kärcher, H.D. Kogelnik, and G. Reinartz, Eds., Raven Press, New York, 1982, p. 387.

CHAPTER 16

Vincristine, Ifosfamide, Peplomycin (VIP): Therapy of Stage D Prostatic Carcinoma

Y. Matsumura

We have achieved favorable results of triple-drug combination chemotherapy (VIP) with vincristine, ifosfamide, and peplomycin for advanced prostatic carcinoma. Ifosfamide single-therapy resulted in a response rate of 26%, and peplomycin single-therapy in a rate of 24%. The triple-drug combination (VIP) therapy resulted in a response rate of 40%, or eight partial remissions in 20 cases of stage D prostatic carcinoma — among the highest reported. The toxicity of peplomycin was mild or moderate.

Material and Method

Based on the results of ifosfamide or peplomycin single therapy (Table 1) and also on the favorable results of triple-drug combination chemotherapy with vinblastine, ifosfamide, and bleomycin for testicular tumors reported by Schmoll[4] we devised the treatment plan for prostatic carcinoma as shown in Table 2. A total of 20 cases of hormone-refractory or relapsing stage D prostatic carcinoma were treated. The patients had a median age of 69 years (Tables 3 and 4).

Results

According to the criteria for evaluation of drug efficacy as proposed by U.S. Na-

Department of Urology, Okayama University Medical School, Okayama, Japan

TABLE 1. Results of Treatment of Prostatic Carcinoma in Japan (Karnofsky's criteria)

Ifosfamide-Monotherapy			
No. of Pts.	I-B	I-A	O-C ~ O-O
19	2	3	14
	(26%)c4)		
Peplomycin-Monotherapy			
Primary cases	I-B	I-A	O-C ~ O-O
42		10	32
	(24%)		
Relapsing cases			
37		13	24
	(35%)		

[a]OO, OC, IB and IA are stages of the disease. Figures indicate numbers of partial remissions.

tional Prostatic Cancer Project,[3] responses have been achieved in eight out of the 20 cases, or a response rate of 40%. The response duration was in the range of 3–24 months, with an average period of 9.5 months or a median period of 5 months (Tables 6 and 7).

Fever, nausea and vomiting, alopecia, and anemia were the relatively frequent

TABLE 2. Treatment Plan of VIP

Induction			
Vincristine:	Ifosfamide:		1 mg I.V., day 1–2
			40~50 mg/kg, I.V. (≦65 y.o.), day 2–4
			30~40 mg/kg, I.V. (<65 y.o.), day 2–4
Peplomycin:	q	3	5 mg I.M., day 1–6
weeks			
Maintenance			
Ifosfamide:			50 mg/Kg, I.V., q 4 weeks

TABLE 3. Patient Characteristics in 20 Cases

Age (Years)	
Median	69
Range	44–78
Performance status (%)	
Median	50
Range	30–90
Prior Therapy	
Endocrine therapy (%)	100
Radiotherapy (%)	30
Chemotherapy (%)	40
Histological grade	
Well-differentiated (%)	30
Moderately well-differentiated (%)	15
Poorly differentiated (%)	55

TABLE 4. Measurable or Evaluable Parameters

Primary lesion	95 (%)
Bone	95
Nodes	20
Lung	10
Penis	10
Liver	5
Acid phosphatase	65
Alc. phosphatase	70

TABLE 5. Effect of VIP (NPCP criteria)

Number of patients	20
Partial regression	8
Stable	6
Progression	6

TABLE 7. Subjective Symptoms

Pain	100 (%)
Bone pain	85
Others	20
Dysuria	85
Gait disturbance	35

TABLE 8. Toxicity of VIP

Number of patients	20 (%)
Fever	11(55)
Nausea/vomiting	12(60)
Anorexia	17(85)
Alopecia	13(65)
Stomatitis	1(5)
Macrohematuria	4(20)
Slight cerebral disorders	3(15)
Pneumonitis	2(10)
Liver function damages	1(5)
Leukopenia, below 2000/cm^3	4(20)
Hemoglobin reduction by more than 2g%	8(40)
Thrombocytopenia, below 50,000/cm^3	1(5)

TABLE 9. Conclusions

1) VIP (Advanced £ relapsed)	
Number of patients	20
Course	1–6
Average	2.6
2) Effective rate	
Shida's criteria	53%
NPCP criteria	40%
3) Toxicity	
mild or moderate	

toxicities. Macrohematuria was also relatively frequent (Table 8).

Pneumonitis was the dose-limiting factor and was severe in one of the cases, while in the other case it remained mild. On the whole, the toxicity of peplomycin was mild but as frequent as that of bleomycin (Table 8).

Conclusion

We performed triple-drug combination chemotherapy with vincristine, ifosfamide, and peplomycin in 20 cases of stage D, advanced prostatic carcinoma and relapsed prostatic carcinoma. A response rate of 40% was achieved according to the

TABLE 6. Relationship between Clinical Effect and Prior Therapy

	Prior Radiotherapy		Prior Chemotherapy	
	Yes (n = 6)	No (n = 14)	Yes (n = 8)	No (n = 12)
Partial regression	1	7	1	7
Stable	1	5	2	4
Progression	4	2	5	1

criteria proposed by NPCP. The toxicities of peplomycin were mild or moderate.

REFERENCES

1. Koiso, K. and Niijima, T.: In *The Prostate* (suppl. 1), A.A. Sandberg, J.T. Karr, Eds., Alan R. Liss, Inc., New York, 1981, p. 103.
2. Matsuda, A., Yoshioka, O., Yamashita, T., Ebihara, K., Umezawa, H., Miura, T., Katayama, I., Yokoyama, M., and Nagai, S.: *Recent Results in Cancer Res, 68: 191, 1978.*
3. Murphy, G.P. and Saroff, J., et al.: *Sem Oncol 3: 103, 1976.*
4. Schmoll, H.J.: In *Proceedings of International Holoxan-Symposium,* H. Burkert, H.C. Voigt, Eds., Dusseldorf, Asta-Werke A.G., 1977, p. 121.
5. Shida, K., Matsumoto, K., Shimazaki, J., Nishimura, R., Takeuchi, H., and Seto, T.: *Nishinihon J Urol 40: 869, 1978.*
6. Yoshimoto, J., Matsumura, Y., Asahi, T., Ozaki, Y., Tanahashi, T., Kaneshige, T., and Ohmori, H.: *Nishinihon J Urol 42: 761, 1980.*

CHAPTER 17

Intermediate-Dose Methotrexate (IDM) for the Treatment of Childhood Acute Lymphocytic Leukemia (ALL)

A.I. Freeman, V. Weinberg, D.M. Green, and M.L. Brecher

Introduction

The cure of children with acute lymphocytic leukemia (ALL) has greatly improved to the point that over 50% of them may be long-term, disease-free survivors. This has been accomplished by the use of central nervous system (CNS) "prophylaxis" and effective multiagent systemic chemotherapy.

In 1968, Cancer and Leukemia Group B (CALGB) employed prophylactic intrathecal methotrexate (I.T. MTX) alone and decreased the incidence of overt CNS leukemia from over 50% to 23%.[14] Cranial radiation (CRT) added to I.T. MTX as CNS prophylaxis further reduced the incidence of CNS disease to approximately 10%.[1,2,3,15,20]

In 1973, a pilot study at Roswell Park Memorial Institute (RPMI) was instituted with the following objectives: 1) to prevent the development of CNS leukemia without employing CRT, and 2) to intensify systemic therapy and thus eradicate leukemic cells in other sanctuaries. This program was based on clinical pharmacologic data demonstrating that I.V. intermediate-dose methotrexate (IDM) at a dose of 500 mg/m^2 given over 24 hours was capable of diffusing across the CNS barrier[29] and, presumably, simultaneously penetrating other sanctuaries. This pilot subsequently led to the randomized study (CALGB Protocol 7611) which compared "standard therapy" utilizing CRT (2400 rads) plus I.T. MTX with IDM × 3 plus I.T. MTX × 6 with respect to their ability to improve the disease-free survival by reducing systemic, CNS, and extramedullary relapses. Results of the IDM RPMI pilot study which preceded the CALGB study indicated that in standard-risk (SR) patients with ALL, IDM was capable of eradicating subclinical extramedullary disease and adding systemic intensification.[29] However, as the original population of pilot patients was observed for a longer period of time, it became apparent that increased-risk (IR) patients had a significant risk of primary CNS relapse.[11,13] Therefore, the original pilot study was further intensified in a second RPMI pilot to provide more aggressive treatment for IR patients. This paper reports the results of these studies.

Materials and Methods

DEFINITIONS AND CRITERIA

Previously untreated children and adolescents less than 20 years old with ALL,

Department of Pediatrics, Roswell Park Memorial Institute, Buffalo, New York and the CALGB Operations Office, Scarsdale, New York

including undifferentiated or stem cell, were eligible for entry after informed consent had been obtained. Spinal taps were performed routinely during the induction and intensification phase. After remaining in continuous complete remission (CCR) for 3 years and prior to cessation of therapy, all patients received a diagnostic spinal tap.

Bone marrow aspirates were examined prior to the onset of induction therapy at day 28 and day 42 (prior to sanctuary therapy) and every 3 months thereafter or at any time that relapse was suspected. Briefly, a remission bone marrow has normal granulopoiesis, thrombopoiesis, and erythropoiesis with fewer than 5% lymphoblasts and less than 40% lymphocytes plus lymphoblasts. Induction failure was defined as those patients not achieving a remission bone marrow by day 42.

Relapse (termination of complete remission) was defined as: 1) bone marrow relapse (greater than 25% blast cells); 2) CNS relapse (definite blast cells on cytologic (cytocentrifuge) preparations of CNS, or 10 mononuclear cells/μl not attributable to chemical meningitis); 3) biopsy-proven leukemic relapse in an extramedullary organ; or 4) death while in complete remission. Patients were stratified according to CALGB risk criteria and were considered to be SR if the initial WBC was less than 30,000/mm^3 and age was after the second and before the eighth birthday. All other patients were classified as IR. Patients were randomized separately from within each risk stratum.

Leukoencephalopathy was defined clinically by the persistent unexplained presence of confusion, somnolence, ataxia, spasticity, focal neurological changes, and seizures. Pathologically, (when applicable) discrete necrotic foci and reactive astrocytosis[16,21] were required for histological confirmation.

The criteria as described above were also utilized for the two RPMI pilots. On the two pilot studies at RPMI, the patients were consecutively entered. Criteria for IR were the same as CALGB, except for age which extended to age 10. Patients with an anterior mediastinal mass or who presented with meningeal leukemia were excluded from entry onto the RPMI studies. Chemotherapy was discontinued in both RPMI pilot studies after 48 months of CCR, whereas it was discontinued after 3 years in CALGB 7611.

TREATMENT

CALGB Study 7611

Figure 1 — Schema.

INDUCTION PHASE

All patients received the same induction therapy, consisting of vincristine 2 mg/m^2/week I.V. for four doses (with a maximum single dose of 2 mg), prednisone 40 mg/m^2 P.O. daily for 4 weeks and then tapered over approximately 10 days, MTX 12 mg/m^2 I.T. for three doses (with a maximum single dose of 15 mg), and L-asparaginase 1000 IU/kg/day I.V. for 10 doses.

SANCTUARY (INTENSIFICATION) PHASE

Intermediate-Dose Methotrexate: IDM was administered at a dose of 500 mg/m^2, 1/3 I.V. push and 2/3 I.V. infusion, over 24 hours given on three occasions at 3-week intervals. A single dose of leucovorin at 12 mg/m^2 was administered 24 hours after completion of IDM. I.T. MTX 12 mg/m^2 (maximum single dose of 15 mg) was given concurrently with IDM on the three occasions.

CNS Radiation: CRT was given over a period of 16 days in 200-rad increments for a total of 2400 rads. External radiation was delivered to the whole brain including the spinal cord down to C2. The radiation field included the entire frontal lobe, posterior half of the eyeball, including the optic disc and nerve. The anterior half of both eyes were shielded. The patients

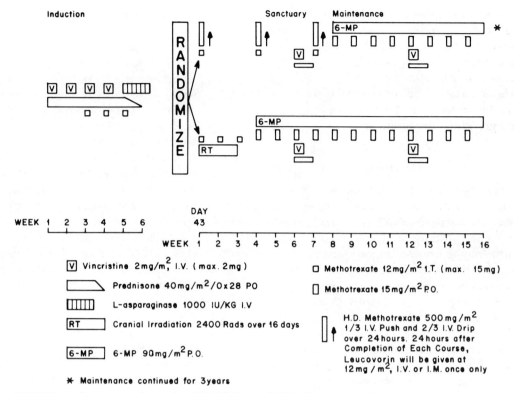

FIGURE 1. Treatment schema for CALGB Protocol 7611 (Treatment of primary untreated acute lymphocytic leukemia in patients under 20 years).

were treated with two lateral parallel opposed fields. I.T. MTX at 12 mg/m² (maximum single dose of 15 mg) weekly for three doses was also administered during the period of CRT.

MAINTENANCE PHASE

Upon completion of the sanctuary phase, all patients received the same maintenance therapy consisting of daily oral 6-mercaptopurine prescribed at 90 mg/m² plus weekly oral MTX at 15 mg/m². Reinforcement courses of vincristine and prednisone were given every 4 weeks for 6 months following the start of sanctuary therapy, and then starting at week 28, two weekly vincristine doses plus 2 weeks of prednisone without tapering were given every 3 months for the duration of maintenance. Following 3 years of maintenance

therapy, patients were completely reevaluated with a bone marrow, diagnostic lumbar puncture, and testicular biopsy to determine their remission status.

RPMI PILOTS

Study I — IDM × 3: Between January 1, 1974 and July 31, 1976, 19 consecutive previously untreated, IR children and adolescents with ALL were entered on a study which was identical to the CALGB IDM (× 3) study, except for an additional year of maintenance therapy (total of 4 years).

Study II — IDM × 6 (Fig. 2): Between August 1, 1976 and December 31, 1978, 22 consecutive previously untreated increased-risk children and adolescents with ALL were entered on a study which differed from the IDM × 3 only in the intensification phase which employed six courses of IDM (3–500 mg/m², and 3–1500 mg/m²), six doses of I.T. MTX plus three additional courses of triple I.T. chemotherapy (MTX, cytosine arabinoside, and hydrocortisone or dexamethasone) for systemic intensification and CNS prophylaxis (Fig. 2). The two pilot groups were comparable in terms of the known risk factors of age, WBC, organomegaly, etc.

Statistics

Remission duration curves were drawn using the actuarial life-table technique to calculate the percent in remission.[8] Differences in patterns of relapse were determined using Breslow's modification of the Kruskal-Wallis test.[5] Differences between treatments in distributions of patient and disease features were examined using the chi-square test for contingency tables.[25] Multivariate regressior. analyses using Cox's regression model for concomitant variables were performed to identify features prognostic of remission duration.[7]

Results

CALGB STUDY 7611

The CALGB Study 7611 accrued 634 patients from November 12, 1976 until July 16, 1979. The current analysis has a median follow-up duration of 40 months. Of the 634 patients entered on study, 600

(95%) were evaluable for response to induction therapy.

Complete remission was achieved by 548 of the 600 evaluable patients (91%). It was higher among the SR patients, where 251/262 (96%) achieved CR, than among the IR patients where 297/338 (88%) achieved CR ($p < 0.01$).

Five hundred and six patients out of 548 were evaluable for the sanctuary phase and 259 were randomized to receive IDM, and 247 to receive CRT as sanctuary therapy. Among SR patients, superior hematologic protection occurred with IDM therapy ($p < 0.01$). In contrast, SR patients had a higher rate of CNS relapse ($p = 0.01$) when treated with IDM, with the resultant overall CCR being similar in both groups (Figs. 3 and 4).

Among IR patients there was no difference in complete remission or in hematologic remission duration (Fig. 5). Again, there was greater CNS protection for IR patients treated with CRT (Fig. 6) ($p = 0.03$).

Eleven males experienced testicular relapse out of the total of 269 males, 10 of which occurred among those who received CRT ($p = 0.01$).

Overall, IDM was quite tolerable, with 94% of the patients having received the full three doses. Overt clinical leukoencephalopathy was not recorded with IDM on this study. Mucositis (generally mild)

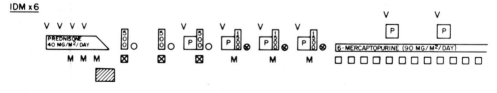

FIGURE 2. Treatment schema for RPMI Pilot 2 (IDM × 6) for IR patients. It differs from IDM × 3 by three additional courses of IDM at 1500 mg/m² and three additional doses of triple I.T. CT.

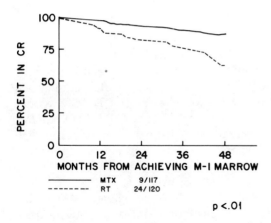

FIGURE 3. CALGB Protocol 7611 — duration of hematological remission in standard risk patients.

was the most common problem and occurred in approximately 30% of the patients.

IDM RPMI PILOT — IR PATIENTS (Fig. 7)

Thirty percent of the IR patients entered on the first RPMI pilot (IDM × 3) remained

in CCR with a median follow-up of 61 months, whereas 57% of the patients entered on the second RPMI pilot (IDM × 6) remained in CCR with a median follow-up of 39 months. The difference in disease-free survival between patients on IDM × 3 and IDM × 6 was statistically significant ($p = 0.046$). However, there was no difference in the incidence of primary CNS relapse between the two studies. Thirty-six percent of patients entered on IDM × 3 had a primary CNS relapse and 30% of the patients entered on IDM × 6 had a primary CNS relapse ($p = 0.44$).

Discussion

The CALGB Study 7611 compared IDM given on three occasions + I.T. MTX with CRT (2400 rads) + I.T. MTX for patients achieving a complete remission. These two treatment features were engrafted on what was considered the best standard induction and maintenance treatment at the time the study was designed.

The clinical basis for testing IDM was:

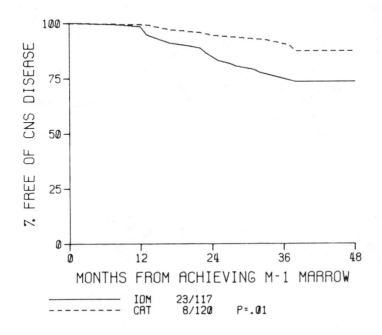

FIGURE 4. CALGB Protocol 7611 — duration of CNS remission in standard risk patients.

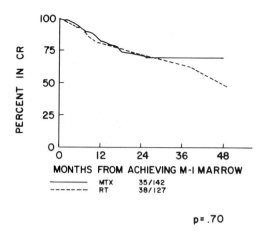

p = .70

FIGURE 5. CALGB Protocol 7611 — duration of hematological remission in increased risk patients.

1) the early work of Djerassi who demonstrated the effectiveness of high doses of MTX in ALL;[9] and 2) the pilot study of IDM conducted at RPMI which indicated, in a nonrandomized fashion, its effectiveness as therapy for ALL, particularly among SR patients.[24] A very similar study was reported by Moe et al. in Norway, again with very promising results.[18]

The pharmacologic basis of this study includes the following: reports showing that intravenous IDM resulted in MTX levels of $10^{-7} M$ reaching the CNS axis and diffusing into the cerebrospinal fluid (CSF).[23,29] The serum MTX levels following 500 mg/m^2 remained at 10^{-5} for the 24-hour infusion period.[29] It was also anticipated that IDM would afford protection to other sanctuary sites such as gonads, liver, and spleen.

An alternative treatment to the utilization of CRT has become particularly important since in recent years there is an increasing number of children surviving their illness and evidence has been reported indicating toxicity to the brain from CRT. Moss et al., recently compared children with ALL treated with CRT plus multiple doses of intrathecal chemotherapy (I.T. CT) to their siblings and showed

a significant mean drop in IQ of approximately 12 IQ points in the patient group.[19]

CALGB assessed CNS toxicity in a large number of patients who had been randomly assigned to three different methods of CNS prophylaxis: 1) I.T. MTX alone, 2) I.T. MTX + CRT, and 3) I.T. MTX + IDM. These patients were disease-free from 1 to 9 years. One hundred-six patients were tested who remained in CCR 1 to 9 years after the completion of their CNS prophylaxis. The parameters tested included psychometric examination, neurological assessment, CT scan, EEG, and evaluation of the neuro-endocrine axis. Significantly more EEG abnormalities were found among the patients who received IDM. Thirty-four percent of the patients receiving IDM had abnormal EEGs as compared to 8% of patients treated with I.T. MTX alone.[6] The clinical significance of this finding is not yet apparent.[6] There was an increased frequency of growth hormone deficiency in the group of children who received CRT, but again it should be noted that all patients maintained consistent linear growth, so that the clinical significance of these findings is not clear.[28] Of importance, however, was the difference in IQ. The mean verbal IQ scores were: I.T. MTX = 107; I.T. MTX + CRT = 95; and I.T. MTX + IDM = 104, ($p < 0.01$). The mean performance IQ scores were: I.T. MTX alone = 104; I.T. MTX + CRT = 91; and I.T. MTX + IDM = 108, $p < 0.01$. Also, school achievement as measured by the Wide Range Achievement Test (WRAT) was significantly lower in the CRT group. The impairments noted in the children receiving CRT appeared more severe in the younger children who were treated at less than 4 years of age.[22]

In the CALGB Study 7611, the pattern of relapse was different according to the therapy they received. SR patients receiving IDM had significantly less bone marrow relapse ($p < 0.01$), but significantly more CNS relapse ($p = 0.01$). IR patients

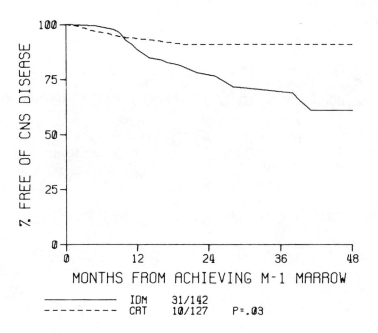

FIGURE 6. CALGB Protocol 7611 — duration of CNS remission in increased risk patients.

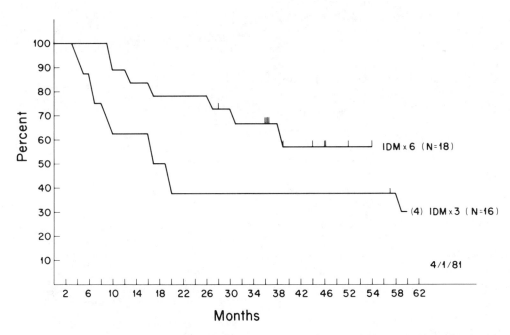

FIGURE 7. Disease free survival. RPMI pilot studies — Comparison of IDM × 3 (RPMI-Pilot 1) with IDM × 6 (RPMI-Pilot 2). There is a statistically significant improvement in duration of CR ($p = 0.046$) for patients receiving IDM × 6.

receiving CRT also showed significantly less CNS relapse ($p = 0.03$). Also noteworthy was the significantly less testicular relapse in male patients receiving IDM ($p = 0.01$). The difference in the pattern of relapse is important because it has been shown that there was a significant salvage rate for children experiencing an isolated CNS relapse.[10] Further, Bowman et al. have observed that an isolated testicular relapse during maintenance is followed by systemic relapse in a median time of 3 months, thereby carrying a poor prognosis; this is in contrast to an isolated testicular relapse after cessation of therapy which has a significant salvage rate.[4] Also, apart from bone marrow transplants,[26] there is virtually no cure rate for children experiencing a bone marrow relapse while receiving CT. Thus while receiving therapy, an isolated CNS relapse does not carry as grave a prognosis as does a bone marrow relapse[2] or a testicular relapse.[4]

Six doses of I.T. MTX along with three doses of IDM appear to be insufficient CNS prophylaxis for patients with ALL. Van Eys et al.[27] and Komp et al.[17] reporting on the Southwest Oncology Group (SWOG) experience, have shown that in both their standard and increased risk ALL group (excluding T-cell ALL), there was no difference between patients receiving CRT + I.T. CT and those receiving multiple repetitive I.T. CT for up to 3 years in terms of CNS protection or in terms of the duration of CR. In the second pilot study conducted at RPMI with IR patients, further intensification of IDM resulted in a statistically superior duration of complete remission because of less systemic relapse.[12]

In a majority of children with ALL, intensive repetitive I.T. CT, along with repetitive IDM, could result in an improved complete remission rate and likely avoid the potential neurotoxicity of CRT. Nonetheless, a segment of IR patients now still require CRT; these probably include those who present with T-cell ALL, or pre-B

ALL, who have a high incidence of extramedullary relapse, or those presenting with a very high WBC.[17,27]

ACKNOWLEDGMENT

This investigation was supported in part by Grant CA 07918, awarded by the National Cancer Institute, DHEW.

REFERENCES

1. Aur, R.J.A., Hustu, H.O., Verzosa, M.S., Wood, A., and Simone, J.S.: *Blood* 42(3): 349–357, 1973.
2. Aur, R.J.A., Simone, J.V., Hustu, H.O., and Verzosa, M.S.: *Cancer* 29: 381–391, 1972.
3. Aur, R.J.A., Simone, J.V., Hustu, H.O., Walters, T., Borella, L., Pratt, L., and Pinkel, D.: *Blood* 37: 272–281, 1971.
4. Bowman, W.P., Aur, R.J., Hustu, H.O., and Rivera, G.: *Proc ASCO* (1): 127, 1982.
5. Breslow, N.: *Biometrika* 57: 579–594, 1970.
6. Cohen, M.E., Duffner, P.K., Brecher, M.L., Diamond, L.S., Glicksman, A.S., and Freeman, A.I.: *Proc ASCO* (1): 135, 1982.
7. Cox, D.R.: *J R Stat Soc* (B)34: 187–220, 1972.
8. Cutler, S.J. and Ederer, F.: *J Chron Dis* 8: 699–713, 1958.
9. Djerassi, I., Farber, S., Abir, E., and Neikirk, W.: *Cancer* 20: 233–242, 1967.
10. Frankel, L.S., Hockenberry, M.J., and Johnston, D.A.: *Proc ASCO* (1): 124, 1982.
11. Freeman, A.I., Brecher, M.L., Wang, J.J., and Sinks, L.F.: In: *Modern Trends in Human Leukemia, III.* R. Neth, R.C. Gallo, P.H. Hofschneider, and K. Mannweiler, Eds., Springer-Verlag, New York, 1979, pp. 115–123.
12. Green, D.M., Brecher, M.L., Blumenson, L.E., Grossi, M., and Freeman, A.I.: *Cancer* 50: 2722–2727, 1982.
13. Green, D.M., Sather, H.N., Sallan, S.E., Nesbit, M.E., Freeman, A.I., Cassady, J.R., Sinks, L.F., Hammond, D., and Frei, E. III: *Lancet* 1: 1398–1402, 1980.
14. Holland, J.F. and Glidewell, O.J.: *N Engl J Med* 294: 440, 1976.
15. Hustu, H.O., Aur, R.J.A., Verzosa, M.S., Simone, J.V., and Pinkel, D.: *Cancer* 32: 585–597, 1973.
16. Kay, H.E.M., Knapton, P.J., O'Sullivan, J.P., Wells, D.G., Harris, R.F., Innes, E.M., Surart, J., Schwartz, F.C.M., and Thompson, E.N.: *Arch Dis Child* 47: 344–354, 1972.
17. Komp, D., Fernandez, C.H., Falletta, J.M., Ragab, A.H., Humphrey, G.B., Pullen, J.M., Moon, T., and Schuster, J.: *Cancer* 50: 1031–1036, 1982.
18. Moe, P.J. and Seip, M.: *Acta Paediatr Scand* 67: 265–268, 1978.
19. Moss, H.A., Nannis, E.D., and Poplack, D.G.: *Am J Med* 71: 47–52, 1981.
20. Pinkel, D., Hustu, H.O., Aur, R.J.A., Smith, K.,

Borella, L.D., and Simone, J.V.: *Cancer 39(2): 817–824, 1977.*

21. Price, R.A. and Jamieson, P.A.: *Cancer 35: 306–318, 1975.*

22. Rowland, J., Glidewell, O., Sibley, J.R., Holland, J.C., Brecher, M., Tull, R., Berman, A., Glicksman, A., Forman, E., Harris, M., McSweeney, J., Jones, B., Black, M., Cohen, M., and Freeman, A.I. for Cancer and Leukemia Group B (CALGB): *Proc ASCO (1): 123, 1982.*

23. Shapiro, W.R., Young, D.F., and Metha, B.M.: *N Engl J Med 293: 161–166, 1975.*

24. Sinks, L.F., Wang, J.J., and Freeman, A.I.: In: *Modern Trends in Human Leukemia IV,* R. Neth, R.C. Gallo, R. Graf, K. Mannweiler, Winkler, Eds., Springer-Verlag, Berlin, Heidelberg, 1981, pp. 99–107.

25. Snedecor, G. and Cochran, W.: *Statistical Methods, 6th ed.,* Iowa State University Press, 1967, p. 228.

26. Thomas, E.D., Storb, R., Clift, R.A., Fefer, A., Johnson, F.L., Neiman, P.E., Lerner, K.G., Glucksberg, H., and Buchner, C.D.: *N Engl J Med 292: 832–843, 895–902, 1975.*

27. van Eys, J., Shuster, J., Boyett, J., Sullivan, M.P., Komp, D., Culbert, S.J., and Vietti, T.J.: In: *Controversies in Pediatric Oncology,* A. Freeman and C. Pochedly, Eds., Masson Publishers, New York, 1981 (in press).

28. Voorhess, M., Brecher, M.L., MacGillivray, M., Hologgitas, J., Harris, M., Dasgupta, I., Vasquez, A., Glidewell, O., and Forman, E.: *Proc ASCO 22: 396, 1981.*

29. Wang, J.J., Freeman, A.I., and Sinks, L.F.: *Cancer Res 36: 1441–1444, 1976.*

CHAPTER 18

Sequential Induction Treatment of Acute Leukemia with Thymidine and Cytosine Arabinoside

R. Zittoun,[a] J. Zittoun,[b] J. Marquet,[b] P. Creaven,[c] Y. Rustum[c]

Cytosine-Arabinoside (Ara-C) is a major drug for remission induction in acute myelogenous leukemia (AML), usually in combination with one anthracycline drug. Many problems are still unsolved in the utilization of Ara-C: the daily doses proposed vary and are usually around 100 mg/m². However, more recently, very high doses have been proposed, up to 3,000 mg/m² b.i.d.[8] With the conventional doses the most usual schedules are either push injections every 12 hours or continuous infusion. A recent trial from the CALGB has shown the superiority of the continuous infusion during induction and the subcutaneous injections during maintenance treatment over the other types of administration.[7]

Ara-C is active in the cells by inhibition of DNA-polymerase after conversion into Ara-CTP.[1] Besides variations of doses and schedules, many methods have been proposed to increase the activity of Ara-C. Trials aiming to increase the number of leukemic cells in S-phase by recruitment and semisynchronization have not been proven superior to empirical treatments.[2]

The intracellular level of Ara-CTP depends on many parameters, among them the activity of the deoxycytine-kinase, and of deaminase which transforms the drug into inactive Ara-U^{2}-.[12] However, recent works trying to correlate Ara-C activity with the ratio kinase / deaminase have led to conflicting results.[10] In fact, it has been shown that resistance to Ara-C correlates mainly with increased levels of intracellular dCTP,[3] the natural nucleoside which competes with Ara-C by feedback inhibition of dC-kinase and Ara-C kinase.[12] Many drugs can modulate the formation of Ara-CTP by decreasing the level of dCTP, mainly pyrazofurin by inhibiting OMP^1-decarboxylase, 3-deazarudine which blocks the conversion of UTP^2 into CTP^{3,6} and thymidine.

Thymidine (TdR) by increasing the level of dTTP,[4] can also decrease the intracellular dCTP. dTTP indeed inhibits the activity of cytidine-reductase, and hence facilitates the formation of Ara-CTP.[1,11] In a phase II study, we have tried to correlate the results of a sequential induction treatment with TdR-Ara-C with some biological parameters involved in the modulation of the drug.

Materials and Methods

TdR was administered by I.V. continuous infusion, 30 g/m² on days 1 and 4 and Ara-C by I.V. continuous infusion, 200

[a]Service d'Hématologie, Hotel-Dieu 1, Place du Parvis Notre Dame, Paris
[b]Service Central d'Hématologie-Immunologie Hôpital Henri Mondor, Creteil, France
[c]Roswell Park Memorial Institute, Buffalo, New York

mg/m[2] on days 2 and 3, and 5 and 6. Plasma nucleosides were assayed using HPLC methods.[4] Plasma and intracellular Ara-C were assayed using a radioimmunological assay described by Pial et al.[5] The intracellular levels of dCTP and dTTP have meen measured using an enzymatic method, according to Lindberg and Skoog.[3] Cell kinetics parameters were evaluated by flow cytophotometry using a Cytofluorograph 4800 A.

Results

Twenty-three acute leukemia patients entered this study; 21 of them were evaluable — 10 AML (six already treated and resistant to conventional treatment or relapsing, and four untreated, with advanced age or cardiac disease not allowing the use of anthracycline drugs), 9 blast crises of CML, 1 blast crisis after myelosclerosis, and 1 ALL.

We observed four complete remissions (three blast crisis of CML, one untreated AML), and two partial remissions (one blast crisis of CML and one AML already treated). The overall clinical results seem poor in primary AML, but promising in blast crisis of CML, with four responders out of nine evaluable patients. Two of the complete remissions in blast crisis of CML were observed in lymphoblastic types with common ALL antigen positive.

The cell kinetics showed some variations of the number of cells in S-phase after TdR infusion; this number increased in some patients and decreased in others. The variation did not correlate with the response to treatment. Plasma nucleoside assays showed the same level of TdR and thymine (T) during TdR infusion in the responders and the nonresponders. The mean value of TdR was 195 μM in the responders and 180 in the nonresponders, and the mean value of T was respectively 621 and 578 μM.

The levels of dCTP and dTTP pools before treatment were not significantly dif-

ferent between the responders and the nonresponders. As expected, the TdR infusion resulted in increased levels of intracellular dTTP. However, on the average, this was accompanied by decreased dCTP levels mainly in responders. The mean intracellular level of Ara-C was also significantly higher in responders (19.1 pmol/10[6] cells) than in the nonresponders (8.4 pmol/10[6] cells) ($p < 0.005$).

Discussion

Our results demonstrate that TdR can modulate the intracellular formation of Ara-CTP via a decrease of the intracellular dCTP. Patients who did not respond to this treatment had sustained levels of dCTP in spite of a markedly increased dTTP pool. This data is in favor of a relative inactivity of dTTP on cytidinereductase in nonresponders, one of the possible mechanisms of resistance to Ara-C associated with resistance to thymidine in some mutants of Chinese hamster fibroblasts.[9] Consequently it appears that the modulation of Ara-C by TdR can be achieved in only a proportion of the patients.

The overall results in our trial were not very good, and do not seem superior to those which could be probably obtained by Ara-C alone. Other doses and schedules could result in higher rates of complete remissions. In a recent trial, Van Echo et al. obtained 47% responses in relapsed AML by continuous and simultaneous infusion of TdR (8 g/m[2]) and Ara-C (250 mg/m[2]).[13] The most promising results were achieved in our trial in blast crisis of CML. This could be explained by some specific biological characters of this type of leukemia as compared to the other types.

ABBREVIATIONS

Ara-C triphosphate = Ara-CTP; Uracile-arabinoside = Ara-U, Deoxycytidine-triphosphate = dCTP. Orotidine 5'-monophosphate = OMP; Uridine triphosphate = UTP; Cytidine triphosphate = CTP; Thymidine triphosphate = dTTP.

REFERENCES

1. Daunhauser, L.L. and Rustum, Y.M.: *Cancer Res 40: 1274–1280, 1980.*
2. Debusscher, L. and Stryckmans, P.: *EORTC Monograph Series, vol. 4, 1978, p. 39.*
3. Linberg, U. and Skoog, L.: *Anal. Biochem 34: 152–160, 1970.*
4. Linssen, P., Drenthe-Schonk, A., Wessels, H., and Haanen, C.: *J Chromatog 223: 371, 1981.*
5. Piall, E.M., Aherne, G.W., and Marks, V.M.: *Eur J Cancer 40: 548–556, 1979.*
6. Plagemann, P.G.W., Marz, R., and Wohlhueter, R.M.: *Cancer Res 38: 978–989, 1978.*
7. Rai, K.R., Holland, J.F., and Glidewell, O.J., et al.: *Blood 58: 1203–1212, 1981.*
8. Rudnick, S.A., Cadman, E.A., Capizzi, R.L., Skeel, R.T., Bertino, J.R., and McIntosh, S.: *Cancer 44: 1189–1193, 1979.*
9. de Saint Vincent, R. and Buttin, G.: *Somatic Cell Gen 5: 67–82, 1979.*
10. Smyth, J.F., Robins, A.B., and Leese, C.L. *Eur J Cancer 12: 567, 1976.*
11. Streifel, J.A. and Howell, S.B.: *Proc Natl Acad Sci USA 75: 5132–5136, 1981.*
12. Tattersall, M.H.N., Ganeshaguru, K., and Hoffbrand, A.V.: *Br J Haematol 27: 39, 1974.*
13. Van Echo, D.A., Markus, S., and Wiernik, P.H.: *Proc Am Soc Clin Oncol 22: 483, 1981.*

CHAPTER 19

A Preliminary Analysis of Prediction of Response of Acute Nonlymphocytic Leukemia to Therapy with High-Dose Cytosine Arabinoside

H.D. Preisler,[a] N. Azarnia,[b] M. Barcos,[b] A.P. Early,[b] A. Raza,[b] G. Browman,[b] J. Brennan,[c] H. Grunwald,[d] J. Goldberg,[e] R. Vogler,[f] and K. Miller[g]

Introduction

Cytosine arabinoside administered at high doses is a promising new therapeutic modality for the treatment of the acute leukemias.[6,16] We have demonstrated its antileukemic efficacy in the treatment of patients with relapsed acute nonlymphocytic leukemia, in the treatment of central nervous system leukemia, and recently in the leukemias which occur secondary to treatment with alkylating agents and/or radiation therapy.[9]

The use of single agent remission induction therapy presents several potential problems. Single agent therapy is theoretically inferior to multiagent therapy since the use of combination chemotherapy makes possible the synergistic interaction of the agents involved and also increases the probability of a successful therapeutic outcome since the leukemic cells are less likely to be simultaneously resistant to two chemotherapeutic agents than to be resistant to one agent. For these reasons, we have attempted to develop methods for recognizing patients for whom high-dose cytosine arabinoside therapy is appropriate remission induction therapy as well as those patients who require therapy with additional agents.

Methods

The patients who were studied had a diagnosis of acute nonlymphocytic leukemia (ANLL) according to the criteria established by the French-American-British Working Party.[1] Patients at all stages of their illness were studied, i.e., previously untreated patients as well as patients in first, second, or third relapse.

The patients were treated with a single course of cytosine arabinoside (ara-C) at 3 g/m^2 q 12 hours for 12 doses.[5] The ara-C was infused over 60 minutes. Patients > 70 years of age were treated with 2 g/m^2 to reduce the likelihood of central nervous system toxicity. Steroid-containing eye drops were administered 4×/day beginning 24 hours prior to the start of ara-C therapy and continuing for 24 hours after the end of therapy to prevent ara-C-induced conjunctivitis. Patients received cotrimoxazole, two regular strength tablets twice a day from day 1 of therapy until their granulocyte count exceeded 500/μl.[13]

[a]From the Roswell Park Memorial Institute, Buffalo, New York
[b]Ontario Cancer Clinic, Ontario, Canada
[c]University of Rochester, Rochester, New York
[d]Queens Hospital Center, New York, New York
[e]Upstate Medical Center, Syracuse, New York
[f]Emory University School of Medicine, Atlanta, GA
[g]New England Medical Center, Boston, Massachusetts

The criteria proposed by Cancer and Acute Leukemia Group B were used to define a complete remission, which was believed to indicate the presence of clinically-documented, ara-C-sensitive disease.[7] Remission induction failures were subdivided into a resistant disease group and an "other" failure group according to previously published criteria.[9,10] In this way, patients whose leukemia failed to enter remission because of the presence of clinically-documented, ara-C-resistant disease could be distinguished from patients who expired too early in their course of therapy to determine if their leukemia was ara-C responsive or ara-C resistant (i.e., these patients were classified as "other" failures).

Bone marrow aspirates and biopsies were obtained prior to the administration of remission induction therapy and 12 hours after the last dose of ara-C was administered. The aspirate differential was determined after Wright-Giemsa stain of the marrow aspirate. The marrow biopsy cellularity was estimated by eye as previously reported.[11] The percent cells in S phase was estimated either on the basis of [3]HTdR labelling index measurements[11] or by DNA histogram analysis.[4,3] For the latter studies, the ethidium bromide-mithramycin technique was used. Histogram generation and analyses were carried out with the ICP[21] component of an Ortho 50H cytofluorograph and its dedicated 2150 computer.

Results

BONE MARROW STUDIES

Sixty-one patients were treated with high-dose ara-C therapy. Of these, 20 patients entered complete remission, 21 had clinically documented drug-resistant disease, and 20 patients were classified as "other" failures. The data presented in Figure 1a demonstrate that the percent of myloblasts + promyelocytes in the pre-therapy bone marrow aspirate was not related to the outcome of remission induction therapy. By contrast, the data presented in Figure 1b suggest that a relationship exists between pretherapy bone marrow biopsy cellularity and the presence of ara-C-sensitive (median cellularity = 46%) or ara-C-resistant disease (median cellularity = 90%). The number of patients studied was small but the data suggest that those individuals with a large tumor load are less likely to enter remission after high-dose ara-C therapy than are patients in whom the tumor load is less.

A bone marrow aspirate was obtained from 50 patients 12 hours after the last dose of ara-C was administered. Figure 2a demonstrates that patients who were destined to enter remission had far fewer myeloblasts + promyelocytes (median = 6%) than did patients who would prove to have drug-resistant disease (median = 40%). The day 6 bone marrow biopsy cellularity was also correlated with the outcome of induction therapy with patients who entered remission having less cellular marrows (median cellularity = 10%) than did patients who proved to have resistant disease (median = 30%). Figure 2c relates the percent marrow myeloblasts in the day 6 marrow aspirate to the biopsy cellularity of the day 6 marrow. These measurements are not significantly correlated, suggesting that bivariate analysis would further increase the predictive ability of a bone marrow examination performed 12 hours after the last dose of ara-C is administered.

PRETHERAPY CELL CYCLE STUDIES

The percent of the pretherapy bone marrow cells which were in S phase and the relationship of this measurement to the outcome of remission induction therapy for 35 patients is illustrated by Figure 3a. Note that not a single patient in whom fewer than 6% of cells were in S phase entered remission, but rather all but one of these patients were drug-resistant treatment failures. It is also of consider-

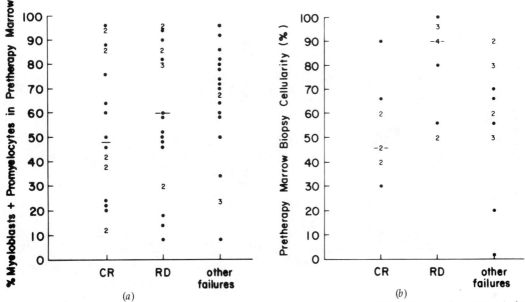

FIGURE 1. Relationship between pretherapy bone marrow characteristics and the outcome of remission induction therapy: (*a*) percent of myeloblasts + promyelocytes in the pretherapy marrow aspirate; (*b*) percent of biopsy cellularity of the pretherapy bone marrow. CR = complete remission, RD = resistant disease, other failures.

able importance that the presence of >6% cells in S phase did not guarantee a successful therapeutic outcome. Figure 3*b* relates the pretherapy percent cells in S phase with the day 6 bone marrow biopsy cellularity. For 10 of the 13 patients, there appears to be an inverse relationship between the percent cells in S phase and the marrow cellularity after 6 days of therapy. These observations are in accord with those presented in Figure 3*a*.

Discussion

Thirty-three percent of patients entered complete remission after a single course of therapy with high-dose cytosine arabinoside. This represents the remission rate for a mixed group of patients and probably does not represent the therapeutic efficacy of high-dose cytosine arabinoside for previously untreated patients with ANLL. For example, we have treated 11 patients with secondary ANLL with this regimen and have achieved eight complete and two partial remissions, the latter accompanied by a return of peripheral

blood counts to normal.[9] Nevertheless, caution should be used before previously untreated patients with spontaneous ANLL are committed to single-agent remission induction therapy.

This paper represents a preliminary report of studies being carried out to define the subsets of patients for whom high-dose ara-C is appropriate or inappropriate therapy. Analysis has been directed solely towards distinguishing drug-sensitive patients from patients who fail to enter remission because of an inadequate antileukemic effect being produced *in vivo* by this form of remission induction therapy since recognition of "other" failure types will be dependent upon the recognition of patient clinical/biological characteristics which determine whether or not a patient will survive remission induction therapy.[15] Analysis of these data are currently in progress and will be reported elsewhere. Reliable pretherapy predictive assays would permit patients who are likely to respond to ara-C alone to avoid the side effects of the anthracycline

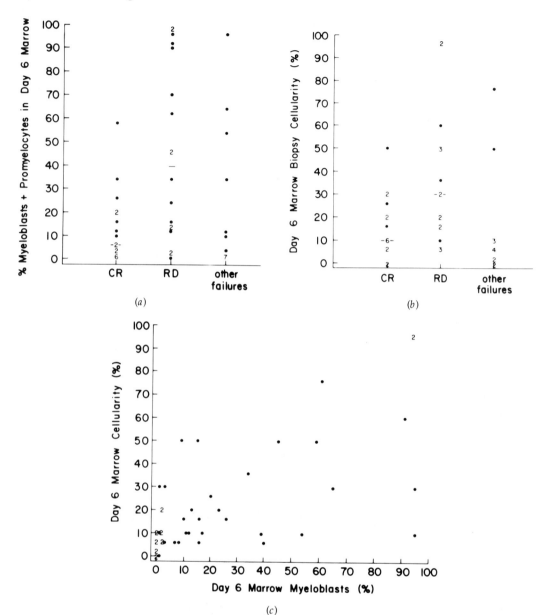

FIGURE 2. Relationship between the characteristics of the day 6 marrow and the outcome of remission induction therapy: (*a*) percent of myeloblasts + promyelocytes in the marrow aspirate; (*b*) percent of bone marrow biopsy cellularity; (*c*) relationship between marrow biopsy cellularity and percent marrow myeloblasts;

antibiotics used in essentially all combination chemotherapy regimens while permitting patients who are not likely to respond to high-dose ara-C therapy to receive an alternate form of therapy. The studies reported here demonstrate that patients who have a very cellular pretherapy bone marrow are less likely to enter remission than are patients who have less cellular bone marrows. Perhaps the addition of another agent to high-dose ara-C, as either simultaneous or sequential therapy, would increase the likelihood that these patients will enter remission. The data also suggest that patients in whom there are few marrow cells in S phase prior to

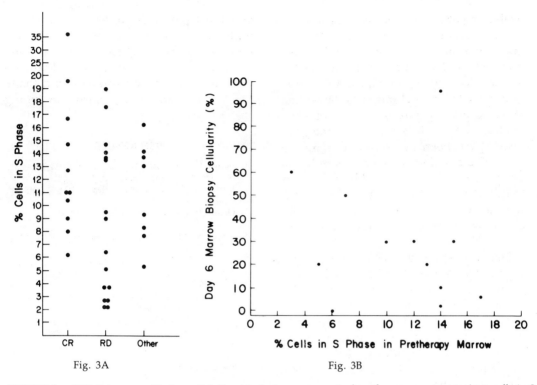

Fig. 3A   Fig. 3B

FIGURE 3. *AML* Intergroup Study — Relationship between percent of pretherapy marrow aspirate cells in S phase and effects of remission induction therapy with high dose ARAC; (*a*) relationship between percent of cells in S phase and outcome of remission induction therapy; (*b*) relationship between percent of cells in S phase and day 6 marrow biopsy cellularity.

the initiation of therapy are unlikely to enter remission. This observation is not surprising since ara-C is an S phase-specific agent. If confirmed, this subset of patients might benefit from a regimen which provides for the administration of several doses of a non S phase-specific agent such as cyclophosphamide, to recruit cells into cycle prior to the administration of the ara-C. Such attempts have been made in the past but were not specifically directed towards this subset of patients,[2] a fact which may have confounded interpretation of the data. A combined analysis of the pretherapy marrow biopsy data and the cell cycle data to enhance the predictive utility of both methods is in progress.

The studies carried out 12 hours after administration of the last dose of cytosine

arabinoside demonstrate that it is not difficult to distinguish between most patients who will enter remission and one half of those who will have drug-resistant disease. The ability to make this distinction will permit testing of the proposition that additional therapy administered to the latter group of patients might be beneficial while avoiding the needless administration of additional therapy (and its consequent side effects) to patients who will enter remission without the additional therapy. The ability to distinguish between potential responders and patients who will prove to have drug-resistant disease will undoubtedly be improved by also taking into consideration the pretherapy measurements described above.

The Intergroup ANLL study is also

evaluating other pretherapy drug sensitivity measurements such as the effects of ara-C exposure on the clonogenic leukemic cells and on the ability of the leukemic cells to phosphorylate ara-C and retain ara-CTP. A preliminary analysis has failed to demonstrate the utility of either *in vitro* assay. Additionally, plasma ara-C levels have been measured in some patients and a wide degree of variability has been noted.[5,6] It is possible that pharmacokinetic measurements of ara-C during therapy will make the pretherapy predictive assays more sensitive and perhaps more reliable.

Taken together, the data suggest that it is possible to identify patients who do or do not have ara-C-sensitive disease. The ability to make this distinction between individuals prior to the initiation of or the conclusion of remission induction therapy should increase the utility of this agent. The addition of clinical estimates of the biological status of the patient per se and therefore of the patient's ability to survive therapy will undoubtedly make decision-making regarding potential remission induction regimens more rational.

ACKNOWLEDGMENTS

The authors thank Dr. Roger Priore for his statistical advice and Dr. George Royer and the Upjohn Company for assistance with these studies. The authors also acknowledge the excellent technical assistance of Ms. Irene Rakowski, Maureen Cannon, and Cathy Costanzo, and thank Ms. J. Barry and Ms. J. Burns for typing the manuscript.

REFERENCES

1. Bennett, J.M., Catovsky, D., Daniel, M.T., et al.: *Br J Haem 33: 451, 1976.*
2. Burke, P.J., Karp., J.E., Braine, H.G., et al.: *Cancer Res 37: 2138, 1977.*
3. Dean, P.N., and Jett, J.H.: *J Cell Biol 60: 523, 1974.*
4. Dosik, G.M., Barlogie, B., Smith, T.L., et al.: *Blood 55: 474, 1980.*
5. Early, A.P., Preisler, H.D., Slocum, H., and Rustum, Y.M.: *Cancer Res 42: 1587, 1982.*
6. Early, A.P., Preisler, H.D., Higby, D.J., Brecher, M., Browman, G., and McBride, J.A.: *Med Ped Oncol (in press) 1982.*
7. Ellison, R.R., Holland, J.F., Weil, M., et al.: *Blood 32: 507, 1968.*
8. Karanes, C., Wolff, S.N., Herzig, G.P., et al.: *Blood 54: 191a, 1979.*
9. Preisler, H.D., Early, A.P., Raza, A., Vlahides, G., Marinello, M.J., Browman, G., and Stein, A.M.: *N Engl J Med 308(1): 21, 1983.*
10. Preisler, H.D.: *Blut 41: 393, 1980.*
11. Preisler, H., Barcos, M., Reese, P., and Pothier, L.: *Leuk Res 7(1): 67, 1983.*
12. Preisler, H.D.: *Med Ped Oncol 4: 275, 1978.*
13. Preisler, H.D., Early, A.P., and Hyrniuk, W.: *Med Ped Oncol 9: 511, 1981.*
14. Preisler, H., and Shoham, D.: *Cancer Res 38: 3681, 1978.*
15. Preisler, H.D.: *Blood Cells 8: 585, 1982.*
16. Rudnick, S.A., Cadman, E.C., Capizzi, R.L., et al.: *Cancer 44: 1189, 1979.*

CHAPTER 20

Treatment of Advanced Colorectal and Gastric Adenocarcinomas with 5-Fluorouracil Combined with High-Dose Folinic Acid: A Pilot Study

D. Machover, L. Schwarzenberg, E. Goldschmidt, J.-M. Tourani, B. Michalski, M. Hayat, T. Dorval, J.L. Misset, C. Jasmin, R. Maral, and G. Mathé

Introduction

The use of 5-fluorouracil (5-Fu) as a single agent in the treatment of advanced colorectal and gastric adenocarcinoma has been disappointing; responses, generally of short duration, have been observed in 20% of the patients with colorectal carcinoma and in 25% of the patients with gastric carcinoma but there has been no proven increase in the overall survival rate.[1,6,8]

We report here a clinical trial, the rationale of which is based on biochemical and cell culture studies performed with various cell lines.[2,5,10,11] The data obtained in these studies demonstrated that an excess of intracellular reduced folates is necessary for optimal inhibition of thymidylate synthetase (TS) and for an increased cytotoxic effect of fluorinated pyrimidines. It was our aim to enhance the activity of 5-Fu in colorectal and gastric adenocarcinomas by simultaneous administration of folinic acid (FA) in high doses.[7]

Patients and Methods

Patients entered in this study had histologically confirmed colorectal or gastric

Service des Maladies Sanguines et Tumorales and I.C.I.G. (INSERM U-50), Hôpital Universitaire Paul-Brousse, Villejuif, France

adenocarcinomas. All had metastatic disease.

COLORECTAL ADENOCARCINOMA PATIENTS

Thirty-five patients were entered in the study. Five of these patients were excluded because their tumors could not be measured accurately. The 30 evaluable patients had measurable disease; 23 had histologically proven metastases, and seven had metastatic tumors as evidenced by radiologic, ultrasonographic, and/or scintigraphic procedures. Patient ages ranged from 30 to 75 years (mean 53.2 ± 11 S.D.). Before entering the trial, 14 patients had been subjected to an ineffective regimen of 5-Fu given either as a single agent or combined with other drugs; the other 16 patients had not received previous chemotherapy.

GASTRIC ADENOCARCINOMA PATIENTS

Six patients were entered in the study; one of them was excluded because neoplastic ascites was the sole indicator of the disease. Five previously untreated patients with measurable disease were evaluated. Their ages ranged from 34 to 71 years (mean 60.8 ± 15 S.D.). The presence of metastases was proved histologically in all cases.

Treatment comprised 5-day courses followed by drug-free intervals of 21 days. Folinic acid was given at a dose of 200 mg/m²/day by I.V. bolus injection, and 5-Fu was given immediately afterwards at a dose of 370 mg/m²/day by I.V. infusion over 15 minutes. In subsequent courses, the daily dose of 5-Fu was raised to 400 mg/m² if toxicity was absent or mild at 370 mg/m²/day. A reduction of the daily dose of 5-Fu by 30 mg/m² was indicated in cases of granulocytopenia <1000 cells/mm³ complicated by fever, thrombocytopenia <50000 cells/mm³, and/or WHO grade 3 or 4 of oral mucositis, or diarrhea.[12] Treatment courses were repeated until failure became evident, or until progressive disease developed in previously responding or previously stable patients. Response was determined quantitatively by comparison of objectively measurable lesions and was categorized as complete (CR), partial (PR), no change (NC), or progressive disease (PD). Duration of response was determined from the start of therapy.

Results

COLORECTAL CANCER PATIENTS (TABLE 1)

Of the 16 previously untreated patients, one achieved CR and eight achieved a PR. The response rate in this group of patients was 56%; responses lasted from 92+ to 258+ days (mean 188 days). Of the 14 patients previously resistant to 5-Fu, one patient attained a CR and two attained a PR. The response rate in this group was 21%; responses lasted 136+, 152+, and 318+ days. The overall objective response rate for the 30 patients with colorectal adenocarcinoma was 40%.

GASTRIC CANCER PATIENTS

Of the five evaluable patients, three reached PRs which lasted for 60+, 90+, and 90+ days. Tumor regression was very

TABLE 1. Colorectal Adenocarcinoma Patients; Results of Therapy in the 30 Evaluable Patients

Results of Therapy	Previously Untreated Patients (n = 16)		Patients Previously Resistant to 5-Fu (n = 14)	
	n	Percent	n	Percent
CR	1	} 56	1	} 21
PR	8		2	
NC	3	19	5	36
PD	4	25	6	43

rapid and resulted in a dramatic reduction of tumor size.

Toxicity

Myelosuppression was studied in 16 patients who had blood counts weekly for 2 months during two consecutive courses at two different dose levels of 5-Fu; the results (Table 2) indicate that myelosuppression was moderate, with rapid recovery. The 35 patients received a total of 207 courses of therapy, of which 198 were evaluable for toxic effects. Of these courses 88 consisted of 370 mg/m²/day × 5 of 5-Fu, and 110 of 400 mg/m²/day × 5 of 5-Fu. The mean number of courses per patient was six, with a range from two to 14. The overall toxicity is indicated in Table 3.

There was no death due to toxicity. Toxic effects required dose reductions in two courses at 370 mg/m²/day of 5-Fu (2%) and in 11 courses of 400 mg/m²/day of 5-Fu (10%).

Discussion

The major action of 5-Fu on cell metabolism is due to its conversion into fluorodeoxyuridylate (FdUMP), which inhibits thymidylate synthetase (TS) resulting in the suppression of DNA synthesis.[4] FdUMP binds tightly to TS in the presence of N5-N10 methylene tetrahydrofolate; this interaction leads to the formation of a slowly dissociating covalent ternary com-

TABLE 2.   Myelosuppression in 16 Patients Who Had Weekly Blood Counts during 2 Months for Two Consecutive Courses at Each Dose Level of 5-Fu

Course and Dose of 5-Fu	Mean Nadir (Range)		Mean Day of Nadir from Day 1 of Treatment	Mean Time of Recovery in Days (Range)
	PNM ($\times 10^2$/mm^3)	Platelets ($\times 10^3$/mm^3)		
I ($n = 16$) (370 mg/m^2/day $\times$ 5)	29,9 (8–80)	296 (140–472)	13 (12–19)	8 (7–9)
II ($n = 16$) (400 mg/m^2/day $\times$ 5)	19,2 (1–64)	238 (120–350)	14 (12–19)	8 (4–14)

plex, resulting in a stable inhibition of the enzyme.[9,10]

In folate-depleted L1210 leukemia cells, both the amount or ternary complex formed and the cytotoxicity of 5-fluorode-oxyuridine are reduced.[10] In mouse sarco-ma S_{180} and in human carcinoma Hep_2 cells, the cytotoxic activity of 5-Fu was potentiated threefold when an excess of FA was added to the medium.[2] Both experiments[2,10] showed that the folate requirement for optimal cell growth was

TABLE 3.   Overall Toxicity in 35 Patients Treated with 5-Fu and High-dose Folinic Acid

Toxic Effect	Degree of Toxicity	Number of Patients Experiencing Toxicity ($n = 35$)	Number of Episodes of Toxicity according to dose of 5-Fu	
			370 mg/m^2/Day: 88 Courses	400 mg/m^2/Day: 110 Courses
PMN	15–20	3	5	1
($\times 10^2$/mm^3)	10–15	4	2	2
	<10	6	1	6
			8/88	9/110
Platelets	100–150	1	1	1
($\times 10^3$/mm^3)	50–100	2	1	1
	<50	1	1	0
			3/88	2/110
Oral Mucositis[a]	1	6	7	4
	2	6	4	5
	3	4	0	4
	4	1	0	1
			11/88	14/110
Diarrhea[a]	1	0	0	0
	2	7	4	5
	3	2	1	1
	4	0	0	0
			5/88	6/110
Fever		6[b]	0	6
Alopecia		4 (partial)		
Skin Rash		2		
Neurologic		0		
Renal		0		

[a]Toxic score according to WHO recommendations.[9]
[b]In five patients, the cause of fever was not documented microbiologically; in one it was due to *Staphylococcus aureus* septicemia.

much lower than that required for maximal cytotoxicity of fluoropyrimidines. In Friend leukemia cells, the growth inhibiting effect of 5-Fu was also increased by addition of FA; this potentiation did not occur in FA transport defective cells.[11] Moreover, in xenografts of human colorectal carcinoma cell lines resistant to fluoropyrimidines, the maximum binding of FdUMP to TS required addition of exogenous folates.[5]

For the above reasons, we assumed that, in some tumors, the amount of naturally occurring intracellular folates may be insufficient to allow optimal cytotoxicity of 5-Fu. We thought that high doses of FA should effectively increase the cellular content of reduced folates, and that they might overcome membrane transport deficiency for these compounds.[3,11]

The objective response data obtained in this study suggest that simultaneous administration of 5-Fu and high doses of FA can enhance the antitumor activity of 5-Fu, and that it also renders some colorectal tumors previously resistant to F-Fu sensitive to this drug. In gastric adenocarcinomas, the results were encouraging in the small number of patients studied during the short follow-up period. In the present trial, toxicity was within acceptable limits. Side effects, when present, were prevented in subsequent courses by a 30 mg/m² decrease in the daily dose of 5-Fu.

The combination of 5-Fu with simultaneous high doses of FA should be tested in all tumors in which 5-Fu has shown some therapeutic effectiveness. Biochemical and pharmacokinetic studies will be necessary for optimization of the doses and schedules of FA combined with 5-Fu and other cytostatic fluoropyrimidines.

REFERENCES

1. Carter, S.K., Slavik, M., and Wasserman, T.H.: J.E. McCay, D.X. Beane, C.S. Spiese, and C.C. Fox, Eds., Year Book Med Publishers, Chicago, 1975, pp. 99–146.
2. Evans, R.M., Laskin, J.D., and Hakala, M.T.: Cancer Res 41: 3283–3295, 1981.
3. Goldman, D.: Cancer Chemother Rep 6: 62–72, 1975.
4. Heidelberger, C.: In Handbook of Experimental Pharmacology, Antineoplastic and Immunosuppressive Agents, Vol. 38,2, A.C. Sartorelli and D.G. Johns, Eds., Springer Verlag, Berlin-Heidelberg-New York, 1975, pp. 193–223.
5. Houghton, J.A., Maroda, S.J., Jr., Philips, J.O., and Houghton, P.J.: Cancer Res 41: 144–149, 1981.
6. Livingstone, R.B., and Carter, S.: IFI/Plenum, New York-Washington-London, 1970, pp. 195–226.
7. Machover, D., Schwarzenberg, L., Goldschmidt, E., Misset, J.L., Maral, R., Jasmin, C., and Mathé, G.: Proc Am Soc Clin Oncol (abstract C-131) 1: 33, 1982.
8. Moertel, C.G.: N Engl J Med 299: 1049–1052, 1978.
9. Santi, D.V.: In Molecular Actions and Targets for Cancer Chemotherapeutic Agents, Vol. 2, A.C. Sartorelli, J.S. Lazo, and J.R. Bertino, Eds., Bristol Myers Cancer Symposia, Academic Press, New York, pp. 285–300, 1981.
10. Ullman, B., Lee, M., Martin, D.W., Jr., and Santi, D.V.: Proc Nat Acad Sci USA 75: 980–983, 1978.
11. Waxman, S., Bruckner, H., Wagle, A., and Schriber, C.: Proc Am Assoc Cancer Res (abstract 596) 19: 149, 1978.
12. WHO Handbook for Reporting Results of Cancer Treatment. World Health Organization, Geneva, 1979.

CHAPTER 21

Improved 5-Year Survival Figures Using Induction Combination Chemotherapy without Cisplatin in Patients with Epidermoid Carcinomas of the Head and Neck

L.A. Price[a] and Bridget T. Hill[b]

Introduction

Traditional treament of head and neck cancer has been surgery and/or radiotherapy. However, the 5-year survival figure for Stages III and IV disease is only approximately 20%.[5] In 1973, we initiated studies using combinations of "standard" antitumor agents to answer the following questions: 1) Using basic principles of stem cell kinetics, derived from the Toronto school[2,6] is it possible to design effective and safe drug protocols? 2) Can such protocols be integrated safely with surgery and radiation therapy?, and 3) Does the resultant combined modality approach prolong overall survival in patients with this group of tumors? The experimental basis of our approach has been described.[9] We have already demonstrated that the answer to the first question is affirmative[14,15] and we now describe results of the application of these principles to questions 2 and 3.

Patients and Methods

All 149 patients entered into the study had squamous cell carcinomas of the head and neck and were ambulatory at the time of their first treatment. Prior therapy of any kind, or the presence of metastases beyond the regional lymph nodes, made the patients ineligible. The following medical precautions were observed in *all* patients receiving drug treatment:

1. No treatment cycles were repeated unless the peripheral white cell and platelet counts had returned to their original level.
2. Patients with impaired renal function receiving methotrexate had an extended folinic acid rescue: if the creatinine clearance was greater than 90 ml/minute the protocol was given as stated; if the creatinine clearance was between 60–90 ml/minute, 12 doses of folinic acid (15 mg) were given; and patients with a clearance below 60 ml/minute were excluded from the study.
3. All patients were adequately hydrated and passed at least two liters of urine during the 24 hours of drug treatment.
4. Patients with a history of pulmonary disease in whom a pulmonary diffusion defect was thought to be present, as shown by a low dCO or radiologic evidence of pulmonary fibrosis, were excluded from the study.

Schedule A chemotherapy consisted of:

[a]Head and Neck Unit, The Royal Marsden Hospital, London, England
[b]The Imperial Cancer Research Fund Laboratories, London, England

vincristine 2 mg I.V. stat. at 0 hours; bleomycin 60 mg as a 6-hour infusion from 12 to 18 hours; methotrexate 100 mg I.V. stat. at 12, 15, and 18 hours; hydrocortisone 500 mg I.V. stat. at 12 and 18 hours; 5-fluorouracil 500 mg I.V. stat. at 18 hours; and folinic acid (calcium leucovorin) 15 mg orally or I.M. at 26, 32, 38, and 44 hours. Patients received two courses of Schedule A on days 1 and 14 and were assessed for chemotherapy response on day 28 when "curative" local therapy was started. Final assessment of response was made 1 month after local treatment finished. Details of local therapies were: 68% radiotherapy only, 6% surgery only, and 36% radiotherapy and surgery. Prior chemotherapy did not compromise subsequent surgery or increase either the immediate complications of surgery or the acute toxicity of radiation therapy. Following local therapy the patients were followed for signs of recurrence but received no further chemotherapy in the absence of relapse.

A response (partial) was defined as a reduction of at least 50% in the product of two perpendicular diameters of all measurable lesions. A complete response (CR) was defined as the absence of clinically detectable disease. Staging was based on the UICC pretreatment clinical classification for head and neck tumors, 1978 edition. Response rates were compared using the Chi-square test with the Yates' correction. Survival was calculated by a life table method and compared using a log rank test.

Results

OVERALL RESPONSE RATES

One hundred thirty-eight patients were assessed for response to schedule A chemotherapy. Ninety-three patients (67%) responded to schedule A chemotherapy. Although only eight patients achieved a CR after chemotherapy alone, this is a difficult figure to estimate since all patients were started on radiation therapy on day 28 even when their tumors were still regressing from chemotherapy. Of the 46 (33%) nonresponders to chemotherapy, a minimal 20–30% response was noted in 13 patients.

Eighty-nine patients (68%) achieved a CR following local therapy. It was particularly significant that patients who responded to two courses of initial schedule A chemotherapy had an increased number of CRs following local therapy (75% vs. 55%, $p < 0.05$).

TOXICITY

The toxicity associated with schedule A chemotherapy is minimal and there was 100% patient compliance. Sixty-two percent of patients had no side effects at all and those observed in the remaining 38% are summarized in Table 1. There was one case of severe myelosuppression following a protocol violation because a patient with impaired renal function was not given an extended folinic acid rescue as specified ("Medical precautions to be observed in all cases," as described in Patients and Methods section).

FACTORS INFLUENCING RESPONSE TO CHEMOTHERAPY

Chemotherapy response was not significantly influenced by sex or histologic tumor grade. Although there were not sufficient numbers for a site by site comparison, it appears from this analysis that oral cavity lesions did better compared with all other sites and that patients 49 years of age or younger were most likely to respond to chemotherapy.

OVERALL SURVIVAL

The overall 5-year survival of this group of patients is 34% compared with an expected approximate 20%. The median survival of all 149 patients is 28 months, that of chemotherapy responders 33

TABLE 1. Incidence of Side Effects from 288 Treatment Cycles of Schedule A Chemotherapy

Side Effects	Number of cycles
Myelosuppression:	
WBC nadir 2500–2000/mm^3	0
<2000/mm^3	1
Platelets nadir <100,000/mm^3	1
Mucositis (mild — no intubation)	8 (3%)
Nephrotoxicity	0
Peripheral neuropathy (mild)	9 (3%)
Pulmonary (chest pains)	1
Cardiovascular (atrial fibrillation)	1
Skin rash/pigmentation	10 (3%)
Alopecia (mild)	8 (3%)
Anorexia, nausea, vomiting	16 (6%)
Malaise or lethargy	8 (3%)
Death from treatment (protocol violation)	1
Others	13
(2, headache; 1, constipation; 1, indigestion; 1, exacerbation of peripheral vascular disease; 1, abdominal distention; 1, earache; 1, pyrexia; 1, muscular ache in inguinal region; 1, weakness in left arm; 1, exacerbation of gout).	

months, and that of chemotherapy non-responders 20 months. Failure to respond to initial chemotherapy is an adverse prognostic sign, therefore. Of particular importance in view of the observation that response to initial schedule A chemotherapy significantly increased the CR rate after local therapy in squamous cell carcinomas of the head and neck is the finding illustrated in Figure 1 that patients who achieved a CR after local therapy live significantly longer ($p < 0.001$) than those who still have residual disease.

Discussion

These results confirm our earlier findings[9–12,14,15] that high response rates can be achieved with complete safety with schedule A combination chemotherapy in previously unirradiated, advanced squamous cell carcinomas of the head and neck, provided that simple medical precautions are always observed. Of major significance was the minimal toxicity as-

sociated with this protocol which insured 100% patient compliance. Our practice of administering drug combinations over approximately 24 hours, based on certain aspects of stem cell kinetics,[2,6] has already been shown in other tumors both by ourselves and others[13] to allow chemotherapy to be given intensively but with minimal side effects. The safety of this approach in the treatment of advanced head and neck cancer has been confirmed by others.[1,8,16] These results contrast with the toxicity and inconvenience that have been a consistent feature of several recent reports involving cisplatin-containing combination schedules for these tumors.[3,4,7,18]

The most important prognostic factors in head and neck cancer are considered to be the initial tumor burden as measured by stage or TNM classification and the site of origin of the disease.[17] In this study, the response rate to chemotherapy was comparable in all patients irrespective of stage.

An important result presented here is that the number of complete remissions following local therapy was significantly greater in patients responding to initial chemotherapy than in chemotherapy non-responders. This achievement of CR is associated with a significantly improved survival ($p < 0.001$) over non-CRs. This finding greatly strengthens the case for using chemotherapy as the treatment of first choice in this group of tumors.

Overall Conclusions

1. The routine use of radiation as first-line treatment in advanced epidermoid carcinomas of the head and neck should be reconsidered.
2. The routine use of cisplatin in initial chemotherapy programs should be reconsidered, since it significantly increases toxicity and the number of days spent in hospital, and to date has failed to produce superior survival data to our

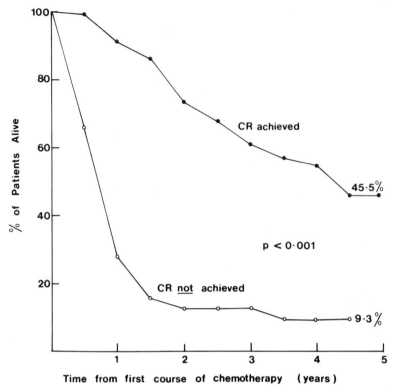

FIGURE 1. Head and neck study: Overall actuarial survival of all patients treated initially with two courses of Schedule A chemotherapy followed by local therapy. Survival was significantly prolonged in patients who achieved a complete remission (CR).

markedly less toxic and more convenient schedule A.

3. Increased cure rates can probably be achieved by adding chemotherapy to radiation and/or surgery, *if the drugs are given first.*

4. There is an urgent need for randomized, prospective, controlled clinical studies to establish firmly the role of chemotherapy in this group of diseases.

Summary

One hundred forty-nine patients with epidermoid head and neck tumors received induction combination chemotherapy, without cisplatin, given over 24 hours on days 1 and 14 prior to local "curative" radiation and/or surgery. Overall response to chemotherapy was 67%. Side effects were minimal. Patient compliance was 100%. Overall complete remission rate (CR) following local therapy was 68% and was significantly higher ($p < 0.05$) in chemotherapy responders (75%) than in nonresponsers (55%). Overall 5-year survival for all patients was 34%, with chemotherapy responders having a significantly longer median duration of survival than nonresponders (33 vs. 20 months). Patients achieving CR after local therapy had the longest median survival (52.5 months) with 45.5% alive at 5 years compared with only 9.3% of non-CRs.

REFERENCES

1. Angers, J.W., Bisi, R.H., and Cole, G.: In *Advances in Medical Oncology, Research and Education,* Proceedings of the XII International Cancer Congress, Buenos Aires, 1978. Vol. XII, A. Canonico, O. Estevez, R. Chacon, and S. Barg,

Eds., Pergamon Press, London, 1979, pp. 645–646.

2. Bruce, W.R., Meeker, B.E., and Valeriote, F.A.: *J Natl Cancer Inst 37: 233, 1966.*

3. Elias, G., Chrétien, P.B., Monnard, E., Khan, T., Bouchelle, W.H., Wiernik, P.H., Lipson, S.D., Hande, K.R., and Zentai, T.: *Cancer 43: 1025, 1979.*

4. Glick, J.H., Marcial, V., Richter, M., and Velez-Garcia, E.: *Cancer 46: 1919, 1980.*

5. Goldsmith, M.A. and Greenspan, E.M.: In *Clinical Interpretation and Practice of Cancer Chemotherapy*, E.M. Greenspan, Ed., Raven Press, New York, 1982, pp. 361–377.

6. Hill, B.T.: *Biochim Biophys Acta 516: 389, 1978.*

7. Hong, W.K., Shapshay, S.M., Bhutani, R., Craft, M.L., Ucmakli, A., Yamaguchi, K.T., Vaughan, C.W., and Strong, M.S.: *Cancer 44: 19, 1979.*

8. Malaker, K., Robson, F., and Schipper, H.: *J Otolaryngol 9: 24, 1980.*

9. Price, L.A. and Hill, B.T.: *Clin Otolaryngol 2: 339, 1977.*

10. Price, L.A. and Hill, B.T.: *J Laryngol Otol 94: 89, 1980.*

11. Price, L.A. and Hill, B.T.: *Cancer Treat Rep 65: 149, 1981.*

12. Price, L.A. and Hill, B.T.: *Med Pediatr Oncol, 10: 535, 1982.*

13. Price, L.A., Hill, B.T., and Ghilchik, M.W., Eds. In *Safer Cancer Chemotherapy*, Bailliere Tindall, London, 1981, pp. 116–120.

14. Price, L.A., Hill, B.T., Calvert, A.H., Shaw, H.J., and Hughes, K.B.: *Br Med J 3: 10, 1975.*

15. Price, L.A., Hill, B.T., Calvert, A.H., Dalley, V.M., Levene, A., Busby, E.R., Schachter, M., and Shaw, H.J.: *Oncology 35: 26, 1978.*

16. Sergeant, R. and Deutsch, G.: *J Laryngol Otol 95: 69, 1981.*

17. Shedd, D.P.: In *Cancer Medicine*, J.F. Holland and E. Frei, Eds., Lea and Febiger, Philadelphia, 1973, pp. 1437–1450.

18. Wittes, R., Heller, K., Randolph, V., Howard, J., Vallejo, A., Farr, H., Harrold, C., Gerold, F., Shah, J., Spiro, R., and Strong, E.: *Cancer Treat Rep 63: 1533, 1979.*

CHAPTER 22

Pre- and Post-Operative Chemotherapy in the Treatment of Acute Breast Cancer

R. Keiling, F. Reiss-Eichler, and H. Calderoli

Introduction

Acute breast cancer has a poor prognosis. Surgery or radiotherapy, or both combined, are unable to cure the systemic subclinical disease which is practically always present, and often even local control cannot be achieved. Donegan[1] published 50 cases treated between 1940 and 1965 by surgery, radiotherapy, or both, with a median survival of 19.7 months. Krutchik et al.[2] found a median survival of 18 months for 32 patients treated by radiotherapy. Preoperative chemotherapy seems logical, and for this reason we started a pilot study of pre- and post-operative chemotherapy.

Materials and Methods

Thirty-nine patients entered this study between January 1, 1980 and November 30, 1981. Ages ranged from 29 to 70 years; median age was 49 years. Criteria for inclusion were: a short clinical course before diagnosis (no longer than 2 months), clinical inflammatory signs (heat, edema, erythema, swelling, and tenderness), and thermographic signs of fast tumor growth. Two of these three criteria were necessary for inclusion.

Service de Radiothérapie et Laboratoire de Cancérologie, C.H.U. de Strasbourg, France

TREATMENT REGIMENS

Treatment began 2 or 3 days after diagnosis. Four courses were given of preoperative chemotherapy: adriamycin 20 mg/m² I.V. day 1; adriamycin 20 mg/m² I.V. + vincristine 1 mg/m² I.V. day 2; and 5-fluorouracil 400 mg/m² I.V. + cyclophosphamide 300 mg/m² I.V. days 3–6. One course was given every 4 weeks. Radical modified mastectomy was performed 4 weeks after the fourth course. The postoperative chemotherapy was adriamycin 20 mg/m² I.V. day 1; adriamycin 20 mg/m² I.V. + methotrexate 2 × 15 mg/m² I.M. day 4; and cyclophosphamide 400 mg/m² I.V. day 5. One course was given every 4 weeks, starting on the second postoperative day. A total of eight courses were given, and after that, patients received three courses of 30 mg melphalan I.V.

Following pretreatment, a drill-biopsy for histopathological diagnosis and for hormonal receptors, a chest X ray, a bone scan, liver ultrasound, CEA, and skin tests were performed. For the response to chemotherapy, the histopathology of operative specimens was studied.

Results

DNCB-TESTS

Acute breast cancer was receptor negative in 34/39 cases. Skin tests with tuberculine and candidine were positive in the

121

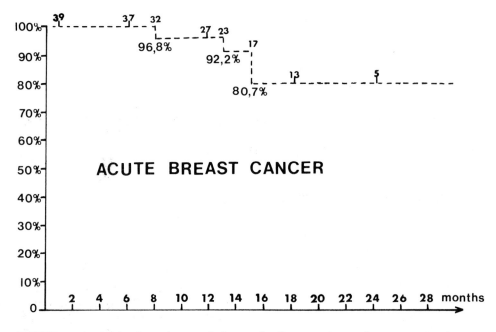

FIGURE 1.   Actuarial, relapse-free survival curve for the present acute breast cancer patients.

same proportion as in ordinary breast cancer. DNCB tests were negative in 35 cases.

TOXICITY

Treatment tolerance was good. Side effects were nausea, vomiting, and alopecia. Cardiac toxicity was closely monitored by isotopic ventricular ejection fractions, and the adriamycin dose was lowered, or the drug discontinued, if the ejection fraction fell below the normal value.

RESPONSE

The histopathological features showed complete sterilization with no cancer cells in the specimen in six cases, persistence of a few pictures in intraepithelial carcinoma in three cases, major alterations — such as necrosis or fibrosis with only a few cancer cells — were seen in 19 cases, and minor modifications in 11 cases. After chemotherapy, 15 nodes were not infiltrated (38%) and 24 were infiltrated (62%).

SURVIVAL AND RELAPSES

Thirty-six patients are alive, 35 in complete remission. Five have relapsed. Two patients with local and general relapses (8 months and 13 months, respectively) are dead (at 21 months and 24 months), and one in general relapse (at 15 months) died also (at 17 months). Two local relapses (15 months and 18 months) are alive, one in CR (18 months) and one with progression (24 months). Actuarial disease-free survival at 2 years is 80%.

These results seem encouraging, and we have started — together with G. Mathé — a randomized trial which compares two regimens of chemotherapy, a 6-day and a 1-day regimen. The cardiotoxicity of epiadriamycin given either in a single injection or for 2 days is being studied.

Discussion

In ordinary breast cancer, DNCB tests are positive in more than 90% of the cases. In acute breast cancer, 35/39 skin tests were negative. DNCB negative skin tests can thus suggest the diagnosis of acute breast cancer. The 80% actuarial survival in acute or inflammatory breast cancer is of interest.

REFERENCES

1. Donegan, W.L., and Spratt, J.S.: *Cancer of the Breast*. W.B. Saunders Co., Philadelphia, 1979.
2. Krutchik, A.N., Buzdar, A.U., Blumenschein, G.R., et al.: *J Surg Oncol 11: 325, 1979.*

CHAPTER 23

Autologous Bone Marrow Transplantation in Acute Leukemia: Use of 4-Hydroperoxycyclophosphamide *in vitro* to Eliminate Occult Leukemia

H. Kaizer, R.K. Stuart, O.M. Colvin, and G.W. Santos

Introduction

The principal obstacle to using autologous bone marrow as a source for transplantation in acute leukemia is the presence of occult residual leukemic cells in remission marrow. The feasibility of using *in vitro* immunologic treatment of marrow-tumor cell mixtures to eliminate all clonogenic tumor cells has been demonstrated in a number of animal models and forms the basis for a number of ongoing clinical trials.[1] An alternative to this approach is the *in vitro* pharmacologic treatment of marrow. At the Johns Hopkins Oncology Center, we have been exploring the use of 4-hydroperoxycyclophosphamide (4HC), a congener of cyclophosphamide, for such treatment. In aqueous solution, 4HC has the same alkylating and cytotoxic effects and the same immunoreactive products as microsomally activated CY.

Our initial studies of this approach utilized a model of acute myelogenous leukemia (AML) in the Lewis-Brown Norway (LBN) hybrid rat. In experiments involving the inoculation of lethally irradiated rats with marrow-tumor cell mixtures which had been treated with varying doses of 4HC, a dose-dependent clearing of tumor cells was demonstrable.[4] Because the LBN–AML model displays an unusual sensitivity to the antitumor effects of CY, we have recently extended these studies to another model of AML in the Wistar-Furth (WFU) rat which is not as sensitive as the LBN–AML to CY. Similar results have been obtained with complete clearing of tumor at optimal concentrations of 4HC. Increasing the concentration beyond 80 nM/ml (24 μg/ml) resulted in the death of a high fraction of rats due to marrow failure.[2]

Methods

Based on these results, we have designed a two-phase study for patients with acute leukemia, either lymphoblastic (ALL) or nonlymphoblastic (ANLL). The goal of the first phase of this study, which is still ongoing, is to determine the maximal concentration of 4HC that can be used for *in vitro* treatment and still achieve hematologic remission. The goal of the second phase of the study will be to determine if treatment with 4HC will eliminate all clonogenic tumor.

The Bone Marrow Transplant Unit, The Johns Hopkins Oncology Center, Baltimore, Maryland

125

TABLE 1. Phase I-4HC Study Patients to June 1, 1982

| Concentration of 4HC | No. of Patients with | |
	ALL	ANLL
40 μg/ml	4	0
60 μg/ml	2	2
80 μg/ml	3	3
100 μg/ml	5	1

Results and Discussion

Thus far, a total of 20 patients with acute leukemia have been treated on this study as shown in Table 1.

The phase 1-4HC study is a dose escalation study. Remission marrow is aliquoted into a treated fraction and a reserve fraction. The latter is only intended for use if the patient does not show evidence of hematologic recovery after reinfusion of the treated marrow. The preparative regimens used are specific for ALL and ANLL and have been previously described.[3] Although morbidity of the procedure is significant, only one of the 20 patients has had a transplant-related death (a heavily pretreated man with AML in sixth remission). Except for the three most recent patients who are still in the process of recovery, all the other patients have been discharged from the hospital in good clinical condition and have been able to resume normal activity. Satisfactory hematologic recovery has been observed in all 19 transplant survivors. This is somewhat surprising since measurements of granulocyte and macrophage progenitor cells in tissue culture (CFU-C) show can almost complete inhibition of assayable CFU-C at the higher 4HC concentrations.

Among the 19 patients evaluable for tumor status, 11 have relapsed. Most of the patients remaining in remission have relatively short observation times, although two of the patients have been in remission for over 14 months. While the ultimate disease-free status of these patients will contribute to our evaluation of the therapeutic efficacy of 4HC incubation, the ultimate test will depend on the results of the second phase of the study which cannot be initiated until the maximal concentration of 4HC is established.

When the maximum safe concentration of 4HC is determined, its therapeutic efficacy will be assessed in a phase II study. In this study, patients with high-risk acute leukemia will have marrow collected in first remission and treated with a maximal concentration of 4HC. Autologous marrow transplantation with such treated marrow will only be carried out in those patients who exhibit hematologic relapse indicating the probable presence of occult tumor in their initial remission marrow.

ACKNOWLEDGMENT

This work was supported in part by DHHS grants CA 06973 and CA 15396.

REFERENCES

1. Kaizer, H. and Santos, G.: I. Ariel, Ed. *Progress in Clinical Cancer 8*, Grune and Stratton, New York, 1982, pp. 31–43.
2. Kaizer, H., Cote, J.P., Sharkis, S., Stuart, R.K., and Santos, G.W.: *Proc Am Assoc Cancer Res 23: 194, 1982.*
3. Santos, G.W. and Kaizer, H.: *Semin Hematol 19: 277–289, 1982.*
4. Sharkis, S.J., Santos, G.W., and Colvin, M.: *Blood 55: 521–522, 1980.*

CHAPTER 24

Bone Marrow Transplantation for Adults over 30 Years of Age with Acute Nonlymphocytic Leukemia (ANLL): A Short Review

H.D. Preisler

Introduction

The advent of histocompatible allogeneic bone marrow transplantation has made possible the long-term survival and perhaps even the cure of end-stage leukemic patients. Approximately 10% of such patients will be significantly benefited by marrow transplantation.[1] Experience suggests that if the leukemia has not recurred within 2 years after transplantation, relapse is unlikely. The other 90%, the patients who expire after transplantation performed in this setting, do so because of the complications associated with the grafting of patients who are quite ill and because of recurrent leukemia.

TRANSPLANTATION IN REMISSION

These data suggested that the results of marrow transplantation would be improved if it were carried out in patients who were not ill and if the number of leukemic cells was minimal. There would then be a decrease in the number of deaths associated with the transplantation procedure, and a reduced likelihood of leukemic relapse. Logically, then, allogeneic marrow transplantation was ad-

vanced to patients in the first complete remission of their acute nonlymphocytic leukemia (ANLL).[2] The initial reports, with several years follow-up of some patients, have been encouraging with a high proportion of survivors and with seemingly little risk of recurrent leukemia. The question now is whether transplantation with histocompatible bone marrow is the treatment of choice for ANLL.

AGE

What is often not appreciated is the significant age dependence of the effects. In the Seattle study, the proportion of survivors at 2 years is different for patients who were <20 years old (70%), 20–30 years of age (52%), or 30–40 years of age (30%).[3] The recurrence of leukemia appears to be uncommon, but death results from transplantation-associated complications during the first year after transplantation. In comparison, the median survival of patients (mean age, 41 years), who entered remission on CALGB protocol 7421 was 19 months[4] and the median duration of *remission* for patients on protocol 7521 was 17 months. In contrast, median *survival* (mean age 41 years) time for the 25 patients >30 years of age transplanted in Seattle while in first remission it was only 6 months.[3]

Roswell Park Memorial Institute, Buffalo, New York

127

CHEMOTHERAPY ALONE VS. TRANSPLANTATION

Twenty-five percent of patients appear to be on the plateau portion of the *remission curve* for chemotherapy patients. The minimal follow-up time was 8 years and 5 years, respectively, for the 125 and 110 patients on each CALGB protocol. The plateau for these patients seemed to begin approximately 2 years after the patient entered remission. Twenty-two percent of the patients were over 60 years of age.

The upper age limit for patients entered onto the transplant study was 50 years. The plateau phase for the *survival curve* of patients >30 years old who were treated in Seattle with marrow allografts seemed to begin at the end of 1 year at approximately 38% (vs. 50% of patients on CALGB 7421 and 60% of patients on CALGB 7521 still in *remission* at the end of 1 year) but a death in the transplant group at 2½ years lowered the projected survival curve to 23%. If there are no deaths in the transplanted patients during the next 2½ years, the *survival* of the transplanted group will be equivalent to the actual proportion of chemotherapy patients still in remission at 5 years.

It should be noted, however, that the "plateau" phase for the patients treated with chemotherapy may not be flat. There may be a low rate of leukemic relapse even after 4 or 5 years of maintenance therapy. The "plateau" phase for the transplanted patients however, appears to be flat. If there were a low rate of relapse it might not be detected because of the small number of patients who have been followed for more than several years after transplantation.

These data demonstrate a clear-cut early survival advantage for patients over 30 years of age who are treated with conventional chemotherapy. After 2 years, the survival curve of the patients transplanted in remission approximates the remission duration curves for the chemotherapy patients. The period of follow-up for the transplanted patients may as yet be too limited to permit any statement to be made regarding its long-term efficacy. If, however, the experience with leukemic patients transplanted during relapse can be extrapolated to patients transplanted in remission, then few relapses would be expected, while relapses may continue to occur in the patients treated with conventional chemotherapy. It is not known as yet whether newer, very aggressive chemotherapy regimens have altered the shape of the relapse curve for the patients treated with chemotherapy.[5]

Discussion

This brief duscussion has not considered the potential long-term problems related to the large doses of whole body radiation, cyclophosphamide, and busulfan which are used to prepare the transplant patient. The incidence of secondary malignancies, late organ failure, and premature aging are unknown because too few patients have been followed for more than a decade after transplantation. It is more likely that these problems would be consequences of marrow transplantation than of chemotherapy but this is now merely conjecture. A review and discussion of the roles of allogeneic bone marrow transplantation and intensive chemotherapy can be found in *Cancer Treatment Reports.*[6]

REFERENCES

1. Thomas, E.D., Buckner, C.D., Banaji, M., et al.: *Blood* 49: 511–530, 1977.
2. Thomas, E.D., Buckner, C.D., Clift, R.A., et al.: *N Engl J Med* 301: 597–599, 1979.
3. Thomas, E.D., Clift, R.A., and Buckner, C.D.: *Cancer Treat Rep (in press)* 1982.
4. Rai, K., Holland, J.F., Glidewell, O.J., et al.: *Blood* 58: 1203–1212, 1981.
5. Preisler, H.D., Brecher, M., Browman, G., et al.: *Am J Hematol* 13(3): 189–198, 1982.
6. Preisler, H.D.: *Cancer Treat Rep* 66(7): 1467–1473, 1982.

CHAPTER 25

Bone Marrow Transplantation in Nonlymphocytic Leukemia without the Use of Total Body Irradiation

H. Kaizer, P.J. Tutschka, R. Saral, and G.W. Santos

Introduction

The use of bone marrow transplantation for patients with acute nonlymphocytic leukemia (ANLL) at a time when they have relapsed and are refractory to conventional chemotherapy (end-stage patients) has resulted in minimal salvage of patients. When this approach is used earlier in the course of ANLL, particularly in first remission, the long-term survival and possible cure rate is dramatically improved.[1] The preparative regimen employed by most centers engaged in these investigations has included total body irradiation (TBI) and cyclophosphamide. Over the past several years, the Johns Hopkins Oncology Center Marrow Transplant Program has developed an alternative preparative regimen which omitted TBI. This regimen employs the combination of very large doses of busulfan (BU) and cyclophosphamide (CY).

The development of this regimen was based on observations made by Drs. Tutschka and Santos[3] in a rat model for marrow transplantation. When marrow is transplanted across a major histocompatibility barrier in the rat, the addition of supralethal doses of BU to CY results in a more rapid rate of engraftment and a

Bone Marrow Transplant Unit, The Johns Hopkins Oncology Center, Baltimore, Maryland

higher percentage of animals displaying full chimerism. The addition of BU also permitted a reduction in the critical number of donor cells required to establish engraftment. Busulfan is not immunosuppressive but can produce irreversible marrow aplasia in the rat as well as in a number of other animal species. These observations suggest that a myelosuppressive "space-making" effect is required in addition to an immunosuppressive effect for efficient allogeneic marrow transplantation. Furthermore, the rather unique myelosuppressive effects of BU and the activity of modest doses of the drug in chronic myelogenous leukemia suggested that BU might have broader applicability in the acute myeloproliferative malignancies.

As a result of these observations, a pilot study of the combination of BU (total doses ranging from 4–20mg/kg) and CY (200 mg/kg total dose) in end-stage patients with ANLL was undertaken. Although the long-term survival of this group of patients was poor, we were encouraged to note that death due to leukemic relapse appeared to be less frequent than in an equivalent group of patients transplanted with CY alone. Furthermore, the kinetics of recovery and development of chimerism was accelerated

129

in the group of patients receiving BU + CY or CY + TBI as compared to CY alone.

Material and Methods

Encouraged by results which showed extended, disease-free survival, a preparative regimen using a fixed total dose of 16mg/kg of BU was employed in a group of 33 patients with ANLL in first, second, or third remission or early relapse (6–15% blasts in the marrow).[2]

Results

The follow-up on these patients ranges from 3+ to 38+ months (median, 16+ months). Only one patient has so far exhibited a leukemic relapse. Actuarial survival curves on these patients show the same trend in long-term survival as that established with CY + TBI preparative regimens, i.e., poorest for end-stage patients and best for first remission patients. The survival plateaus for the various groups of patients is statistically no different for the BU + CY preparative regimen as compared to the published results with CY + TBI. The principal causes of failure in this group of 33 patients are related to graft vs. host disease, interstitial pneumonitis (most commonly of viral etiology), other viral infections, or some combination of these factors. There are now some promising approaches to the

reduction of these complications of allogeneic marrow transplantation which may result in even better long-term survival rates.

Discussion

The availability of a regimen that does not involve radiation therapy has several advantages. First, not all institutions that may wish to undertake investigations of allogeneic marrow transplantation have facilities for TBI. Second, should interinstitutional collaborative studies prove desirable, problems of dose standardization are much simpler without TBI. Finally, the long-term complications of TBI may be more significant than those associated with BU + CY. If these early results are confirmed, large-scale prospective studies may be required.

ACKNOWLEDGMENT

This was supported in part by DHHS grants CA 06973 and CA 15396.

REFERENCES

1. Santos, G.W. and Kaizer, H.: *Semin Hematol 19: 277–289, 1982.*
2. Santos, G.W., and Tutschka, P.J., Beschorner, W.E., et al.: *Blood 58(Suppl 1): 176a, 1981.*
3. Tutschka, P.S. and Santos, G.W.: *Transplantation 29: 52–62, 1977.*

PART III

Biological Response Modifiers
and Hormones

CHAPTER 26

The New Concept of Biological Response Modifiers

S.A. Sherwin and R.K. Oldham

Introduction

The term biological response modifiers (BRM) is a term recently developed to describe agents and approaches to the treatment of cancer that involve augmentation of the host immune response or biological modification of the tumor cell itself. Agents or approaches that depend on augmentation of the host immune response include the broad category of immunoaugmenting and immunorestorative agents, interferons and other lymphokines, thymic factors, and modifiers of tumor antigen, cell surface components. Agents which act through biological modification of the tumor cell itself include various growth factors and maturation factors. In certain instances, BRM may be directly toxic to the tumor cell. Examples of this mechanism of action include antitumor monoclonal antibodies and antitumor effector cells. In addition, certain lymphokines and cytokines (e.g., interferons) may have a direct, toxic, or antiproliferative effect on the tumor cell itself.

The Biological Response Modifiers Program (BRMP) was recently established within the Division of Cancer Treatment of the National Cancer Institute in order to provide a comprehensive approach to the preclinical and clinical development of potential BRM. This program, situated in the NCI's Frederick Cancer Research Facility in Frederick, Maryland, includes both extramural contract and grant support for research in this area as well as an intramural laboratory and clinical research program to complement the activities of extramural investigators. A key component of the BRMP is the Preclinical Screening Program which is responsible for identifying from the many hundreds of biologicals with potential antineoplastic activity those BRM most worthy of clinical development. The screening program consists of a series of Common Tract assays involving *in vitro* and *in vivo* tests of B cell, T cell, NK cell, and macrophage function as well as screening for antitumor activity *in vivo* and in spontaneously metastasizing animal models systems. In addition, various Specific Tract screens for specific lymphokines, cytokines, growth factors, and antitumor monoclonal antibodies are being developed. During the first 2–3 years of operation of the preclinical screening program, an attempt will be made to define those assays which are most predictive of antitumor effect in patients. Therefore, agents currently being tested in the screen include those currently undergoing or having recently completed clinical trials. Some of the assays in the preclinical screening program may therefore be modified if they are not found to predict clinical activity.

A high priority of BRMP in both its extramural and intramural research programs is to develop an approach to phase I trials of these agents which will allow not

Biological Response Modifiers Program, Division of Cancer Treatment, National Cancer Institute, Frederick, Maryland

only the determination of a maximum tolerated dose but also, where possible, the identification of an optimal biological response modifying dose. Therefore, as patients are monitored carefully for toxicity and tolerance, they will also be monitored simultaneously through a variety of immunologic assays for evidence of biological response modification. It is hoped that for most of the agents tested in this fashion, a dose which is optimal biologically may be identified and it is clearly possible that this dose may be well below the maximum tolerated dose for the agent. Wherever possible, this optimal BRM dose will be correlated with antitumor response. Initially there may be a problem in determining which immunologic assays to use for the various agents being tested. However, there is considerable flexibility in the choice of assays and, with time, it should be possible to refine the immunologic monitoring to reflect an increasing knowledge of the mechanism of action of the agent being tested.

An example of this approach to the early clinical development of biological response modifiers is provided by the recently completely phase I trials of recombinant leukocyte-A interferon conducted by the Intramural Clinical Research Program of the BRMP. In this trial, more than 80 patients were treated with increasing doses of recombinant interferon ranging from $1-136 \times 10^6$ units given by I.M. injection three times weekly for 28 days. The recombinant interferon employed represented a highly purified, single molecular species of alpha-interferon with a specific activity of $2-4 \times 10^8$ u/mg and was prepared by Hoffman LaRoche Inc., (Nutley, NJ) in collaboration with Genentech, Inc., (San Francisco, CA). All patients on this trial were carefully examined for evidence of antitumor effect and toxicity and were also monitored extensively for serum interferon activity and biological response modification in a panel of immunologic assays. The results of this trial indicate that recombinant leukocyte-A interferon can be given safely in doses up to 118×10^6 units three times weekly for 28 days. At higher doses, mild reversible hepatic transaminase elevation occurs in most patients. However, at lower doses considerable systemic toxicity including fever, chills, fatigue, anorexia, gastrointestinal disturbances, and flu-like symptoms are encountered. Objective evidence of antitumor effect was seen in 9/76 evaluable patients with measured partial remissions occurring in five patients with non-Hodgkin's lymphoma and one patient each with chronic lymphocytic leukemia, Hodgkin's disease, malignant melanoma, and breast cancer. The results of the immunologic assays performed in these patients indicate that distinct immunomodulatory effects are seen. The majority of patients had no change or decrease in natural-killer-cell-mediated cytotoxicity, perhaps as a result of inhibitory factors present in the serum. In contrast, the majority of patients (greater than 80%) had evidence for increased monocyte function as judged by a growth inhibition assay. Lymphocyte blastogenesis was decreased in the majority of patients. Although these distinct immunomodulatory effects were easily reproducible, it was impossible to determine whether any of these effects correlated with dose and/or tumor response. Therefore this trial indicates in a preliminary way that we are as yet unable to identify an optimal biological response modifying dose for recombinant leukocyte-A interferon of this type. Nonetheless using the information gathered in this extensive phase I trial, phase II efficacy trials in a variety of malignancies have been instituted by the BRMP and other investigators throughout the United States. The results of these trials are forthcoming.

In other clinical trials recently initiated or soon to begin, the BRMP will continue to emphasize the need to identify optimal biological response modifying doses for the agents being tested, as well as the need for determination of a maximum tolerated dose in the usual manner. These trials will include early clinical testing of other highly purified, recombinant and non-recombinant interferons (including beta and gamma interferons) as well as antitumor monoclonal antibodies and other selected biological response modifiers. It is hoped that, as these trials proceed, further insights will be gained into the biological response modifying effects of these agents which will guide the determination of optimal biological dosing in the future.

CHAPTER 27

Effects of BCG on the Biological Response to Tumors: A Short Review

P. Reizenstein,[a] C. Ogier, and G. Mathé[b]

BCG, The Model Substance

After Coley's vaccine,[38] and together with immunodepressants like corticosteroids, cytostatics, and possibly other drugs, BCG belongs to the first generation of substances intended to modify the immunological and biological response to tumors. Even though the first generation is never the last one, and although better-defined substances like bacterial extracts and synthetized molecules (Table 1) have appeared, BCG remains the model substance and perhaps the only immunomodulator of which a sufficient number of experimental and clinical studies have been published to permit another evaluation, in addition to those published earlier.[5,6,9,28]

Activity Against Experimental Tumors

There is no doubt that in some, but not in all, of the frequently quite immunogenic experimental tumors, immunoprophylaxis is possible. The original experiments by Old and Benacerraf[40] have been confirmed repeatedly.[29,43,46,48,64]

Nor is there any doubt that, in certain models, a regression of certain experimental tumors can be achieved with intralesional BCG,[25,46,48,56,64] but also with intracutaneous or intravenous administration.[19,29,41–43]

Effects are Controversial

The effects are controversial, however. Only some animal tumors can be prevented or treated with BCG.[40] Variations in BCG strains, treatment duration and dosage schedules[18,27,29,50,56] and in administration forms (I.V., I.P., I.D., etc.)[31,37] have been assumed to explain the differences in results in animals.

In man, however, similar results have been described despite different administration forms and different BCG strains.[51,62] Here, the treatment duration seems more important. Prolonged treatment seems to reduce the T-cell mitogen response, whereas a normal response is seen during the first month of treatment.[50]

The clinical results are also controversial, even in the best-studied diseases which are acute myelogenous leukemia,[61] bronchial carcinoma,[32,33] non-Hodgkin's lymphoma[22] and acute lymphatic leukemia.[61] However, in these four patient groups, at least tentative explanations for the discrepancies can be found (Table 2). Differences in the composition of the patient groups studied, in part due to therapeutic progress, could be one of several alternative explanations of the contradic-

[a]Division of Hematology, Karolinska Hospital, Stockholm, Sweden; Visiting Professor at the Institute of Cancerology, University of Paris-Sud
[b]Institute of Cancérology and Immunogénétics (INSERM U 50), Hôpital Paul-Brousse, Villejuif, France

137

TABLE 1.   Second Generation Biological
Response Modifiers

Interferon[7,8,17]
Interferon inducers (poly A–poly U)
Cytokines (interleukines, tumor necrotizing factor,
  etc.)
Bacterial extracts (MER, LTA, lipopolysaccharides,
  endotoxin, muramyl dipeptide, pertussis toxin,
  etc.)[15]
Thymus extracts ("thymostimulin" or TP-1, TPF,
  TS, etc.)[12,39]
Levamisole[2,26,44,52,53]
Azimexon[20]
Tuftsin
Retinoids[30]
Transfer factor[16]

tory results. For instance, in the original studies of acute lymphatic or myeloid leukemia, the frequencies of complete remission were only about one half those of the later studies (Table 2). Therefore, it can not be excluded that the population of subjects who entered remission and thus began BCG-therapy in the early studies was different from that in the later ones. Speculatively this group could, like the young, female, stage I non-Hodgkin lymphomas, represent "rapid chemotherapy respond-ers" who respond better to BCG than the patients who achieve remission with greater difficulty. This speculation, however, does not in any obvious way explain why blood — and HLA — groups affect the apparent efficacy of BCG (Table 2).

The controversies about the therapeutic effect of BCG are even greater in melanoma,[57] in colon carcinoma,[8,52] chronic myelocytic leukemias, advanced breast cancer[45,54] and bladder cancer.[36] In general, the conclusion at present is that, in these latter diseases, the BCG-effects is either still controversial or not yet confirmed.

Possible Mechanisms of the Possible BCG Effect

Some of the conclusions above are based on studies combining BCG and tumor cells. While in some[29,64] but not all[42] animal tumors, the specific antigen appears to add something, and although some claims for effective specific immunization in melanoma have been made,[23] no additional benefit of the tumor cell administration was seen in acute leukemia.[51,62] For

TABLE 2.   Subgroups of Patients and the Response to Nonspecific Adjuvant Therapy

Diagnosis	Patient Group with a Significant Effect	Patient Group with No Significant Effect	Reference
Acute myelogenous leukemia	A group with 35% remissions	A group with 65% remissions	51
Non-Hodgkin's lymphoma	Young, or Stage I, or women, or in initial phase of the disease	Old, or Stage II–IV, or men, or in the relapse phase	22
Bronchial carcinoma	Non-small cell carcinoma or blood groups A, B, AB, Rh+	Small cell carcinoma, or blood groups O, Rh–	1, 32, 33
Acute lymphatic leukemia	First patients treated 1962. Patients who had, without neuroprophylaxis, survived over 2 years and who frequently had HLA BW 17 and AW 33	First patients treated 1972. Patients who had received neuroprophylaxis and had survived for 2–3 months	21a, 23a, 26a, 59, 61
	Approximate remission frequency 80%. Some patients induced with prednisone alone	Remission frequency 93%. All patients given combination chemotherapy	

the present purpose, therefore, it will be assumed that the biological effects discussed below are due to the BCG.

Among the mechanisms of the possible BCG effect, cross-reactivity between BCG and some hepatoma[11] and melanoma cells[34] and controversial effects on B and T cells have been discussed.

The effect on non-T, non-B cells may be more convincing, however. A null cell increase after BCG treatment has been found[10] as has a NK-cell-restoration,[3,4,14,21,58,63] a local macrophage accumulation[47,53] and an activation of several macrophage functions,[60] such as the production of colony stimulating activity,[49] the helper-function,[3,35] and the cytotoxicity.[13] The regression of animal tumors after BCG treatment seems correlated both to autoreactive cells and to autoreactive serum factors.[24]

Conclusions

It is highly probable that BCG can lead to prevention and regression of certain animal tumors, particularly if the tumor is antigenic and the BCG is applied locally. This regression is in part mediated by T-cell cytotoxicity, but non-T-cell cytotoxicity and antibody formation may play a part.

In certain subgroups of patients with AML, non-Hodgkin's lymphoma, and bronchial carcinoma, a temporary clinical effect of BCG has been described by several authors. These BCG-sensitive subgroups seem to be defined by host factors (blood and HLA groups) and by factors characterizing the tumor (possibly high sensitivity to cytostatic treatment or other factors characteristic of a good prognosis indicate sensitivity to BCG as well). In human tumors, however, there is little confirmed evidence that the effect is mediated by T-cell-cytotoxicity. There is more evidence, although still very circumstantial, that several of the functions of the non-T non-B cells, possibly the OKM$_1$

positive macrophages and NK-cells, are stimulated by certain modes of administering BCG.

In view of the marginal and temporary effect of BCG, the meaning of continued experiments has been justly questioned. However, if it can be confirmed in man that cytotoxic cells can attack "resting" G$_0$-tumor cells, which are refractory to most cytostatics, and that tumor cells are more sensitive to cytotoxic attack than normal cells, then possibilities to modify the macrophage and NK-cell activities in a better-defined way would be of interest. There may be, in man, after all, a certain defense against tumors.

REFERENCES

1. Anthony, H.M.: *Cancer Immunol Immunother 11:* 287, 1981.
2. Amery, W.K., Losemans, J., Gooszen, H.C., Lopes Cardozo, E., Louwagie, A., Stam, J., Swierenga, J., Vanderschueren, R.G., and Veldhuizen, R.W.: *Cancer Immunol Immunother 7: 191,* 1979.
3. Arends-Merino, A., Giscombe, R., Ogier, C., Reizenstein, P., Sjogren, A.M., and Wasserman, J.: *Cancer Immunol Immunother 14: 32, 1982.*
4. Arends-Merino, A., Sjogren, A.M., and Reizenstein, P.: *Cancer Immunol Immunother (in press).*
5. Baldwin, R.W., and Pimm, M.V.: *Natl Cancer Inst Monograph 39: 11, 1973.*
6. Baldwin, R.W., and Pimm, M.V.: *Adv Cancer Res 28: 91, 1978.*
7. Balkwill, F.R.: *Cancer Immunol Immunother 7: 7,* 1979.
8. Bancewicz, J., Calman, K.L., Macpherson, S.G., McArdle, C.S., McVie, J.G., and Soukop, M.: *J Soc Med 73: 197, 1980.*
9. Bast, R.C., Zbar, B., Borsos, T., and Rapp, H.J.: *N Engl J Med 290: 1413–1420, 1458–1469, 1974.*
10. Belpomme, D., Joseph, R., and Lelarge, N.: *Cancer Immunol Immunother 1: 113–114, 1976.*
11. Borsos, T., and Rapp, H.J.: *J Natl Cancer Inst 51:* 1085, 1973.
12. Davis, S.: In *Immunomodulation and Thermotherapy in Cancer,* H. Fudenberg, P. Pontiggia, C. Ogier, Eds., Field International, Rome, 1983.
13. Eccles, S.A.: *Immunological Aspects of Cancer,* J.E. Castro, Ed., MIP Press, England, 1978.
14. Florentin, I., Huchet, R., Bruley-Rosset, M., Halle-Pannenko, O., and Mathé, G.: *Cancer Immunol Immunother 1: 31, 1976.*
15. Friedman, H. In *Immunomodulation and Thermotherapy in Cancer,* H. Fudenberg, P. Pontiggia, C. Ogier, Eds., Field International, Rome, 1983 (in press).
16. Fudenberg, H.: *Immunomodulation and Thermotherapy in Cancer,* H. Fudenberg, P. Pontiggia,

C. Ogier, Eds., Field International, Rome, 1983 (in press).

17. Gutterman, J.U.: *Cancer Bull* 33: 271, 1981.

18. Halle-Pannenko, O., Bourut, C., and Kamel, M.: *Cancer Immunol Immunother* 1: 17, 1976.

19. Hanna, M.G., Pollack, V.A., Peters, L.C., and Hoover, H.C.: *Cancer,* 49: 659–664, 1982.

20. Heim, M.E., Mabner, B., Knebel, L., Stosier, U., Boerner, D., and Bicker, U.: *Cancer Immunol Immunother* 12: 87, 1981.

21. Herberman, R.B., Nunn, M.E., Holden, H.T., Staal, S., and Djeu, J.Y.: *Int J Cancer* 19: 555, 1977.

21a. Heyn, R.M., Joo, P., Karon, M., Nesbit, M., Shore, N., Breslow, N., Weiner, J., Reed, A., and Hammond, D.: *Blood* 46: 431, 1975.

22. Hoerni, B., Durand, M., Eghbali, H., Hoerni-Simon, G., and Lagarde, C.: In *Adjuvant Therapy of Cancer, III,* S.E. Salmon and S.E. Jones Eds., Grune & Stratton, New York, 1981, pp. 99–106.

23. Hollinshead, D.A., Arlen, M., Yonemoto, R., Cohen, M., Tanner, K., Kundin, W.D., and Scherrer, J.: *Cancer* 49: 1387–1404, 1982.

23a. Jacquillat, C., Weil, M., Auclerc, M.F., Chastang, C., Flandrin, G., Izrael, V., Schaison, G., Degos, L., Boiron, M., and Bernard, J.: *Cancer Chemother Pharmacol* 1: 113, 1978.

24. Killion, J.J., and Baker, J.R.: *Cancer Immunother* 12: 111, 1982.

25. Kleinschuster, S.J., Rapp, H.J., Lueker, D.C., and Kainer, R.A.: *J Natl Cancer Inst* 58: 1807, 1978.

26. Lehtinen, M.: *Cancer Immunol Immunother* 9: 137, 1980.

26a. Leukaemia Committee and the Working Party on Leukaemia in Childhood. *Br Med J* 4: 189, 1971.

27. Mackaness, G.B., Auclair, D.J., and Lagrange, P.H.: *J Natl Cancer Inst* 51: 1655–1667, 1973.

28. Mathé, G.: *Recent Results in Cancer Research,* vol. 55, Springer Verlag, New York 1976.

29. Mathé, G., Amiel, J.L., Schwarzenberg, L., Schneider, M., Cattan, A., Schlumberger, J.R., Hayat, M., and De Vassal, F.: *Lancet* 2: 697, 1969.

30. Mathé, G., Gouveia, J., Hercend, T., Gros, F., Dorval, T., Hazon, J., Misset, J.L., Schwarzenberg, L., Ribaud, P., Lemaigre, G., Santelli, G., and Reizenstein, P.: Presented at the International Symposium on Prevention and Detection of Cancer, San Paolo, 1982. *Cancer Detection and Prevention (in press).*

31. McKneally, M.F., Maver, C., and Kausel, H.W.: *Lancet* 1: 593, 1977.

32. Mikulski, S.M., McGuire, W.P., Louie, A.C., Chirigos, M.A., and Muggia, F.M.: *Cancer Treat Rev,* 6: 177–190, 1979.

33. Mikulski, S.M., McGuire, W.P., Louie, A.C., Chirigos, M.A., and Muggia, F.M.: *Cancer Treat Rep* 6: 125–130, 1979.

34. Minden, P., Sharpton, T.R., and McClatchy, J.K.: *J Immunol* 116: 1407, 1976.

35. Mokyr, M.B., and Mitchell, M.S.: *Cell Immunol* 15: 264, 1975.

36. Morales, A. *Cancer Immunol Immunother* 7: 7, 1979.

37. Nathanson, L. *Cancer Chemother Rep* 56: 659–665, 1972.

38. Nauts, H.C.: *The Beneficial Effects of Bacterial Infections on Host Resistance to Cancer. End Results in 449 Cases.* Cancer Res. Inst., 1980, Monograph. No. 8.

39. Ogier, C.: Effect of thymic factors on the phenotypic modulation of leukemic cells. In: *Immunomodulation and Thermotherapy in Cancer.* H. Fudenberg, P. Pontiggia, C. Ogier, Eds. Field International, Rome, 1983, (in press).

40. Old, L.J., Clarke, D.A., Benacerraf, B.: *Nature* (London) 184: 291, 1959.

41. Olsson, L., Ebbesen, P.: *Biomedicine* 28: 88, 1978.

42. Olsson, L., Florentin, I., Kiger, N., Mathé, G.: *J. Natl Cancer Inst* 59: 1297, 1977.

43. Parr, I.: *Br J Cancer* 26: 174, 1972.

44. Paterson, A.H.G., Nutting, M., Takats, L., Edwards, A.M., Schinnour, D., McClellan, A.: *Cancer Clin Trials* 3: 5, 1980.

45. Pinsky, C.M., De Jager, R.L., Wittes, R.E., Wong, P.P., Kaufman, R.J., Mike, V., Mansen, J.A., Oettgen, H.F., and Krakuff, I.H.: In *Immunotherapy of Cancer: Present Status of Trials in Man,* W.D. Terry and D. Windhorst, Eds., Raven Press, New York, 1978, p. 647.

46. Rapp, H.J.: *Israel J Med Sci* 9: 366, 1973.

47. Rappaport, H., and Khalil, A.: *Cancer Immunol Immunother* 1: 45, 1976.

48. Ray, P.K., Poduval, T.B., and Sundaram, K.: *J Natl Cancer Inst* 58: 763–767, 1977.

49. Reizenstein, P., Anderson, B., and Beran, M.: EORTC Plenary session, Paris, June 23–27, 1980. To be published in *Rec Res Cancer Research,* Springer Verlag.

50. Reizenstein, P., Ogier, C., and Sjögren, A.M.: *Rec Res Cancer Research* 75: 29, 1980.

51. Reizenstein, P., Andersson, B., Bjorkholmm, M., Brenning, G., Engsted, T.L., Gahrton, G., Hast, R., Holm, G., Hornsten, P., Killander, A., Lantz, B., Lindemalm, C., Lockner, D., Lonnqvist, B., Mellstedt, H., Palmblad, J., Paul, C., Simmonsson, B., Sjogren, A.M., Stalfelt, A.M., Uden, A.M., Wadman, B., Oberg, G., and Osby, E.: In *Immunotherapy of Cancer,* W.D. Terry and D. Windhorst, Eds., Raven Press, New York, 1982, p. 17.

52. Robinson, E., Bartal, A., Cohen, Y., Haim, N., Mohilever, J., and Mekori, T.: *Cancer Chemother Pharmacol* 8: 35–40, 1982.

53. Rosenthal, M., Trabert, U., Muller, W.: *Clin Exp Immunol* 25: 493, 1976.

54. Smith, G.V., Morse, P.A., Deraps, G.D., Raju, S., Hardy, J.D.: *Surgery* 74: 59, 1973.

55. Spitler, L.E., Sagebiel, R.W., Glogau, R.G., Wong, P.P., Malm, T.M., Ohase, R.H., and Gonzalez, R.L.: In *Immunotherapy of Cancer, Present Status of Trials in Man,* W.D. Terry and D. Windhorst, Eds., Raven Press, New York, 1978, p. 73.

56. Tanaka, T.: *Gann* 65: 145, 1974.

57. Terry, W.D.: *N Engl J Med* 303: 1174, 1980.

58. Thatcher, N., Swindell, R., and Crowther, N., *Clin Exp Immunol* 35: 171, 1979.

59. Tursz, T., Hors, J., Lipinski, M., and Amiel, J.L.: *Br Med J* 1: 1250, 1978.

60. Unanue, E.R., Askonas, B.A., and Allison, A.C.: *J Immunol* 103: 71, 1969.

61. Vogler, W.R.: *Cancer Immunol Immunother 9: 15, 1980.*

62. Whittaker, J., Bailey-Wood, R., and Hutchins, S.: *Br J Haematol 45: 389, 1980.*

63. Wolfe, S.A., Tracey, D.E., and Henney, C.S.: *Nature (London) 262: 584, 1976.*

64. Zbar, B., Bernstein, I.D., and Rapp, H.J.: *J Natl Cancer Inst 46: 831, 1971.*

CHAPTER 28

Experimental Data on the Aromatic Retinid, Ro 10-9359, Etretinate, Tigason®

W. Bollag

Introduction

Retinoids (vitamin A and analogs, natural and synthetic ones) are a class of compounds possessing a marked influence on prevention as well as on therapy of tumors. In organ cultures, they prevent and reverse hyperplasia and metaplasia induced by carcinogenic agents. Many investigations have shown that retinoids prevent and reverse malignant transformation in cell cultures and many chemically or virally induced tumors are influenced by retinoids. The development of tumors at various organ sites (e.g., skin, oral cavity, stomach, intestine, colon, pancreas, trachea, bronchus, urinary bladder, cervix, and mammary gland) and induced by different carcinogens is prevented or retarded. Some tumors even regress under treatment with retinoids.[3–5,8–10]

Material and Methods

CHEMISTRY

Ro 10-9359, etretinate, Tigason® is ethyl all - trans - 9 - (4 - methoxy - 2,3,6 - trimethyl - phenyl) - 3,7 - dimethyl - 2,4,6,8 - nonatetra - enoate.

Pharmaceutical Research Department, F. Hoffmann-La Roche Co. Ltd., Basel, Switzerland

BIOLOGY

Chemically Induced Papillomas and Carcinomas

Papillomas or carcinomas were induced by painting the skin of the backs of mice with the initiating agent dimethylbenzanthracene (DMBA) and the promoting agent croton oil.[1]

Prevention. Mice received 30 mg/kg of etretinate orally daily (5 × per week) during the promotion phase.[2]

Therapy. Mice with established papillomas or carcinomas were treated during a 2-week period either orally or intraperitoneally, weekly or daily, with various doses. The treated mice were compared with controls concerning papilloma diameters and carcinoma volumes.[1]

Organ Cultures

Prevention. Tracheal explants of neonatal rats and explants of fetal mouse lungs (bronchial epithelium) were grown for 14 days with either 3,4-benzpyrene or cigarette smoke condensate alone or combined with etretinate.

Therapy. Explants of both tissues were first exposed for 14 days to benzpyrene or cigarette smoke condensate and then transferred to control medium or medium containing etretinate for a further 4 days. At the end of the experiments the number of mitoses was determined and secretory activity as well as ciliary function were evaluated.[7]

Results

PREVENTION OF CHEMICALLY INDUCED PAPILLOMAS AND CARCINOMAS[2]

The daily oral administration of 30 mg/kg etretinate during the promotion phase of carcinogenesis delayed the appearance and retarded the growth of papillomas and reduced the incidence of carcinomas. Three hundred days after the beginning of the experiment, etretinate — in comparison with controls — reduced the mean number of papillomas per mouse from 12.4 to 1.1, the mean volume of papillomas per mouse from 426.3 to 6.8 mm³, and the incidence of carcinomas from 46 to 4.

THERAPY OF CHEMICALLY INDUCED TUMORS[1]

Papillomas (Table 1)

In a 14-day therapeutic experiment with established papillomas, the controls showed a progression of growth by 23.2%, whereas in the animals treated with etretinate once a week the papillomas regressed dose-dependently: 200 mg/kg I.P. led to a regression of 74.1% and even 25 mg/kg still reduced the papilloma diameters by 48.8%. Oral daily doses of 40 mg/kg provoked a 76.4% regression and 10 mg/kg still led to a regression of 46.7%.

Carcinomas

The therapeutic effect on chemically induced squamous cell carcinomas of the skin was also pronounced. Whereas the mean carcinoma volume of the controls increased by 92.7%, the carcinoma volumes of the animals treated with 200 mg/kg daily I.P. for 14 days regressed by 53.4% and with 400 mg/kg by 72.2%.

TABLE 1.   Therapy of Chemically Induced Papillomas: Results of Treatment of Established Skin Papillomas during 2 weeks with Different Dosage Schedules of the Retinoid Etretinate

Dose (mg/kg)	Average Sum of the Papilloma Diameter/Animal (mm)		Percent Change in the Average Sum of the Papilloma Diameter/Animal
	Day 0	Day 14	
Controls	21.1	26.0	+23.2%
Etretinate			
200 1 × weekly i.p.	25.5	6.6	−74.1
100	28.0	8.5	−69.6
50	20.4	9.1	−55.4
25	24.4	12.5	−48.8
12.5	24.8	17.3	−30.2
400 1 × weekly p.o.	22.0	4.8	−78.2
200	23.7	9.8	−58.6
100	21.5	14.3	−33.5
50	21.0	16.5	−21.4
25	16.0	14.2	−11.3
40 daily p.o.	19.5	4.6	−76.4
20	16.6	7.4	−55.4
10	18.4	9.8	−46.7
5	16.5	13.7	−17.0

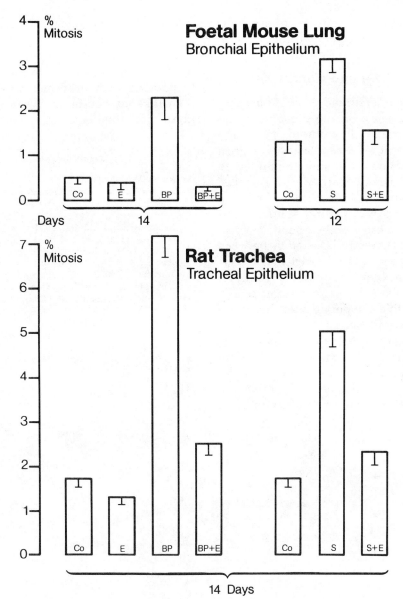

FIGURE 1. Prevention of benzpyrene (BP) and cigarette smoke condensate (S) induced mitotic stimulation of bronchial and tracheal epithelium in organ culture by etretinate (E), control medium (Co).

ORGAN CULTURES

In both tissues, tracheal and bronchial epithelium, benzpyrene as well as cigarette smoke condensate induces a striking increase in epithelial mitosis.

Prevention (Figure 1)

Etretinate combined with benzpyrene or smoke condensate inhibits the increase

in cell division (hyperplasia) and prevents the loss of secretory activity or ciliary function (metaplasia).[7]

Therapy

In explants pretreated with benzpyrene or smoke condensate and transferred to a medium containing etretinate, the carcinogen- or smoke condensate-induced rise in mitotic activity is reduced to normal levels and the secretory differentiation and ciliary function restored.[7]

Discussion and Conclusion

Etretinate is a retinoid possessing a very marked influence on the prevention and therapy of chemically induced benign and malignant epithelial neoplasias. The great handicap of vitamin A and vitamin A acid was their marked toxicity, the so-called hypervitaminosis A syndrome. The goal of our efforts was to find synthetic retinoids with a broader therapeutic margin, i.e., with a marked dissociation between therapeutic activity and toxicity. The therapeutic index of etretinate is 10 times more favorable than that of retinoic acid.[1,4] Therefore, this compound was chosen for clinical trials in oncology and dermatology. Its marked preventive and therapeutic effect in animal experiments on preneoplastic and neoplastic epithelial lesions and its pronounced preventive and therapeutic influence in organ cultures on hyperplasia and metaplasia of tracheal and bronchial epithelium, in combination with a favorable therapeutic index, made it a preferable candidate for clinical trials in patients with bronchial metaplasia, a premalignant condition eventually leading to bronchial carcinoma.[6]

REFERENCES

1. Bollag, W.: *Eur J Cancer 10: 731–737, 1974.*
2. Bollag, W.: *Eur J Cancer 11: 721–724, 1975.*
3. Bollag, W.: *Cancer Chemother Pharmacol 3: 207–215, 1979.*
4. Bollag, W., and Matter, A.: *Annals NY Acad Sci 359: 9–24, 1981.*
5. DeLuca, L.M., and Shapiro, S.S., Eds.: *Annals NY Acad Sci 359: 1–430, 1981.*
6. Gouveia, J., Mathé, G., Hercend, T., Gros, F., Lemaigre, G., Santelli, G., Homasson, J.P., Gaillard, J.P., Angebault, M., Bonniot, J.P., Lededente, A., Marsac, J., Parrot, R., and Pretet, S.: *Lancet 1: 710–712, 1982.*
7. Lasnitzki, I., and Bollag, W.: *Cancer Treat Rep 66: 1375–1380, 1982.*
8. Lotan, R.: *Biochim Biophys Acta 605: 33–91, 1980.*
9. Mayer, H., Bollag, W., Hänni, R., and Ruegg, R.: *Experientia 34: 1105–1119, 1978.*
10. Sporn, M.B., Dunlop, N.M., Newton, D.L., and Smith, J.M.: *Fed Proc 35: 1332–1338, 1976.*

CHAPTER 29

New Data on Interferon Action: Long-Term Treatment with Interferon Leads to the Reversion of the Transformed and Tumorigenic Phenotype of Cells in Culture

D. Brouty-Boyé and I. Gresser

Introduction

We have previously shown that cloned murine C3H/10T1/2 cells transformed by x-irradiation reverted to a normal phenotype under certain conditions of culture. Furthermore, it has been shown by ourselves and by others that interferon could modify to some extent the phenotypic expression of certain cells. To determine whether interferon could induce reversion of the transformed and tumorigenic phenotype, we undertook a systematic analysis of the effects of interferon on the phenotype of cloned x-ray transformed 10T1/2 cells.

Material and Methods

The origin of x-ray transformed 10T1/2 cells and the conditions of culture with interferon have been previously described in detail.[1] In brief, transformed cells were serially passaged once every week in the continuous presence of 640 units of mouse C-243 cell interferon. At different passage levels the phenotype of the cells was determined according to the criteria of cell proliferation, morphology, structure, and tumorigenicity as previously reported.[1,2]

Laboratory of Viral Oncology, Institut de Recherches Scientifiques sur le Cancer, Villejuif, France

Results

The long-term cultivation of transformed and tumorigenic C3H/10T1/2 cells with interferon leads to a progressive change towards a nontransformed and nontumorigenic phenotype. As summarized in Table 1, transformed cells reached low cell densities after one passage with interferon. Their morphology changed from a spindled shape to a flat conformation after 5–7 passages in the presence of interferon. Concomitant with this morphologic change there was a highly organized distribution of actin microfilaments. Finally, we observed a decrease in tumorigenicity of these cells, exemplified first by a delay in the growth of tumor cells and then a delay in the appearance of the tumors and a decrease in the number of mice bearing tumors. After more than 10 passages, none of the mice injected with interferon-treated cells developed tumors.

Conclusion and Discussion

The salient points of these results may be summarized as follows:

1) The reversion of the transformed and tumorigenic phenotype induced by in-

147

TABLE 1. Phenotypic Characteristics of Parental and Interferon-treated Transformed Cells

	Parental Transformed Cells	Interferon-treated Transformed Cells
Transformed phenotype		
Cell saturation density	High	Reduced (1)[a]
Morphology	Fibroblastic-like	Flat (5–7)[a]
Fibronectin expression	High	High
Cytoskeleton		
Microtubules	Organized	Organized
Microfilaments	Poorly organized	Organized
Tumorigenic phenotype	Expressed	Not expressed (>10)[a]

[a]Number of *in vitro* passages with interferon at which the observed effect was fully expressed.

terferon is not immediate but progressive.

2) The reversion is reversible. Thus, although the revertant phenotype was expressed as long as the transformed cells were maintained in the presence of interferon, the transformed phenotype did reappear when interferon was removed from the cultures and the cells then passaged in the absence of interferon [the proliferation increased, the morphology became "transformed," and tumorigenicity was reexpressed much later].

Until now, therapy of cancer has been directed to the search of agents able to kill and eliminate tumor cells. Although the reversion of tumor cells to the normal state has been mostly described in *in vitro* models, it is conceivable that a similar process can be induced *in vivo*. It is worthwhile, then, to look for substances (i.e., interferon) capable of inducing the reversion of the neoplastic state.

REFERENCES

1. Brouty-Boyé, D., and Gresser, I.: *Int J Cancer 28:* 165, 1981.
2. Brouty-Boyé, D., Cheng, Y.E., and Chen, L.B.: *Cancer Res 41: 4174, 1981.*

CHAPTER 30

LHRH Superactive Agonistic Analogs for Prostate Cancer: An Alternative to Orchidectomy and Estrogen Therapy

G. Tolis and M. Koutsilieris

Introduction

Prostatic and colorectal cancer rate second after lung cancer as causes of death in the male. The age-adjusted death rate from prostatic cancer per 100,000 population for U.S.A. and Europe (1976–1977) has been estimated to be between 22.3–32.3 per 100,000 inhabitants. Cancer deaths for all sites account for 213.6 per 100,000.[3] Presently, the annual mortality rate for prostatic cancer is 20,000 for the U.S.A. and the annual morbidity rate is 60,000.

The high mortality rate may be secondary to the fact that prostatic cancer is diagnosed in the advanced stages C and D. In these stages, radiotherapy, chemotherapy, castration, and/or estrogens are the usual therapeutic modalities. The use of estrogens is probably the single most responsible factor for augmenting morbidity or mortality in patients with prostate cancer. Estrogen side effects include: 1) Cardiovascular, 2) Vasculogenic–hemostatic, 3) gastrointestinal, 4) hematologic — edema, sodium retention, thrombophlebitis, and vascular insults to the myocardium are dangerous and not infrequent complications. Finally, painful gyne-

comastia is bothersome to two-thirds of all patients receiving high-dose estrogens.

It should be pointed out however that a large segment (60–70%) of patients with such bone pains secondary to metastatic disease experience great reduction of cancer growth when castration or large doses of estrogens are administered. These early observations were the milestones for developing the concept of hormone-sensitive prostate cancer. Yet, there are at least two main questions to be answered. If we consider castration to be a successful treatment modality for 60–70% of patients, then the remaining 30–40% will undergo an unnecessarily mutilating experience which undoubtedly carries a psychological burden. On the other hand, if there are many side effects of estrogen, usually intolerable to the patient with previous cardiovascular disease, and if many patients show no improvement despite this treatment, the high morbidity and mortality[6] from the treatment may be unjustified.

If we accept that estrogens, like castration, arrest prostatic cancer growth mainly by their ability to induce chemical castration, then the development of a substance which could selectively suppress Leydig cell function without affecting other endocrine glands or other organs,

McGill University, Royal Victoria Hospital, Montreal, Quebec, Canada

should be welcomed. Such a substance, at present, seems to be the agonist analog of the gonadotropin-releasing hormone (LHRH-A).

LHRH is a decapeptide synthesized primarily in the mammalian hypothalamus. It is released in a pulsatile fashion and is responsible for maintaining the synthesis and release of follicle-stimulating hormone (FSH), and luteinizing hormone (LH) from the pituitary in a well-programmed fashion. This allows the normal function of the target endocrine glands, the ovaries or testes. If LHRH is administered in large doses continuously, then a regulation process begins which leads to cessation of the response of the pituitary and subsequently of the target glands. A similar phenomenon occurs with the use of LHRH-agonistic analogs. These differ from the native decapeptide in that they usually have a D aminoacid residue in position 6, *i.e.*, tryptophan, leucine, or serine. They may or may not have the glycine of position 10 removed and an ethylamide chain annexed. These analogs are much more potent than the native decapeptide in stimulating FSH and LH release. Daily administration of such agonistic analogs, even for a short time, *i.e.*, 1 week, will render the pituitary unresponsive to further stimulation and will lead to a significant decrease of sex steroid plasma levels.[11]

Materials and Methods

We have used two superactive long-acting LHRH-analogs so far — the decapeptide D-tryptophan 6 (pyro-Glu-HIS - TRP - SER - TYR - D - TRP - LEU - ARG - PRO-GLY-NH$_2$, D-tryp-6) and the nonapeptide D-serine (Bu^t)/HOE-766 (pyro-GLU-HIS-TRP-SER-TYR-D, SER (Bu^t)-LEU-ARG-PRO-ethylamide). Extensive investigations have shown these materials to be devoid of adverse effects; both of them result in reversible inhibition of reproductive function.[1,4,8,10,11]

The D-tryp-6 analog was provided by Dr. A.V. Schally and HOE-766 from the Medical Department, Hoechst Canada, Montreal; the latter was provided in both injectable and intranasal forms.

The dosage schedule for D-tryp-6 was 50–100 μg daily subcutaneously. The HOE-766 is now given at 500 μg three times daily subcutaneously for 6 days and 400 μg three times daily intranasally thereafter, without interruption. All patients treated underwent a thorough, complete clinical and laboratory examination.

The size of the prostate was evaluated with transabdominal ultrasonography at bimonthly intervals. The kidney function and the residual urinary volume were evaluated with isotopic renal scanning, pelvic ultrasonography, and intravenous pyelography when indicated; the bone metastases were assessed by bone scanning and bone radiography every 3 months. Urinalysis, hemogram, electrolytes, liver enzymes, 5' nucleotidase, alkaline phosphatase, and prostatic acid phosphatase by RIA were done at monthly intervals. Plasma testosterone was determined every 2 weeks for 2 months and monthly thereafter. Cortisol, thyroxine, FSH, LH, and prolactin levels were determined every 3 months.

Results

Fifteen evaluable patients with advanced metastatic disease were treated with LHRH superagonistic analogs for up to 18 months. In all patients, plasma testosterone and estradiol levels fell and they remained at castrate levels in 11 patients treated for more than 2 months. Plasma testosterone (T) and estradiol (E$_2$) levels in ng/dl prior to treatment were T:612.1 (360–1000) E$_2$:2.7 (1.5–4.1); during treatment the corresponding values were T:33.4 (15–45) E$_2$:0.64 (0.3–1.1) (means and ranges, respectively). Note that normal range for T is 300–1200 ng/dl and for

E_2 1–4ng/dl. In no patient was any escape phenomenon seen during pretreatment. This includes the patient in Figure 1 who was treated for 22 months continuously.

If, despite the fall of plasma testosterone to castrate levels, there was no improvement in bone pain or lowering of acid and alkaline phosphatases, the patient was felt to bear a hormone-insensitive cancer and was referred without delay (within 3 months) for radiotherapy and/or chemotherapy. A typical profile of a patient bearing a hormone-sensitive tumor is given in Figures 1–3. In this patient, following the decrease of plasma testosterone, a gradual lowering of prostatic acid phosphatase and alkaline phosphatase were seen. These biochemical changes were associated with an improvement in performance status, decrease of bone pain, and amelioration of the bone scan.[9] In patients with stage C cancer, a decrease in prostatic size was documented ultrasonographically.[7,9] Practically all patients complained of a decreased libido, and some developed "hot flushes".

Discussion

The present results document and extend previous observations.[2,5,7,9,11,12] Chronic administration of LHRH-agonistic analogues leads to medical castration within a few weeks from initiation of treatment. The paucity of side effects from this new therapeutic modality makes these agents superior to estrogens. Furthermore, the observed drop in circulating estrogens suggests that tumor growth inhibition can be achieved in the absence of elevated estrogens. The ability of estrogens to act upon the tumor independently of their androgen lowering capacity thus becomes questionable. The inability of LHRH-A to improve patients who do not respond to castration or estrogens[5] indicates that LHRH-A should not be given to patients whose pituitary–testicular axis is not intact. On the other hand, our data strongly indicate that the chronic administration of LHRH analogues can replace orchidectomy and estrogens as means for castration. Finally, for the future, we be-

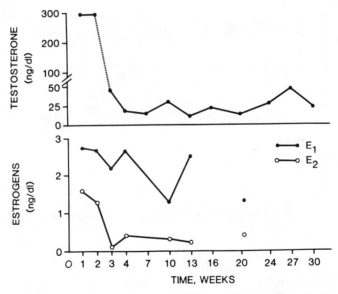

FIGURE 1. Effect of daily administration of D-SER(TBU)[6]LHRH on hormonal and biochemical variables in a patient with Stage D prostatic carcinoma. Administration of LHRH-A led to a fall of plasma testosterone to the castrate range within three weeks. Note the decline also of plasma estrone (E_1) and estradiol (E_2).

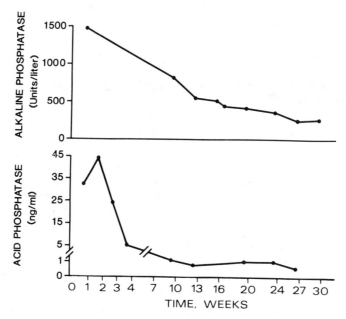

FIGURE 2.   Effect of daily administration of D-SER(TBU)⁶LHRH on hormonal and biochemical variables in a patient with Stage D prostatic carcinoma. Note the lowering of alkaline phosphatase and the normalization of the acid phosphatase in the patient in Figure 1.

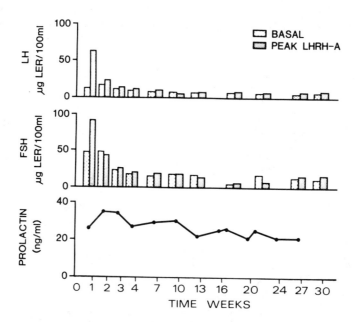

FIGURE 3.   Effect of daily administration of D-SER(TBU)⁶LHRH on hormonal and biochemical variables in a patient with Stage D prostatic carcinoma. Chronic administration of LHRH-A resulted in a gradual lowering of basal FSH and LH and in a rapid (within 2 weeks) decrease of the pituitary gonadotropin response to LHRH-A; serum PRL levels remained practically unchanged during the chronic administration of LHRH-A.

lieve that determinations of the sex steroid receptor content in prostatic tumors and assessment of the clinical response to LHRH-A will represent the sine qua non dual strategy to predict hormone sensitivity in prostatic tumors, and thus to avoid unnecessary treatment modalities.

REFERENCES

1. Bergquist, C., Nillius, S.L., Bergh, T., Skarin, G., and Wide, L.: *Acta Endocr (Copenhagen) 91: 601, 1979.*

2. Borgmann, V., Hardt, W., Schmidt-Gollwitzer, M., Adenauer, H., and Nagel, R.: *Lancet 1: 1097, 1982.*

3. *Cancer Around the World, 1976–1977.* World Health Statistics Annual 1979–1980.

4. Coy, D.H., Vilchez-Martinez, J.A., Coy, E.J., and Schally, A.V.: *J Med Chem 119: 423, 1976.*

5. Glode, L.M.: Eighteenth Meeting of the American Society of Clinical Oncology, St. Louis, Missouri, April 25–27, 1982.

6. Hedlund, P.O., Gustafson, H., and Sjogren, S.: *Scand J Urol Nephrol (Suppl) 55: 103, 1980.*

7. Patton, R., and Tolis, G.: Program Canadian Society of Clinical Investigation Quebec, September 14, 1982.

8. Sandow, J., Von Rechenberg, W., Jerzabek, G., and Stoll, W.: *Fertil Steril 30: 205, 1978.*

9. Tolis, G., Ackman, D., Stellos, A., Mehta, A., Labrie, F., Fazekas, A.T.A., Comaru-Schally, A.M., and Schally, A.V.: *Proc Natl Acad Sci USA 79: 1658, 1982.*

10. Tolis, G., Chapdelaine, A., Roberts, K., Papandreou, N., Papacharalambous, M., Golematis, V., and Friedman, N.: In *Endocrinological Cancer,* H. Adelcruetz, E.D. Bulbrook, H. J. van der Molen, A. Vermeulen, and F. Sciarra, Eds. Excerpta Medica Series, 1981, p. 79.

11. Tolis, G., Mehta, A., and Chapdelaine, A.: In *Frontiers of Hormone Research,* K. Ruf and G. Tolis, Eds., Karger Verlag, 1982, p. 43.

12. Tolis, G., Mehta, A., Comaru-Schally, A.M., and Schally, A.V.: *J Clin Invest 68: 819, 1981.*

CHAPTER 31

Progesterone Receptor as an Indicator of the Tumor Response to an Antiestrogen
I: Postmenopausal Endometrial Carcinoma
II: Metastatic Breast Cancer

P. Robel,[a] R. Mortel,[b] M. Namer,[c] and E.E. Baulieu[a]

Introduction

Target tissues contain specific intracellular receptors for steroid hormones, and receptor concentrations in tumors might be possible indicators of hormone responsiveness.[16,27] Some attempts were made to demonstrate directly the effects of hormones on tumors, using incubations or cultures of tumor explants in presence of steroid hormones.[39,46] This *in vitro* approach suffers from serious limitations and therefore we have tried to set up an *in vivo* biochemical approach to relate receptors and hormonal response in endometrial and breast cancers.

Several compounds of the triphenylethylene series exhibit both estrogenic and antiestrogenic properties. This is the case of tamoxifen which, in the rodent uterus, has been shown to increase progesterone receptor concentration, while it counteracts estrogen-induced uterine growth.[17] Since the hormonal control of progesterone receptor in human endometrium[1] seems to follow the same principles as in

animal models,[28] we decided to give tamoxifen to postmenopausal patients with endometrial carcinoma.[30,40] Moreover, tamoxifen has been widely used for the treatment of breast cancer patients with good results, and we consequently found it appropriate to test this drug in metastatic breast cancers.[32] In endometrial and breast cancer patients, two tumor samples could be obtained under acceptable ethical conditions, the first one before, and the second one after, administration of tamoxifen. It was anticipated that the exposure of tumor cells to the drug would be indicated by the decrease of available cytoplasmic sites and the increase of nuclear receptor. The tumor response to tamoxifen, on the other hand, would be demonstrated by increase of progesterone receptor.

Material and Methods

RECEPTOR MEASUREMENTS

Estradiol and progesterone receptors were measured in fresh biopsy samples of *endometrial cancers* collected in ice-cold medium and processed less than 1 hour after removal. The technique utilized allowed measurements of total (filled and unfilled) estradiol and progesterone recep-

[a]ER 125 CNRS and U 33 INSERM, Department of Biochemistry, University Paris-Sud, Laboratory Hormones, Bicêtre, France
[b]Present address: Milton S. Hershey Medical Center, Hershey Pennsylvania
[c]Centre A. Lacassagne, Nice, France

tor sites in the cytosol and nuclei as reported in detail by Bayard et al.[1] The measurement of nuclear receptor sites has been improved recently by the use of a glass-fiber filter exchange technique.[24]

Aliquots of the homogenate and nuclear suspensions were measured for DNA using the technique of Burton.[3] All results were expressed in pmol of hormonal binding sites per mg of DNA. Assay sensitivity was such that any value <0.09 pmol of nuclear receptors and <0.11 pmol of cytosol receptors per mg of DNA was considered zero and reported as such in the tables.

In *skin metastases of breast cancers,* estradiol and progesterone receptors, readily labeled by radioactive ligands at $0-4°C$, were measured only in cytosol fractions, otherwise using a procedure similar to the one of Bayard et al.[1] Results were expressed in fmol/mg cytosol protein. Assay sensitivity was such that any value <5 fmol/mg cytosol protein was considered zero and reported as such in the tables. In several cases, measurements were made on biopsies from adjacent nodules, and receptor concentrations were not significantly different.

ORNITHINE–DECARBOXYLASE

Ornithine–decarboxylase (ODC) activity was assayed in endometrium samples according to Kaye et al.[20] with minor modifications. The results were expressed in pmol of CO_2 produced per hour per mg of DNA.

RADIOIMMUNOASSAY OF SERUM HORMONES

Serum samples were extracted with ethyl acetate, defatted, and chromatographed on small celite columns (1 g) soaked with formamide (1:2 v/w) and prepared in hexane. Progesterone, estrone, and estradiol were recovered in hexane: benzene (85/15), hexane: ethyl acetate (90/10), hexane: ethyl acetate (80/20), respectively. The appropriate fractions were then processed for radioimmunoassay. Antiestrone, antiestradiol, and antiprogesterone antibodies were provided by Roussel-Uclaf. All results were expressed in pg/ml of serum.

CALCULATIONS

Means are presented with a standard error of the mean as the index of dispersion. The nonparametric rank correlation coefficient of Spearman was used to compare data.

Part I: Endometrial Carcinoma

Endometrial carcinoma occurs most frequently in postmenopausal women, and epidemiological studies have shown an increased risk in women exposed to prolonged unopposed estrogenic stimulation.[12,38,43] It is equally well accepted that progestational agents achieve objective remission in 30–35% of patients with advanced or metastatic endometrial cancer.[21,37,43] Numerous investigators have reported the presence of estradiol and/or progesterone receptors in human endometrial carcinoma and quantitative estimates have been published.[4,7,13,35,45,47] However, based on clinical criteria or receptor assays, it is not possible to select those patients likely to benefit from hormonal therapy.

PATIENTS

Forty-three patients with histologically proven adenocarcinoma of the endometrium were seen in consultation and treated at the Institut Gustave Roussy, Villejuif, France. Their age ranged from 43 to 75 years with a mean of 62. All patients menopaused spontaneously for at least three years; only three had a known history of exogenous hormone ingestion after menopause. Two partial outpatient uterine curettages were performed on 25 patients, the first at the time of referral, the second during surgery or immediately before radiotherapy. The degree of tumor differentiation was recorded: Grade 1 — well differentiated, Grade 2 — moderately differentiated, and Grade 3 — anaplastic tumors. After the first biopsy, 15 patients took 40 mg of tamoxifen orally daily for 5–7 days (Group 1) and the second endometrial sampling was performed 12–18 hours after the last dose. Ten patients ingested 10 mg, 8 and 4 hours prior to the second biopsy (Group 2). The interval between the 2 samplings in this last group varied from 1 to 6 days. Receptor concentrations were determined in all biopsy samples and, in addition, the activity of ODC and serum hormones were evaluated before and after tamoxifen treatment.

Results of Part I

ESTRADIOL AND PROGESTERONE

Receptor amounts were undetectable or insignificant (<0.3 pmol/mg DNA) in three tumors examined for estradiol and

10 tumors assayed for progesterone (Fig. 1). Although the difference was not statistically significant among the groups, there was a clear tendency for the more differentiated grade 1 tumors to contain higher levels of estradiol and progesterone receptors than the grade 2 carcinomas. The small number of grade 3 cases allowed no comparison.

HORMONAL CORRELATIONS OF RECEPTORS

The values for serum estradiol remained lower than those for estrone (Table 1). Estradiol values did not change with the degree of tumor differentiation. The observed mean estrone values were lower than the plasma levels reported by Korenman et al.[22] and Benjamin and Deutsch,[2] but they correlated well with those published by Judd et al.[18] A highly significant difference ($p < 0.01$) was observed in the mean estrone levels of

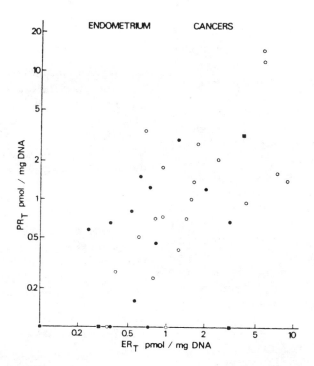

FIGURE 1. Total estradiol (ER_T) and progesterone receptors (PR_T) in endometrium cancers (●, Grade 1 tumors; ○, Grade 2 tumors; ■, Grade 3 tumors).

patients from well- to moderately-differentiated cancers. it may be related to a difference in body weight (63.6 ± 13.6 in grade 1 versus 76.6 ± 16.0 kg in grade 2 patients). Serum progesterone levels were low as in normal postmenopausal women, and the mean progesterone values were identical in the three histologic grading groups.

We found no significant correlation between estradiol or progesterone receptor and serum levels of estrone, estradiol, or progesterone, even within the histologically defined groups, with the exception of well-differentiated tumors, in which a positive correlation at the limit of statistical significance ($0.05 < p < 0.10$) was observed between serum estradiol and progesterone receptor concentration.

EFFECTS OF TAMOXIFEN ON RECEPTORS

Following tamoxifen administration, no statistically significant increase in estrogen receptor concentration was demonstrable in either group of patients. However, in group 2, where tamoxifen administration immediately preceded biopsy, the ratio of cytoplasmic to nuclear receptors shifted in favor of nuclear receptors as previously observed in animal model experiments.[44] In group 1, progesterone receptor sites increased more than two-fold in all but four samples (Fig. 2), and the difference was statistically significant at $p < 0.05$. Interestingly, a substantial elevation in progesterone receptor concentration was noted in two tumors in which the receptor had not been measurable or had not been present at very low concentration in the samples assayed before tamoxifen treatment. In group 2 patients, no increase of progesterone receptor was generally observed.

EFFECTS OF TAMOXIFEN ON ORNITHINE DECARBOXYLASE

Activity of ODC was measured along with receptor concentration in 13 tumors

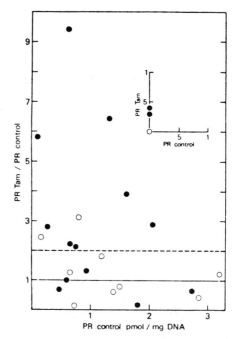

FIGURE 2. Total progesterone receptors (PR) in endometrial cancers before and after tamoxifen (Tam). The concentration of PR in control sample is given on abscissa, and the ratio of tamoxifen treated over control samples on ordinate (●, Group 1 patients; ○, Group 2 patients). *Insert:* responses of three PR negative cases.

and was determined before and after tamoxifen in nine other tumors where receptors could not be measured due to limited sample size. The administration of tamoxifen in these additional patients was similar to that of group 2 patients. The mean value (± sem) was 8.1 ± 2.8 nmol CO_2/hour/mg DNA, about 10 times larger than in proliferative endometrium (1.3 ± 0.3, $n = 4$). No statistical difference was observed in enzyme activity before and after tamoxifen treatment in either group. We also found no correlation between tumor grading and ODC activity before or after tamoxifen treatment.

EFFECTS OF TAMOXIFEN ON SERUM ESTROGENS AND PROGESTERONE

The serum levels of estrone, estradiol, and progesterone showed no significant changes in the values at the schedules and doses of tamoxifen used in this study.

Discussion of Part I

ESTRADIOL AND PROGESTERONE RECEPTORS

Widespread variations in the concentration of estradiol receptors were measured in 36/37 tumors examined. The mean values observed in this study support the findings of Tseng and Gurpide[45] that, in postmenopausal endometrial carcinoma, the level of estradiol receptors is similar to that in the endometrium of normal women in the proliferative phase of the cycle. Crocker et al.[4] and Pollow et al.[35] found estradiol receptors in all endometrial cancer samples, but Grilli et al.[10] and Muechler et al.[31] reported estrogen receptor in 67–92% of the specimen assayed. Therefore, it appears that estradiol receptors are present in a large majority of endometrial adenocarcinomas.

Of 38 tumors assayed for progesterone receptors, 10 contained undetectable or insignificant amounts of receptors (<0.3 pmol/mg DNA). In six cases, the concentration was comparable to that of the proliferative phase; in the majority of samples, as reported by Pollow et al.,[36] the range and mean values were similar to those observed in late secretory endometrium. Consequently, the estrogen/progesterone receptor ratio in these postmenopausal adenocarcinomas was generally greater than in normal premenopausal endometrium.

When present, most estradiol and progesterone receptors were found in the cytosol. This was not surprising considering the low levels of circulating estrogen and progesterone in these women. However, five more tumors would have been classified as "estradiol receptor-negative" and two more as "progesterone receptor-negative" on the basis of cytoplasmic receptor measurements alone. Our findings are in keeping with the recent observations suggesting that unoccupied estrogen receptor sites are present in the nuclei of normal endometrium[9,25] as well as in malignant breast tissue and established breast cancer cell lines.[33,48]

The relationship between receptor levels and the degree of tumor differentiation has been the subject of conflicting reports.[7,8,13,35,45,47] Nevertheless, as reported by other investigators,[13,35,48] our study showed a clear tendency for well-differentiated tumors to contain higher levels of both estrogen and progesterone receptors. Our findings disagree with those of Pollow et al.[36] who reported a progressive increase of estradiol receptor concentration from well- to poorly-differentiated tumors.

HORMONAL CORRELATIONS OF TUMOR DIFFERENTIATION

Siiteri et al.[42] has suggested the possibility that estrone plays an important role in the development of postmenopausal endometrial carcinoma. In this respect, we have observed that the concentration of serum estrone was significantly higher in patients with less differentiated cancers than in those with well-differentiated tumors. This difference may well be related to a difference in body weight among the two groups of patients. However, it remains to be explained how the level of serum estrone is related to the degree of tumor differentiation.

EFFECTS OF TAMOXIFEN

The level of receptors at which a tumor will respond to hormone or antihormone treatment is still unknown. Thus, a test that allows us to evaluate directly the response to a hormonal challenge is desirable. Gurpide and Tseng[11] and Pollow et al.[34] proposed a method based on the measurement of 17 β-hydroxysteroid dehydrogenase (E_2DH) before and following medroxyprogesterone acetate administration to patients with endometrial carcinoma. They reported up to four-fold increase in enzyme activity and a reduction of estrogen receptor levels in those tumors responsive to progestins. These findings suggest that measurement of E_2DH before and after progestin along with determination of sex steroid receptor concentrations may provide a reliable means to select those tumors that are likely to respond to progestogen therapy.

The role played by estrogens in the etiology of endometrial cancer and the high estradiol receptor to progesterone receptor ratio found in carcinoma samples prompted us to investigate the biochemical changes following antiestrogen administration as a test of *in vivo* tumor sensitivity. Contrary to the test with medroxy-progesterone acetate which acts via the progesterone receptor, tamoxifen is active via the estrogen receptor of the tumor, whereas progesterone receptor is assayed as a biochemical marker of the estrogenic response. We have confirmed our preliminary results[40] and now have evidence that in human endometrial carcinoma, tamoxifen given at a dose of 40 mg daily for 5–7 days induces or increases progesterone receptor concentration in most tumors (11/15).[30]

Following a single dose of estradiol to immature rats, ODC activity starts to rise in the uterus by 2 hours, but after prolonged treatment, it returns to basal

values.[20] Accordingly, we observed no changes in ODC activity in our Group 2 patients and postulated that a rapid or transitory increase may have been missed. We then administered 10 mg of tamoxifen 8 and 4 hours prior to the second biopsy and again no increase in ODC activity was observed. These results are in keeping with observations that in the rat uterus and cultured mouse L cells, tamoxifen cannot induce cell division.[17,19]

Part II: Breast Cancer

Sixty to seventy percent of postmenopausal breast cancers are estradiol receptor (ER) "positive." Of those, about 50% respond to hormonal manipulation whether it be ablative surgery or administration of androgen, estrogen, progestagen, and, more recently, antiestrogen.[5]

Approximately 50% of postmenopausal cancers have measurable concentration of progesterone receptor (PR), and of these, >90% belong to the ER positive group. There are no experimental data demonstrating the hormonal regulation of progesterone receptor concentration in breast tissue *in vivo*. Therefore, it was interesting to check whether the increase observed after tamoxifen in endometrial cancer would also be seen in mammary tumors.

TABLE 1.   Serum Levels of Estrone, Estradiol, and Progesterone in Patients with Postmenopausal Endometrial Carcinoma[a]

Endometrial Carcinoma	Estrone	Estradiol	Progesterone
Whole series	(43)[b]	(42)	(42)
	33.8	23.6	435.6
	± 2.5	± 1.5	± 48.6
Grade 1	(24)	(23)	(23)
	29.3	22.0	439.9
	± 2.9	± 1.6	± 55.9
Grade 2	(15)	(15)	(15)
	43.0[c]	25.6	451.0
	± 4.0	± 2.9	± 102.0
Grade 3	(4)	(4)	(4)
	57.2	27.2	361.0
	+ 15.3	± 7.7	± 10.3

[a]pg/ml serum, mean ± sem.
[b]Number of cases.
[c]$p < 0.01$ (nonparametric rank correlation coefficient of Spearman between Grade 1 and Grade 2 groups).

PATIENTS

Twenty-one postmenopausal women with advanced metastatic breast cancer were investigated at the Centre Lacassagne, Nice, France. None of them had received any adjuvant therapy. Biopsies were performed on adjacent hypodermic nodules. After the first biopsy, patients received 30 mg of tamoxifen for 7 days until the second sample was obtained.

Results of Part II

ESTRADIOL AND PROGESTERONE RECEPTORS

Estradiol receptor was absent or low (<20 fmol/mg protein) in nine cases. All but one ER negative cases were also PR negative. Among the 12 remaining ER positive cases, only two were PR negative (Table 2). A significant positive correlation was observed between the concentrations of PR and ER in untreated tumors.

EFFECT OF TAMOXIFEN

Whenever present, available ER sites were greatly decreased after tamoxifen. This decrease probably resulted from tamoxifen binding to estrogen receptor and transfer of the receptor complexes into the nucleus. No PR receptor change was recorded in cases where ER was <20 fmol/mg cytosol protein. Seven of the twelve remaining cases showed an increase of PR of more than 100 fmol/mg cytosol protein.

General Discussion and Conclusions: Response to Hormones and Prospects of Hormone Therapy

When measurements are made on a small specimen of a malignant tumor, it is assumed that the results are representative of the whole tumor. It is quite likely that several samples of the same tumor may differ in terms of differentiation, relative amounts of epithelial and stromal elements, proportion of malignant cells, inflammatory or necrotic changes, and so forth. We were, however, reassured by the fact that receptor measurements performed on adjacent skin metastases of breast cancer gave closely similar results. Also, the constancy of ODC activities and ER concentrations in endometrial cancer before and after tamoxifen is worth mentioning. The possibility that the response of progesterone receptor to tamoxifen might reflect the response of normal cells interspersed in the biopsy samples is a critical point. However, careful histologic evaluation could be performed on most biopsies, and has generally shown that

TABLE 2. Estradiol and Progesterone Receptors in Breast Cancer Metastases[a]

Id[b]	Age (y)	Before Tamoxifen		After Tamoxifen	
		ER	PR	ER	PR
1	71	0[c]	0	0	0
2	85	0	0	6	0
3	60	0	0	0	0
4	54	0	30	n[d]	0
5	58	0	0	0	0
6	72	7	0	0	0
7	59	11	0	n	0
8	71	13	0	0	11
9	72	20	7	0	13
10	72	25	20	n	50
11	63	53	92	12	1120
12	70	80	110	17	980
13	80	85	60	7	50
14	69	92	34	11	605
15	77	120	105	0	0
16	57	120	1030	12	1600
17	65	185	190	25	440
18	57	225	0	8	0
19	70	350	65	9	205
20	67	430	n	11	30
21	75	n	0	25	770

[a]fmol/mg cytosol protein.
[b]Id = identification number.
[c]Values < 5 fmol/mg cytosol protein were considered as not different from zero.
[d]n = not determined for technical reasons.

most, if not all, of the cells were indeed malignant. It should also be recalled that sensitivity of breast cancer cells to hormones has been directly demonstrated in cultures of established cell lines.[14,26]

In addition, complex hormonal changes may be elicited at the pituitary, adrenal, or ovarian level, following administration of an antiestrogen. However, such changes are likely not very prominent in postmenopausal women, and no change of plasma sex steroids has been recorded.

In metastatic breast cancer, our results confirm the predictive value of estradiol receptor. Estradiol receptor negative cases were also generally progesterone receptor negative, and they did not respond to tamoxifen. The same was true for cases with ER < 20 fmol/mg cytosol protein, and the tamoxifen test might prove useful to determine objectively the set-point of "receptor negative" cases. About one half of estradiol receptor positive cases respond to tamoxifen by an increase (or induction) of progesterone receptor. An improved predictive value has been shown for the combined measurement of both estradiol and progesterone receptors, compared to estradiol receptor alone.[5,6] Further improvement might result from the tamoxifen test, although the limited number of cases investigated precludes definitive conclusions. It should be performed systematically when available metastases are present. In the future, the development of microassays, which will be performed on needle biopsies of primary tumors, might lead to an extended use of *in vivo* hormonal challenge.

ACKNOWLEDGMENTS

The authors thank B. Eychenne and M. Synguelakis for their expert technical assistance, and D. Drouet for statistical evaluation. This work was supported by contract no. 76.5.478.A. INSERM.

REFERENCES

1. Bayard, F., Damilano, S., Robel, P., and Baulieu, E.E.: *J Clin Endocrinol Metab* 46: 635–648, 1978.
2. Benjamin, F., and Deutsch, S.: *Am J Obstet Gynecol* 126: 638–647, 1976.
3. Burton, K.: In *Methods of Enzymology*, Vol. 12B, L. Grossman and K. Moldave, Eds., Academic Press, New York, 1968, pp. 163–166.
4. Crocker, S.G., Milton, P.J.D., and King, R.J.B.: *J Endocrinol* 62: 145–152, 1974.
5. De Sombre, E.R., Carbone, P.P., Jensen, E.V., McGuire, W.L., Wells, S.A., Wittliff, J.A., and Lipsett, M.B.: *N Engl J Med* 301: 1011–1012, 1979.
6. Edwards, D.P., Chamness, G.C., and McGuire, W.L.: *Biochim Biophys Acta* 560: 457–486, 1979.
7. Evans, L.H., Martin, J.D., and Hähnel, R.: *J Clin Endocrinol Metab* 38: 23–32, 1974.
8. Feil, P.D., Mann, W.J., Mortel, R., and Bardin, C.W. *J Clin Endocrinol Metab* 48: 327–374, 1979.
9. Fleming, H., and Gurpide, E.: *J Steroid Biochem* 13: 3–11, 1980.
10. Grilli, S., Ferrari, A.M., Gola, G., Rochetta, R., Orlandi, C., and Prodi, G.: *Cancer Letters* 2: 247–258, 1977.
11. Gurpide, E., and Tseng, L.: In *Endometrial Cancer*, M.G. Brush, R.J.B. King, and R.W. Taylor, Eds., Bailliere Tindall, London, 1978, pp. 252–257.
12. Gusberg, S.B.: *Am J Obstet Gynecol* 126: 535.
13. Gustafsson, J.A., Einhorn, N., Elfstrom, G., Nordenskjold, B., and Wrange, O.: In *Progesterone Receptors in Normal and Neoplastic Tissues*, W.L. McGuire, J.P. Raynaud, and E.E. Baulieu, Eds., Raven Press, New York, 1977, pp. 299–312.
14. Horwitz, K.B., and McGuire, W.L.: *J Biol Chem* 253: 8185–8191, 1978.
15. Jänne, O., Kauppila, A., Kontula, K., Syrjälä, P., Vierikko, P., and Vihko, R.: In *Steroid Receptors and Hormone Dependent Neoplasia*, J.L. Wittliff and I. Dapunt, Eds., Masson Publishing, USA, Inc., New York, 1980, pp. 37–44.
16. Jensen, E.V., De Sombre, E.R., and Jungblut, P.W.: In *Endogenous Factors Influencing Host–Tumor Balance*, R.W. Wissler, T.L. Dao, and S. Wood, Eds., University of Chicago Press, Chicago, 1967, pp. 15–30.
17. Jordan, V.C. and Dix, C.J.: *J Steroid Biochem* 11: 285–291, 1979.
18. Judd, H.L., Lucas, W.E., and Yen, S.S.C.: *J Clin Endocrinol Metab* 43: 272–278, 1976.
19. Jung-Testas, I. and Baulieu, E.E.: *Exp Cell Res* 119: 25–85, 1979.
20. Kaye, A.M., Icekson, I., and Lindner, H.R.: *Biochem Biophys Acta* 252: 150–159, 1971.
21. Kohorn, E.I.: *Gynecol Oncol* 4: 398–411, 1976.
22. Korenman, S.G., Perrin, L.E., and McCallum, T.P.: *J Clin Endocrinol Metab* 29: 879–883, 1969.
23. Lerner, H., Band, P.R., Israel, L., and Leung, B.S.: *Cancer Treat Rep* 60: 1431–1435, 1976.
24. Levy, C., Eychenne, B., and Robel, P.: *Biochim Biophys Acta* 630: 301–305, 1980.
25. Levy, C., Mortel, R., Eychenne, B., Robel, P., and Baulieu, E.E.: *Biochem J* 185: 733–738, 1980.
26. Lippman, M., Bolan, G., and Huff, K.: *Cancer Res* 35: 4595–4601, 1976.
27. McGuire, W.L., Raynaud, J.P., and Baulieu, E.E., Eds.: *Progesterone Receptors in Normal and Neoplastic Tissues*. Raven Press, New York, 1977.
28. Milgrom, E., Thi, L., Atger, M., and Baulieu, E.E.: *J Biol Chem* 248: 6366–6374, 1973.
29. Morgan, L.R., Schein, P.S., Woolley, P.V., Hoth, D., McDonald, J., Lippman, M., Posey, L.E., and Beasley, R.W.: *Cancer Treat Rep* 60: 1437–1443, 1976.
30. Mortel, R., Levy, C., Wolff, J.P., Nicolas, J.C., Robel, P., and Baulieu, E.E.: *Cancer Res* 41: 1140–1147, 1981.
31. Muechler, E.K., Flinckinger, G.L., Mangan, C.E., and Mikhail, G. *Gynecol Oncol* 3: 244–250, 1975.
32. Namer, M., Lalanne, C., and Baulieu, E.E.: *Cancer Res* 40: 1750–1752, 1980.
33. Panko, W.B., and McLeod, R.M.: *Cancer Res* 38: 1948–1951, 1978.
34. Pollow, K., Boquoi, E., Lubbert, H., and Pollow, B.: *J Endocrinol* 67: 131–132, 1975.
35. Pollow, K., Lubbert, H., Boquoi, E., Kreuzer, G., and Pollow, B.: *Endocrinology* 96: 319–328, 1975.
36. Pollow, K., Schmidt-Gollwitzer, M., and Nevinny-Stickel, J.: In *Progesterone Receptors in Normal and Neoplastic Tissues*, W.L. McGuire, J.P.

Raynaud, and E.E. Baulieu, Eds., Raven Press, New York, 1977, pp. 313–338.

37. Reifenstein, E.C.: *Gynecol Oncol 2: 277–414, 1974.*

38. Richardson, G.S., and McLaughlin, D.H.: In *Hormonal Biology of Endometrial Cancer,* Vol. 42, UICC Technical Report Series, 1978, pp. 13–14.

39. Saez, S., Martin, P.M., and Chouvet, C.D.: *Cancer Res 38: 3468–3473, 1978.*

40. Robel, P., Levy, C., Wolff, J.P., Nicolas, J.C., and Baulieu, E.E.: *CR Acad Sci Paris 287: 1353–1356, 1978.*

41. Sherman, A.I.: *Obstet Gynecol 28: 309–314, 1966.*

42. Siiteri, P.K., Schwarz, B., and McDonald, P.C.: *Gynecol Oncol 2: 228–238, 1974.*

43. Smith, D.C., Prentice, R., Thomson, D.J., and Hermann, W.L. (1975): *N Engl J Med 293: 1164–1187, 1975.*

44. Sutherland, R., Mester, J., and Baulieu, E.E.: In *Hormones and Cell Regulation,* J. Dumont and J. Nunez, North Holland Publishing Company, Amsterdam, 1977, pp. 31–48.

45. Tseng, L., and Gurpide, E.: *Am J Obstet Gynecol 114: 995–1001, 1972.*

46. Tseng, L., Gusberg, S., and Gurpide, E.: *Ann NY Acad Sci 286: 190–198, 1977.*

47. Young, P.C.M., Ehrlich, E., and Cleary, R.E.: *Am J Obstet Gynecol 125: 353–360, 1976.*

48. Zava, D.T., Chamness, G.C., Horwitz, K.B., and McGuire, W.L.: *Science 196: 663–669, 1977.*

CHAPTER 32

T-Cell Depletion to Prevent Acute Graft-vs.-Host Disease (GVHD) in Allogeneic Bone Marrow Transplantation

H. Ozer, M. O'Leary, T. Han, H. Preisler, D. Thompson, B. Dadey, N. Cohen, M. Marinello, and D.J. Higby

Introduction

GVHD continues to be one of the most serious complications of bone marrow transplantation in patients over the age of 18 years, occurring in more than 60% of these patients despite compatibility of sibling donors and recipients at the major histocompatibility complex and in virtually all patients lacking full histocompatibility with their donors. Immunosuppressive regimens, of which the most promising is cyclosporin A,[10] have been used to prevent GVHD,[1,14] but add to the already high risk of fatal infectious complications in the posttransplant period.

Because T lymphocytes in donor marrow are thought to be the mediators of acute GVHD,[4] a variety of methods aimed at selectively reducing or inactivating the contaminating T-cell population have been attempted. *In vitro* depletion of immunocompetent T cells from donor marrow in animal transplantation experiments has been shown to prevent GVHD mortality without interfering with bone marrow regeneration.[5,13,16,17] Recently, the monoclonal antibody OKT3 that binds to peripheral immunocompetent T lymphocytes[6] has been employed to opsonize contaminating T cells in whole marrow inoculae, but this technique has achieved only limited success in reducing GVHD.[2,11] As an alternative, we have employed a rosetting technique which results in virtually complete TCD of large volumes of harvested marrow, allows manipulation of the stem cell-enriched mononuclear population for 24–48 hours, restores durable hematopoiesis with as few as 5×10^6 cells/kg body weight, and may reduce GVHD morbidity or mortality in histoincompatible transplants.

Material and Methods

PATIENTS

Three consecutive patients, ages 23–26, undergoing bone marrow transplantation with MLC mismatched donors for hematological malignancy or aplastic anemia received TCD bone marrow. Clinical details, preparative regimens, and total mononuclear cells and CFUc infused are shown for each patient in Figure 1.

BONE MARROW PREPARATION

Approximately 1200 ml of bone marrow aspirated from posterior iliac crests of transplant donors was diluted 1:2 with

Department of Medical Oncology, Roswell Park Memorial Institute, Buffalo, New York

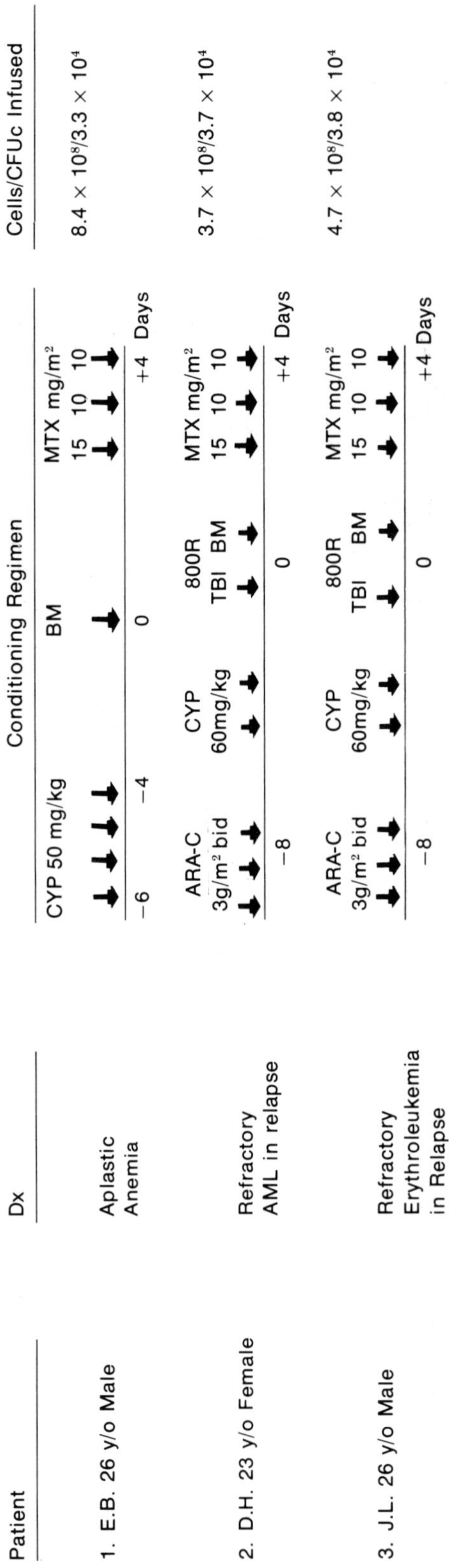

Patient	Dx	Conditioning Regimen				Cells/CFUc Infused
1. E.B. 26 y/o Male	Aplastic Anemia	CYP 50 mg/kg −6 ... −4	BM 0		MTX mg/m² 15 10 10 10 +4 Days	$8.4 \times 10^8/3.3 \times 10^4$
2. D.H. 23 y/o Female	Refractory AML in relapse	ARA-C 3g/m² bid −8	CYP 60mg/kg	800R TBI BM 0	MTX mg/m² 15 10 10 10 +4 Days	$3.7 \times 10^8/3.7 \times 10^4$
3. J.L. 26 y/o Male	Refractory Erythroleukemia in Relapse	ARA-C 3g/m² bid −8	CYP 60mg/kg	800R TBI BM 0	MTX mg/m² 15 10 10 10 +4 Days	$4.7 \times 10^8/3.8 \times 10^4$

FIGURE 1.   Clinical status and transplant conditioning. CYP = cyclophosphamide; BM = marrow infusion; MTX = methotrexate; R = rad.

heparinized Hank's medium and filtered through a Nitrex nylon mesh, then layered on Ficoll Hypaque and centrifuged for 40 minutes at 400 xg. An overall outline of the separation methods is illustrated in Figure 2. Specific methods for the rosetting procedure, monoclonal antibody staining, and flow cytometry on the FACS-II cell sorter have been previously described.[7,8] CFUc were assayed by the method of Pike and Robinson.[9]

ASSESSMENT OF ENGRAFTMENT AND GVHD

The day of engraftment was defined as the third consecutive day the WBC count was $> 1 \times 10^9/l$ and by the presence of donor karyotype in blood and marrow metaphases when there was a sex difference between donor and recipient. The clinical and histological criteria for GVHD defined by the Seattle marrow transplant team[15] were used throughout.

Results

CELL RECOVERY, VIABILITY AND CFUc CAPACITY

The separation steps with cell recoveries are indicated in Figure 2. Although as many as 2×10^{10} nucleated cells were obtained by iliac crest aspiration, the initial Ficoll gradient yielded only 5–10% of that number as mononuclear cells at the interface, with the balance of nucleated erythrocytes and granulocytes passing through the gradient. The mononuclear cell population was rosetted for 18 hours at 4°C after which the nonrosetting mononuclear cell recovery was reduced to 4–8 $\times 10^8$ total cells. During each stage of the isolation procedure, a cell aliquot was set aside for enumeration of E-rosetting cells, CFUc, and for FACS analysis with monoclonal antibodies. The initial contaminating percentage of E+ T cells ranged from 10 to 55% of the mononuclear fraction and could be reduced to <2% follow-

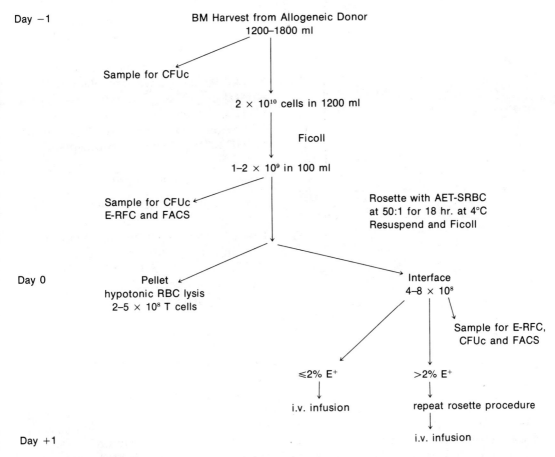

FIGURE 2. T cell depletion

ing TCD. The TCD mononuclear population was >99% viable by trypan blue dye exclusion and CFUc recovery from the initial bone marrow harvest was 45–65% of the total harvested CFUc measured in parallel cultures.

ASSESSMENT OF TCD

In order to verify depletion of contaminating T cells, the mononuclear E⁻ fraction was re-rosetted and stained with a panel of monoclonal antibodies for cytofluorographic analysis. Repeat E-rosette proportions were <2% and, in two instances, <0.5% of the infused mononuclear population. Table 1 independently confirms significant T cell depletion by demonstrating a reduction in the $OKT3^+$, $Leu4^+$ T population from 50% to <1% although both the OKIa and OKM1 populations (B cells, null cells, and monocytes) were either unaffected or slightly enriched. Functional assays further confirmed TCD by demonstrating a complete loss of PHA, Con A, and mixed lymphocyte culture responses in the T-depleted population whereas the mononuclear population responded vigorously in all three assays prior to TCD.

MONONUCLEAR CELL INFUSION AND CLINICAL OUTCOME

The TCD mononuclear population could be safely reinfused by the intravenous route in sterile RPMI 1640 containing antibiotics and 10% human AB serum. Reinfused total cell numbers ranged from 3.7–8.4 × 10⁸ of which 3.3–3.8 × 10⁴ were

TABLE 1. BM T-Cell Contamination Pre- and Post-Depletion by FACS-II Analysis Patient J.L.—Percent of Mononuclear Cells

Percent of Cells Reactive with Monoclonal Ab/Surface Marker	BM Ficolled Buffy Coat	BM after TCD
Ab brand		
E-RFC (2 hours)	41.3	<1
Ortho		
OKT3	49.0	<2
OKT4	41.9	<1
OKT6	10.2	<1
OKT8	14.5	<1
OKT8	14.5	<1
OKT 11a	13.7	<1
OKIa	11.8	13.8
OKM1	14.4	18.2
B-D		
Leu 1	50.1	<1
Leu 2	14.8	<1
Leu 3	36.9	<1
Leu 4	47.8	<1
Leu 5	44.0	<1
Leu 7	<1	<1

Ab = Antibody; B-D = Becton Dickinson; BM = Bone marrow; TCD = T-cell depletion.

CFUc. Despite these relatively low cell numbers, engraftment occurred within 18–35 days (Table 2). Engraftment was confirmed by conversion of MLC reactivity in patient E.B. (whose donor was of the same sex) and by conversion of karyotypes in patients D.H. and J.L. Leukemic relapse occurred in both D.H. and J.L., with return of recipient karyotype in the bone marrow 1 week after relapse in patient J.L. The two relapsed leukemic patients died 52 and 92 days after transplant with no clinical or pathological evidence of acute GVHD. Patient E.B. remains alive and well without evidence of acute or chronic GVHD at 16 months post-transplant.

Discussion

Although these data are preliminary and require confirmation in larger numbers of patients with regard to efficacy in reducing morbidity or mortality from GVHD, they do allow three important conclusions. First, TCD by these methods can be applied easily and effectively to the large volumes obtained in routine marrow harvests. This method results in depletion of >99% of T cells contaminating the mononuclear fraction of harvested marrow, whether measured by repeat E-rosetting or by cytofluorography with multiple anti-T-cell monoclonal antibodies. This degree of T-depletion is the equivalent of those employing specific anti-T-cell monoclonal antibodies either in the absence[2,11] or presence[3] of complement, and is less complicated than meth-

TABLE 2. Post-transplant Course

Patient	Course	Day	Outcome
1) E.B.	Fever duration	5–23	Alive and
	Polys >1000	34	well at 16 months
	Platelets >20,000	35	
2) D.H.	Fever duration	3–21	
	Oropharyngeal candidiasis		
	S. epidermidis bacteremia		
	BM karyotype XY,		Died day 92
	Polys >1000	28	
	Platelets >20,000	30	
	Leukemic relapse in BM,		
	BM karyotype XX	84	
3) J.L.	Fever duration	5–52	
	Platelets >20,000	14	
	Polys >600, karyotype XX,		
	leukemic relapse	23	Died day 52
	BM karyotype XX,		
	increased BM blasts	31	

ods employing lectin column fractionation.[12] The second conclusion which can be drawn from these results is that prolonged manipulation of the bone marrow mononuclear fraction, including overnight rosetting at 4°C, Ficoll gradient passage and repeated washing does not apparently affect viability or engraftment potential of the transplanted stem cell population. This result emphasizes the potential for applying additional treatment or separation procedures over a period of at least 24, and possibly 48 hours, allowing the possibility of utilizing T-subset-specific monoclonal antibodies or drugs *in vitro* to block the differentiation of GVHD-precursors selectively.

The third conclusion provided by these data is that complete engraftment can be achieved in the allogeneic setting with as few as $3-4 \times 10^8$ total cells infused, providing that they represent a stem-cell-enriched population of mononuclear cells. Again, this represents a technical advantage in that it affords the opportunity to deplete other nucleated cell components fully prior to manipulations designed to deplete T cells, or more selective techniques aimed at the GVHD precursors. It is therefore possible to T-deplete the large volume of marrow obtained for transplant by simple rosetting techniques over an extended period of time with significant removal of contaminating T cells and with complete retention of engraftment potential.

Whether this method of T-depletion can potentially reduce or eliminate GVHD remains to be determined. It is encouraging that, in these three MLC-mismatched patients, one of whom was also disparate at the HLA-B locus, no clinical or histological evidence of GVHD was observed. These results would suggest that this technique is more effective than *in vitro* exposure of bone marrow to the monoclonal antibody, OKT3.[2,11] However, the small patient numbers and short duration of survival (due to leukemic relapse) in two of the patients preclude more than cautious optimism with regard to amelioration of GVHD. Nonetheless, further trials of these techniques, possibly in a controlled, randomized, HLA-matched trial, are clearly warranted.

ACKNOWLEDGMENT

The authors thank Dr. Noel Warner of Becton-Dickinson for providing the Leu monoclonals.

REFERENCES

1. Blume, K.G., Beutler, E., Bross, K.H., et al.: *N Engl J Med 302: 1041, 1980.*
2. Filipovich, A., Ramsay, N.K.C., Warkentin, P.I., et al.: *Lancet 1: 1266, 1982.*
3. Granger, S.M., Janossy, G., Francis, G., et al.: *Br J Haematol 50: 367, 1982.*
4. Kersey, J.H., Meuwissen, H.J., and Good, R.A.: *Human Pathol 2: 389, 1971.*
5. Kolb, H.J., Rieder, I., Rodt, H., et al.: *Transplantation 27: 242, 1979.*
6. Kung, P.C., Goldstein, G., Reinherz, E.L., and Schlossman, S.F.: *Science 206: 347, 1979.*
7. O'Malley, J., Nussbaum-Blumenson, A., Sheedy, D., Grossmayer, B.J., and Ozer, H.: *J Immunol 128: 2522, 1982.*
8. Ozer, H., Cowens, J.W., Colvin, M., et al.: *J Exp Med 155: 276, 1982.*
9. Pike, B.L., and Robinson, V.A.: *J Cell Physiol 76: 77, 1970.*
10. Powles, R.L., Clink, H.M., Spence, D., et al.: *Lancet 1: 327, 1980.*
11. Prentice, H.G., Janossy, G., Skeggs, D., et al.: *Lancet 1: 700, 1982.*
12. Reisner, Y., Kirkpatrick, D., Dupont, B., et al.: *Lancet 1: 327, 1981.*
13. Rodt, H., Thierfelder, S., and Eulitz, M.: *Eur J Immunol 4: 25, 1974.*
14. Thomas, E.D., Storb, R., Clift, R.A., et al.: *N Engl J Med 292: 832, 1975.*
15. Thomas, E.D., Storb, R., Clift, R.A., et al.: *N Engl J Med 292: 895, 1975.*
16. Vallera, D.A., Soderling, C.C.R., Carlson, G.J., and Kersey, J.H.: *Transplantation 31: 218, 1974.*
17. Wagemaker, G., Heidt, P.J., Merchav, S., and vanBekkum, D.W.: *Exp Haematol 9: 95, 1981.*

CHAPTER 33

DTC, a T-Cell-Specific Agent in *Nu/Nu* Mice

G. Renoux and M. Renoux

Introduction

DTC (sodium diethyldithiocarbamate) was selected from a large series of sulfur-containing drug in an attempt to obviate the ambivalent effects of levamisole and also to obtain an agent devoid of the sensitizing influence of thiazole or benzol ring structures. Available data show that DTC fulfills safety requirements and exerts a unique influence on the T-cell lineage.[4-8] Current studies also show that this influence is under the control of the brain neocortex. Table 1 summarizes some of the main findings. The present report is evidence that a single administration of DTC to *nu/nu* mice induces the appearance of functionally active T (Thy-1$^+$) cells without affecting B cells.

Materials and Methods

Healthy *nu/nu* (C57B1/6 or BALB/c background), 4–6 weeks of age, were employed throughout these studies. Each group comprised four to six animals. DTC (Institut Merieux, Table 1) was administered subcutaneously at a dose of 25 mg/kg; controls were treated with pyrogen-free saline. The acquisition of a specific (Thy-1$^+$) marker by precommitted precursor cells was evaluated in a semi-automated, enzyme cytotoxicity test[6] and B (CR$^+$) cells were enumerated by the technique described by Scheid et al.[7] DNA synthesis in

Laboratoire d'Immunologie, Faculté de Médecine, 37032 Tours, France

the presence of T-cell mitogens (PHA or Con A) and B-cell mitogen (PWM) were assessed in triplicate cultures for 3 days, where 0.5 μCi tritiated-thymidine was added for the last 18 hours of incubation, and labeled thymidine incorporation was determined by liquid scintillation spectrometry.

Assay of antibody-secreting spleen cells (PFC) was evaluated 4 days after an intravenous injection of 1×10^8 SRBC. Direct (IgM) or indirect (IgG) PFC were counted by techniques already described.[10,11]

Results

Since the results of administering 25 mg/kg DTC to *nu/nu* mice were very similar whatever might have been the background (BALB/c or C57 B1/6), the data obtained are compiled in Figure 1.

Untreated, healthy *nu/nu* mice have low percentages of spleen cells with the specific Thy-1 cytotopic marker (4 ± 3) as well as with the specific CR$^+$ marker of B cells (18 ± 1.8), confirming the findings of Scheid et al.[13] As shown in Figure 1, a single administration of DTC elicited the presence of 24% Thy-1$^+$ spleen cells, and did not modify the percentage of B cells. Induction of T (Thy-1$^+$) cells was accompanied by *de novo* T-cell functional activities. Indeed, more than a 2,000-fold increase in lymphoproliferative responses to the T-cell mitogens, PHA, or Con A, was observed in *nu/nu* spleen cells, 4 days after treatment with DTC, without effect on background

TABLE 1.   Sodium Diethyldithiocarbamate, DTC: Mean Features

I. Pharmacology
   Low acute or chronic toxicity: $LD_{50} > 2.5$ g/kg
   Nonantigenic or sensitizing agent
   Possesses antibiotic activity
   Protects against chemically-induced cancers
   No untoward side effects in man
II. Immunologic Activities
A unique influence on the T-cell lineage, without affecting B cells.
   In man as in animals, DTC:
   • increases lymphoproliferative responses to T-cell mitogens and alloantigens,
   • increases IgG-antibody levels and delayed hypersensitivities,
   • augments NK activity, without production of endogenous interferon,
   • restores responses abrogated by chemotherapies and prevents immunodepression associated with surgical trauma; regulates T-cell subsets,
   • no effect on: PWM-induced responses or ADCC to chicken erythrocytes,
   • decreases circulating IgM-antibody levels and immediate hypersensitivity.
III. Mechanism of Action
   • No significant *in vitro* influence. Acts through the increased synthesis of a factor specific for T cells (synthesized by the liver).
   • Replaces a signal missing in *nu/nu* mice allowing maturation of functionally active T cells, without effect on B cells.
   • The influence of DTC on T cells is controlled by the brain neocortex.

(spontaneous cpm in absence of mitogens) counts which were $2,460 \pm 40$ in control and $2,508 \pm 193$ in DTC-treated samples. Similarly, an important IgG-PFC response, a T-cell-associated event, was obtained (107 IgG-PFC/10^6 spleen cells), which response was always negative in control athymic mice. In sharp contrast, and confirming all data from euthymic mice, B-cell-associated responses, such as PWM-induced lymphoproliferation and IgM-PFC, were found diminished in treated *nu/nu* mice, in comparison with saline-treated controls (Fig. 1).

Discussion

The data obtained in this investigation show a unique influence of DTC on the immune system. Although it is a sulfur compound, DTC does not act through the elaboration of a general lymphocyte activator such as is produced by 2-mercaptoethanol and related thiols, including levamisole. Indeed, the general lymphocyte activator is described as a mitogenic factor which enhances preexisting events and acts not only on T cells but also on B cells.[2] DTC has no direct influence on B cells or mitogenic activities; the agent recruits T cells from precommitted precursors, and induces functional activities. Strikingly enough, these influences are obtained following a single administration.

It has been demonstrated that the third branchial pouch of the nude mouse embryo involutes after the first $11\frac{1}{2}$ days instead of continuing to develop,[1] and that the so-called thymus-like organs of adult *nu/nu* mice do not have the structure of thymic tissue but that of lymph nodes.[1,3] The present data, therefore, show that thymic activities are not a prerequisite for the elaboration of an inducer of T-lymphocyte recruitment and activation. Current studies attempt to identify the site of synthesis and the nature of the inducer, and also to elucidate the role displayed by the thymus; preliminary data suggest that DTC replaces a signal from the thymus. Other studies evidence that the cerebral neocortex controls the T-cell lineage activities as well as the inducing capacity of DTC.[12]

Taken together, these findings are consonant with the hypothesis that DTC does not act directly to differentiate T cells but, through stimulation of the central nervous system network, influences the endocrinal network for the synthesis of a hormone specific for T cells. In other words, a thymusless animal treated by DTC can generate T cells, but an animal deprived of the right neocortex and then treated by DTC cannot increase the number and activity of its T cells.

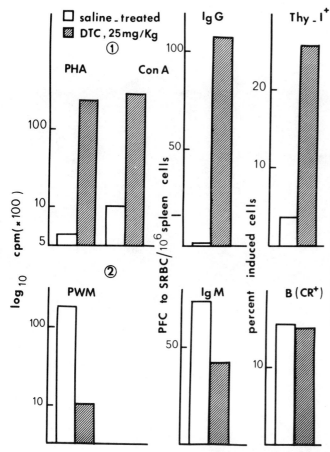

FIGURE 1. DTC induces functionally active T cells but not B cells in congenitally athymic mice. Five *nu/nu* mice per group were treated subcutaneously with 25 mg/kg DTC (shaded columns) or pyrogen-free saline as controls. Spleen T (Thy-1+) and B (CR+) cell percentages were evaluated 24 hrs after treatment, as were responses to mitogens. Sheep red cells, SRBC (1×10^8) were injected I.V. and the numbers of specific direct (IgM) and indirect (IgG) antibody-plaque-forming spleen cells (PFC) evaluated 4 days later. Vertical bars indicate S.E.M. (DTC: A T cell specific agent in *nu/nu* mice.)

Conclusions

DTC satisfies the criteria for an agent devoid of untoward side effects, carcinogenicity, and antigenicity, and with recruiting and regulating abilities on a set of immunocompetent cells. Its unique activity on the T-cell lineage, and even after a single administration, suggests that it would be an effective agent for treatment of syndromes and disease states where the underlying defect is a T-cell deficiency or dysfunction.

REFERENCES

1. Cordier, A.C., and Haumont, S.M.: *Am J Anat* 157: 227, 1980.
2. Hewlett, G., Opitz, H.G., and Schlumberger, H.D.: In *Lymphokines*, E. Pick and Landy, Eds., vol. 4, Academic Press, New York, 1981, pp. 89–105.
3. Hsu, Ch.K., Whitney, R.A., and Hansen, C.T.: *Nature* 257: 681, 1975.
4. Renoux, G., and Renoux, M.: *J Immunopharmacology* 1: 247, 1979.
5. Renoux, G.: In *Trends in Human Immunology and Cancer Immunotherapy*, B. Serrou and C. Rosenfeld, Eds., Doin, Paris, 1980, pp. 986–994.
6. Renoux, G., and Renoux, M.: *Thymus* 2: 139, 1980.
7. Renoux, G., and Renoux, M.: In *Augmenting Agents in Cancer Therapy*, E.M. Hersh, M.A. Chirigo, and M.J. Mastrangelo, Eds., Raven Press, New York, 1981, pp. 427–440.
8. Renoux, G.: *J Pharmacol (Paris)* 13: 95, 1982.
9. Renoux, G., Gyenes, L., Guillaumin, J.M., and Jean, B.: *J Immunol Meths* 36: 71, 1980.
10. Renoux, G., and Renoux, M.: *J Immunol* 113: 779, 1974.
11. Renoux, G., and Renoux, M.: In *Control of Neoplasia by Modulation of the Immune System*, M.A. Chirigos, Ed. Raven Press, New York, 1977, pp. 67–80.
12. Renoux, G., Bizière, K., and Renoux, M.: *Bull Acad Med* 166: 88, 1982.
13. Scheid, M.P., Goldstein, G., and Boyse, E.A.: *J Exptl Med* 147: 1727, 1978.

PART IV

Mechanism of Action
and Toxicity

CHAPTER 34

A Review of the Role of DNA Repair Processes in the Initiation of Carcinogenesis

A. Sarasin and C. Sarasin

Introduction

It is frequently said that most human malignancies are caused by environmental factors such as irradiation, chemicals, or drugs. Almost all these agents cause direct or indirect effects on the DNA molecule. Several lines of evidence suggest that DNA alterations are among the early events leading to the carcinogenic process.[12]

Repair

All living cells are well equipped with several specific repair processes acting on various types of DNA lesions (Fig. 1). Several enzymatic pathways have been described both in prokaryotes and in eukaryotes.[7] DNA lesions are repaired either by a direct removal of the lesions without any change in the integrity of the DNA molecule (photolyase for pyrimidine dimers or methyltransferase for O^6-methyl-guanine) or by the excision of a piece of DNA containing the lesion (excision repair pathway). During the replication process, some tolerance pathways are able to bypass DNA lesions without a direct repair of these lesions. These pathways are either error-free (daughter strand gap repair) or error-prone. The latter lead to a high mutation frequency in the surviv-

Institut de Recherches Scientifiques sur le Cancer, Villejuif, France

ors (translesion synthesis or SOS repair) (Fig. 1).

Poor Repair

Xeroderma pigmentosum (XP) was the first human example showing the fundamental role of DNA repair in cancer etiology.[2] XP is an autosomal recessive human skin disease in which affected individuals exhibit sunlight hypersensitivity associated with the occurrence of multiple skin cancers in the exposed areas. These patients can be classified into several complementation groups indicating that the XP disease can have a multigenic origin. In 1968, J. Cleaver discovered that XP cells were unable to carry out the excision repair pathway after treatment with UV light or with various chemical carcinogens. This result shows for the first time that unrepaired DNA lesions are directly responsible for initiating the carcinogenic process in humans.[2] Since that discovery, several other human diseases, characterized by a DNA repair deficiency and a cancer predisposition, have been described and analyzed in molecular terms. Cells isolated from ataxia telangiectasia patients are very sensitive to ionizing radiations and to alkylating agents; cells isolated from Fanconi's anemia are very sensitive to cross-linking agents such as mitomycin C.[7]

ENZYMATIC PROCESSING OF DAMAGED DNA

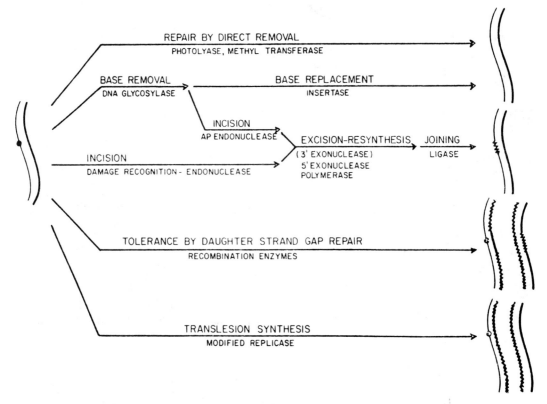

FIGURE 1.   General scheme of the DNA repair pathways. (Reproduced from M. Defais, P.C. Hanawalt and A. Sarasin, Viral probes for DNA repair processes. *Adv Radiat Biol* **10:** 1, 1982,)

Mutations

The studies of these human diseases which cause high susceptibility to cancer suggest that some mutations, and particularly those induced by UV light, are carcinogenic in humans. Similarly, the DNA lesion O⁶-methyl-guanine induced by methylating agents is apparently carcinogenic, but only in cells unable to repair it. The important event for carcinogenesis initiation is the balance between the level of DNA lesions and the efficiency of our various repair pathways. DNA lesions should be removed before the onset of DNA replication or the fork of replication is blocked by the unrepaired lesions, leading to an arrest in DNA synthesis. In that case, several possibilities exist, such as recombination, postreplication repair, or discontinuities in the newly-synthesized DNA. It is also possible that some new repair pathways are induced in order to permit a bypass of the lesions. Such a translesion synthesis is mutagenic per se and belongs to the SOS repair pathways described in bacteria.[10] In that case, the "repair" of DNA lesions is more mutagenic than the DNA lesion itself (Fig. 1). Such an error-prone repair pathway has been shown to be induced in monkey kidney cells treated with UV light or various chemical carcinogens.[11,13] Detection of mutagenic pathways is important in understanding the mechanism of mutation induction in mammalian cells.

During the last decade, the discovery

that almost all carcinogens are mutagens and almost all mutagens are carcinogens, has led scientists to think that mutations are a general cause of cancers. However, several lines of evidence indicate that a localized change in the DNA sequence alone may not be enough to give rise to tumors, but that larger changes in the genome are necessary to express the transformed phenotype.[1] For example, Bloom's syndrome is an autosomal recessive human disease associated with a very high frequency of chromosomal rearrangements and aberrations and a high level of spontaneous sister chromatid exchanges. The exact molecular biology of this disease is still unclear. It has been shown, however, that a high level of free radicals and active oxygen species are observed in the cultured cells, leading to DNA damages and, probably, to this chromosome breakage syndrome.[4] The medical consequence of this extreme chromosomal instability is a large increase of the incidence of all common cancers without any specific localization or any specific tumor type. The death rate from cancers is increased about 100-fold for carcinomas, leukemias, or lymphomas. It seems that in this disease the usual process leading to carcinogenesis is strongly accelerated, with a shortening of the long latency period usually observed in human cancers. This shortening of the latency period is probably due to the high chromosomal instability which rapidly disorganizes the cell genome and rapidly expresses any localized mutations induced by contact with conventional mutagens and carcinogens. Other inherited diseases with a predisposition to cancer present a spontaneous chromosomal instability pattern, as in Fanconi's anemia, ataxia telangiectasia, and even XP cells after treatment with DNA-damaging agents. It is interesting to notice that some tumor promoters, such as 12-O-tetradecanoyl-phorbol-13-acetate (TPA), induce chromosomal rearrangements and specific recombination.[6,8] By definition, the effect of tumor promoters is to shorten the latent period for cancer occurrence, as is the case in Bloom's syndrome. This similarity strongly supports the hypothesis that genome rearrangements and gene transposition are essential in the initiation of carcinogenesis, as already pointed out by Cairns.[1]

Oncogenes

It was recently shown that some cellular genes which are normally repressed during the adult state could be abnormally expressed, leading to the expression of a transformed phenotype. These cellular oncogenes are almost identical to some transforming genes from retroviruses[5] and they can induce cell transformation of NIH 3T3 cells after DNA transfection.[3] The expression of these oncogenes may be obtained either by a localized mutation on the gene itself or on its regulatory unit, or by a specific translocation or transposition which would permit these oncogenes to be under the control of an active viral or cellular promoter. These genes are present both in normal and transformed cells but they could be expressed at a higher level in the latter. Consequently, the high incidence of cancer in the human chromosome breakage syndromes and after tumor promoter-treatment could be due to the high probability to express mutated genes, important for cell regulation, or oncogenes which could either be cellular or viral ones. In that hypothesis, the initial mutation obtained by contact with mutagens is a silent one, until a transposition or a chromosomal rearrangement permits its expression.

Conclusions

If "abnormal" expression of cellular oncogenes represents a common pathway for initiation of carcinogenesis by many carcinogens, several implications for cancer therapy should be underlined. First, the design for rational therapeutic strategies may be very difficult, since the same genes and therefore closely related protein activities are both potentially present in normal and tumoral cells. These oncogenes are probably very important for the life of normal cells during specific physiological states and therefore it is improbable that a therapeutic strategy can be designed to inhibit this specific activity constantly. Second, most of the antitumor agents used in cancer chemotherapy have the DNA molecule as target, which they damage. They also induce chromosomal aberrations and sister chromatid exchanges, as do many carcinogens.[9] Therefore, it is important for clinical purposes to determine exactly the mechanism of action of these drugs, in order to discover whether therapeutic activity can be associated with minimal long-term effect on DNA mutagenesis and DNA recombination, and to analyze their carcinogenic properties before using them extensively in the human population.

REFERENCES

1. Cairns, J.: *Nature 289: 353, 1981.*

2. Cleaver, J.E. and Bootsma, D.: *Ann Rev Genetics 9: 19, 1975.*

3. Copeland, N.G. and Cooper, G.M.: *Cell 16: 347, 1979.*

4. Emerit, I. and Cerutti, P.: *Proc Natl Acad Sci USA 78: 1868, 1981.*

5. Eva, A., et al.: *Nature 295: 116, 1982.*

6. Gentil, A.: In *Sister Chromatid Exchange,* A.A. Sandberg, Ed., A.R. Liss, Inc., New York, 1982, p. 535.

7. Hanawalt, P.C., Cooper, P.K., Ganesan, A.K., and Smith, C.A.: *Ann Rev Biochem 48: 783, 1979.*

8. Kinsella, A.R. and Radman, M.: *Proc Natl Acad Sci USA 76: 6149, 1978.*

9. Raposa, T.: In *Sister Chromatid Exchange,* A.A. Sandberg, Ed., A.R. Liss, Inc., New York, 1982, p. 579.

10. Sarasin, A.: In *Mechanisms of Chemical Carcinogenesis,* C. Harris and P. Cerutti, Eds., A.R. Liss, Inc., New York, 1982, p. 461.

11. Sarasin, A. and Benoit, A.: *Mutation Res 70: 71, 1980.*

12. Sarasin, A. and Meunier-Rotival, M.: *Biomedicine, 24: 306, 1976.*

13. Sarasin, A., Bourre, F., and Benoit, A.: *Biochimie 64: 815, 1982.*

CHAPTER 35

Mechanisms of Resistance to Anthracyclines

H. Tapiero,[a] A. Fourcade,[a] E. Goldschmidt,[a] and G. Zwingelstein[b]

Introduction

Anthracyclines have been previously described as incorporated in cells and distributed mainly in nuclei.[2,6] Since the cytotoxic effect is correlated with an interaction with DNA altering the DNA-dependent DNA and RNA polymerase activities,[1,12,14] cellular uptake and the cell ability to retain the drug could be a decisive factor for the biological and therapeutic effect of drugs belonging to this group. The exact mode of cellular uptake, drug retention, and the mechanism by which these parameters could be altered *in vitro* and *in vivo* are not known.[4,8,10,11,13,17,19] The possibility of changes in the dynamic structural organization of the cell surface occurring during the development of cell resistance cannot be excluded. The present study was undertaken to determine the relationship between cellular uptake, efflux, and membrane composition changes.

Materials and Methods

CELL CULTURE

Friend leukemia cells (FLC) were derived from a clone of Friend virus-transformed cells 745A. Cells were grown in modified Eagle's spinner medium lacking calcium and containing 10mM sodium phosphate and nonessential amino acids (Gibco, Grand Island, NY). Medium was supplemented with 10% fetal calf serum (Gibco, lot K3862015) and antibiotics. All cell cultures were incubated at 37°C in a CO_2 incubator. Cell densities were determined by repeated cell counts using a hematocytometer and cell viability was measured by counting the cells excluding 0.1% trypan blue.

The highly-resistant cell variants, resistant to adriamycin (ADM-RFLC) and daunorubicin (DNR-RFLC) were derived from FLC 745A by continuous exposure to increasing concentrations of each drug over a period of 9 months and maintained at 8 µg/ml of adriamycin (ADM) and daunorubicin (DNR) for 3 months. The resistant cell variants were then transferred for more than 70 passages without a drug. Under these conditions, resistance was maintained.

CHEMICALS

All chemicals were of analytical grade. Adriamycin (Doxorubicine hydrochloride) was provided by the Roger Bellon Lab. (Paris, France) and daunorubicin (Daunorubicin hydrochloride) by Rhône Poulenc (Paris, France).

LIPID EXTRACTION AND PURIFICATION

Lipids were obtained from cells by several extractions with a chloroform–

[a]Département de Pharmacologie Cellulaire et Moléculaire et de Pharmacocinétique, Unité Simone et Cino Del Duca de Pharmacologie Humaine des Cancers, Institut de Cancérologie et d'Immunogénétique (INSERM U-50), Hôpital Paul-Brousse, Villejuif, France
[b]Groupe CNRS 33, Unité de Virologie, INSERM U-51, Lyon, France

methanol mixture (1:1, v/v). The extract was taken to dryness, dissolved in chloroform–methanol (2:1, v/v) and filtered. The combined filtrates were subsequently washed once with 0.2 vol. of 0.9% KCl in water and once with 0.5 vol. of methanol–water (10:6, v/v). The washed extract was then evaporated to dryness under vacuum at 45°C and made up to a known volume of chloroform–ethanol (2:1, v/v).

PHOSPHOLIPIDS

Phospholipids were separated by two-dimensional thin-layer chromatography as already described.[15] Quantification was measured by determining the phosphorus content[3] in each spot after staining with a specific spray reagent.[5] Total lipid phosphorus was quantified by a modification of Bartlett's method.[3]

The HPLC conditions were similar to those already described,[9,16] with minor modifications. The HPLC was achieved with a Waters associate liquid chromatograph on radial microbondapakphenyl column. The solvent was a mixture of acetonitrile and formate buffer (32/68, v/v). The formate buffer was prepared with 0.17% ammonia adjusted to pH 4.00 with

pure formic acid. This solvent was used isocratically at a flow rate of 2 ml/minute. Detection of the peaks was accomplished with a Schoeffel fluorometer with an excitation wavelength of 254 nm and an emission cut-off filter at 550 nm.

Results and Discussion

Sublines of Friend leukemia cells resistant to adriamycin (ADM-RFLC) and to daunorubicin (DNR-RFLC) were developed in our laboratory. The increase in resistance up to 100-fold was obtained and cross-resistance was observed between ADM and DNR.[18] The relationship between resistance and cellular uptake was investigated by exposing 5×10^6 cells in 1-ml growth medium containing 1 and 10 μg ADM. After incubation at 37°C for different time periods, cells were washed twice with cold Hanks saline buffer, and the incorporated ADM was extracted and analyzed by HPLC. When cells were exposed to a high concentration of ADM (10 μg/ml), the amount detected into the cells, increased with time, according to the cell variant. From 15 minutes to 4 hours, it increased five- and two-fold in sensitive cells and DNR-RFLC cells, respectively, but it was lower in ADM-RFLC cells.

TABLE 1. Comparative Uptake of Adriamycin into Sensitive and Resistant Friend Leukemia Cells

Treatment	Time of Incubation (minutes)	Adriamycin Incorporation (ng/5 × 10⁶ Cells)			Ratios	
		FLC	ADM–RFLC	DNR–RFLC	FLC/ADM–RFLC	FLC/DNR–RFLC
ADM	15	118	112	116	1.05	1.02
(1 μg)	30	159	117	152	1.36	1.05
	60	245	123	208	1.99	1.18
	120	356	199	311	1.80	1.14
	240	419	378	414	1.11	1.01
ADM	15	640	380	560	1.68	1.14
(10 μg)	30	1 261	390	720	3.23	1.75
	60	1 859	390	770	4.77	2.41
	120	2 720	400	900	6.80	3.02
	240	3 185	440	1 020	7.24	3.12

Exponentially growing FLC were exposed to 1 and 10 μg ADM/ml growth medium. After incubation at 37°C for different time periods, aliquots of 5×10^6 cells were taken, washed with Hanks saline. The incorporated ADM was extracted and injected onto HPLC as described in Materials and Methods.

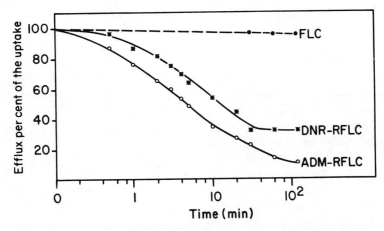

FIGURE 1. Aliquots of 5×10^6 sensitive Friend leukemia cells (FLC), adriamycin-resistant (ADM-RFLC) and daunorubicin-resistant cells (DNR-RFLC) were exposed to 1 µg adriamycin/ml of growth medium. After 15 minutes of incubation at 37°C, cells were washed twice with Hanks saline, resuspended in growth medium and incubated at 37°C. At different times, 5 × 10^6 cell samples were washed, and ADM was extracted and injected onto HPLC as described in Materials and Methods.

According to these results, the ratio of the amount incorporated into sensitive cells to that incorporated into ADM-RFLC cells varied from 1.68 to 7.24 and on that incorporated into DNR-RFLC cells from 1.14 to 3.12 (Table 1). Since these ratios were about the same when sensitive and resistant cells were exposed to a low concentration of ADM (1 µg/ml) we suggest, therefore, that resistance is not due to the ease with which ADM crosses the cell membrane but rather to the ability of the cell to retain the drug. This assumption is supported by exposing cells to 1 µg ADM/ml for a very short time (less than 5 minutes). In those conditions, the amount detected in resistant cells was unexpectedly higher than that in sensitive cells. Moreover, the efflux of ADM from resistant cells is shown to be a very rapid process. While it did not occur in sensitive cells after 2 hours, it was about 70%

TABLE 2. Phospholipid Composition of Friend Leukemia Cells and of Adriamycin- and Daunorubicin-resistant FLC

	FLC	ADM–RFLC	DNR–RFLC
Sphingomyelin (SPH)	4.6 ± 0.4	3.0 ± 0.1	3.2 ± 0.3
Phosphatidyl choline (PC)	50.9 ± 1.2	68.8 ± 0.4	66.1 ± 0.4
Phosphatidyl serine (PS)	3.0 ± 0.3	3.5 ± 0.2	2.4 ± 0.2
Phosphatidyl inositol (PI)	8.2 ± 0.2	4.9 ± 0.4	5.0 ± 0.1
Phosphatidyl ethanolamine (PE)	25.2 ± 1.3	13.8 ± 0.9	17.3 ± 1.3
Diphosphatidyl glycerol (DPG)	8.1 ± 0.7	5.1 ± 0.3	5.2 ± 0.1
Molar Ratios			
−PC:PE	2.0 ± 0.2	5.0 ± 0.2	3.8 ± 0.1
−PC:SPH	11.6 ± 1.4	23.1 ± 0.9	20.6 ± 1.8
−PI:PS	2.7 ± 0.3	1.4 ± 0.3	2.1 ± 0.2

Cells which were cultured for 4 days were washed four times with NaCl 0.15 *M*, Tris 0.01 *M* pH 7.2. The last pellets are resuspended in 20 volumes of chloroform–methanol (2:1) and the analysis carried out as described in Materials and Methods (results are expressed as percentage of the total lipid phosphorus).

and 40% of the incorporated amount in ADM-RFLC and DNR-RFLC cells, respectively (Fig. 1).

The mechanism by which cellular uptake and drug efflux occur is still unclear. In previous studies, we have reported that uptake is a passive process and efflux an active one.[7,18] Both processes could be related to the membrane structure. Changes in the cell membrane will probably alter these processes. In order to investigate the nature of these changes, the phospholipid composition of sensitive and resistant cells was undertaken. As compared to sensitive cells, the phospholipid composition of resistant cells was characterized by an increase in phosphatidyl choline (PC) and a decrease in sphingomyelin (SPH) and phosphatidyl ethanolamine (PE). As a result of these changes, the ratios PC/SPH and PC/PE increased by about 100% in the resistant cells (Table 2). The significance of these changes and their relations to cell resistance are under investigation in our laboratory.

ACKNOWLEDGMENTS

The authors thank Professeur G. Mathé, Nicole Vriz, and Roger Bellon Laboratories for their help. This work was supported by contracts from INSERM, CNRS and ADRC.

REFERENCES

1. Atassi, G., Tagnon, H.S., Bournonville, F., and Wynands, M.: *Eur J Cancer* 10: 339–403, 1974.
2. Bachur, N.R., Hildebrand, R.C., and Jaenke, R.S.: *Pharmacol Exp Ther* 191: 331–340, 1974.
3. Bartlett, G.R.: *J Biol Chem* 234: 466–468, 1959.
4. Bhuyan, B.K., McGovern, J.P., and Crampton, S.L.: *Cancer Res* 41: 882–887, 1981.
5. Ditmer, J.C. and Lester, R.L.: *J Lipid Res* 5: 126–131, 1964.
6. Egorin, B.K., Hildebrand, R.C., Cimino, E.F., and Bachur, N.R.: *Cancer Res* 34: 2243–2245, 1974.
7. Fourcade, A., Farhi, J.J., Bennoun, M., and Tapiero, H.: *Cancer Res* 42: 1950–1954, 1982.
8. Inaba, M. and Johnson, R.K.: *Biochem Pharmacol* 27: 2123–2130, 1978.
9. Israel, M., Pegg, W.J., Wilkinson, P.H., and Garniek, M.B.: *J Liquid Chromatogr* 1: 795–801, 1978.
10. Krishan, A., Israel, M., Modest, E.J., and Frei, E. III: *Cancer Res* 36: 2114–2116, 1976.
11. Landos-Gagliardi, D., Aubel-Sadron G., Maral, R., and Trouet, A.: *Eur J Cancer* 16: 849–854, 1980.
12. Meriwether, W.D., and Bachur, N.R.: *Cancer Res* 32: 1137–1142, 1972.
13. Noel, G., Peterson, C., Trouet, A., and Tulkens, P.: *Eur J Cancer* 14: 363–368, 1978.
14. Pigram, W.J., Fuller, W., and Hamilton, L.D.: *Nature New Biol* 235: 17–19, 1972.
15. Portoukalian, J., Meister, R., and Zwingelstein, G.: *J Chromatogr* 152: 569–574, 1978.
16. Robert, J.: *J Liquid Chromatogr* 3: 1561–1572, 1980.
17. Skovsgaard, T.: *Biochem Pharmacol* 26: 215–222, 1977.
18. Tapiero, H., Fourcade, A., Vaigot, P., and Farhi, J.J.: *Cytometry* 2: 298–302, 1982.
19. Yesair, D.W., Thayer, P.S., McNitt, S., and Teague, K.: *Eur J Cancer* 16: 901–907, 1980.

CHAPTER 36

Variable Patterns of *in vitro* Drug Responses between Vincristine- and Vindesine-Resistant Murine Cell Lines

B.T. Hill

Introduction

Vindesine, a newer semisynthetic vinca alkaloid, is now undergoing clinical evaluation in Phase I–II studies. This drug is likely to prove a valuable addition to cancer chemotherapy if it is shown: 1) to have superior antitumor effectiveness with reduced toxic side effects; and/or 2) to have a different spectrum of antitumor activity from the other vinca alkaloids; and/or 3) to be effective against vincristine-resistant cells. This study was designed to investigate this third possibility. We have developed drug-resistant, murine cell lines *in vitro* and established their patterns of response to the various vinca alkaloids and several other clinically useful antitumor agents.

Materials and Methods

Full details of the materials, including all the antitumor drugs and methods used have been provided previously.[1,2] The procedure used to establish drug-resistant sublines of L5178Y murine lymphoblasts has been described in detail.[2] Briefly, cell clones were isolated from soft agarose following a 24-hour drug exposure of the

Laboratory of Cellular Chemotherapy, Imperial Cancer Research Fund, Lincoln's Inn Fields, London, England

parent lines to 200 ng/ml of either VCR or VDS. Cell lines were subsequently established and have been fully characterized and their mechanisms of resistance have been studied.[2] The VCR-resistant neuroblastoma line was established using similar techniques, except that a concentration of 1 μg/ml of VCR was employed for the 24-hour drug exposure.

Results

STUDIES WITH MURINE LYMPHOMA L5178Y CELLS

The VCR-resistant and VDS-resistant sublines exhibit an approximate 40-fold order of resistance under conditions of continuous drug exposure. For a 24-hour exposure period, ID_{50} values for the parent and -resistant lines differ only by a factor of approximately 5. However, it should be noted that for a 24-hour drug exposure, resistance in these lines cannot be overcome by increasing the drug concentration since plateaus in the survival curves occur at $\geq$50% cell survival in both resistant lines, contrasting with the approximately 30% level for the parent lines (for VCR, see top left hand panel of Figure 1).

The presence or absence of cross-resistance between VCR and VDS appears to be dependent on the drug concentration used for a 24-hour exposure, as shown for the VCR-resistant line in Figure 1 (top panels). Using drug concentrations of <0.5 ng/ml, VCR-resistant cells were cross-resistant to either VCR or VDS. However, at concentrations ≥1 ng/ml, cross-resistance was *not* expressed and VDS proved equally effective at reducing survival of parent and VCR-resistant cells. Comparable results were obtained with the VDS-resistant line.

Patterns of responses of these drug-resistant lines to various other antitumor drugs are summarized in Table 1. Both lines showed very similar responses to all the drugs, with the exception of actinomycin D and *m*-AMSA. VDS-resistant cells exhibited cross-resistance to both drugs, while VCR-resistant cells showed only

slight resistance to actinomycin D and proved sensitive to *m*-AMSA. This result therefore provides further evidence that these resistant cells do not exhibit *identical* drug responses.

STUDIES WITH MURINE NEUROBLASTOMA CELLS

The VCR-resistant subline established exhibits an approximate 25-fold order of resistance to VCR under conditions of continuous drug exposure. For a limited 24-hour exposure, the ID_{50} values for parent and -resistant lines differ by a factor of 5. Figure 1 (lower left hand panel) shows that the pattern of response to VCR in this -resistant subline differs from those of the lymphoblasts, since resistance to VCR in these cells may be overcome by *either* in-

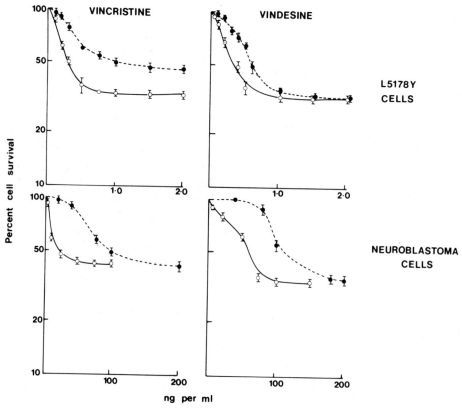

FIGURE 1. The lethal effects of treatment with VCR (left-hand panels) or VDS (right-hand panels) for 24 hours on the colony-forming ability of logarithmically-growing L5178Y lymphoma cells (top panels) or murine neuroblastoma cells (bottom panels). ●- - -● = VCR-resistant lines; ○ —— ○ = parent lines. Each point represents the mean and each bar the SEM of four assays.

TABLE 1.   A Summary of Patterns of *in vitro* Drug Responses[a]

Drugs Tested	Cell Lines		
	VDS$_R$-L5178Y	VCR$_R$-L5178Y	VCR$_R$-Neuroblastoma
5-fluorouracil	S[b]	S	S
Methotrexate	S	S	S
VM26	S	S	S
VP-16-213	S	S	S
m-AMSA	R$^+$	S	R^{++}
Actinomycin D	R^{++}	R	R^{++}
Vinblastine	[c]R$^+$	[c]R$^+$	R$^+$
Vindesine	[c]R^{++}	[c]R^{++}	R^{++}
Formyl-leurosine	R^{++}	R^{++}	—[d]
Adriamycin	R^{+++}	R^{+++}	R^{+++}
4'-Epiadriamycin	R^{+++}	R^{+++}	—
4'-Deoxyadriamycin	R^{+++}	R^{+++}	—
4'-O-methyl-adriamycin	R^{+++}	R^{+++}	—
7-O-methylnogarol	R^{+++}	R^{++}	—
Dianhydroanthracenedione	R^{+++}	R^{++}	—
Quelamycin	R^{++}	R^{++}	—

[a]Drug exposures were for 24 hours and cell survival was assessed by colony formation in soft agarose.
[b]S = sensitive: order of resistance: R^{+++} > +R^{++} > R$^+$ > R.
[c]Dose-dependent responses were noted with resistance being most marked at "low" concentrations and negligible at "high" concentrations.
[d]Not studied.

creasing the drug concentration for a fixed 24-hour exposure *or* by increasing the exposure duration. These data therefore suggest that there may be more than one mechanism of resistance to VCR which may be differentially expressed in particular cell types. Figure 1 also shows that the VCR-resistant cells are completely cross-resistant to VDS (lower right hand panel). Again dose-dependency is exhibited, with resistance being overcome at the higher drug concentrations.

Patterns of responses to the other antitumor drugs are listed in Table 1. A comparison of these data with those obtained using the lymphoblast lines shows essentially similar responses, with the exception of *m*-AMSA. VCR-resistant neuroblastoma cells are resistant to *m*-AMSA, contrasting with VCR-resistant L5178Y cells which retain full sensitivity. Therefore, these *in vitro* studies, while indicating a close similarity in patterns of drug resistance or sensitivities between these vinca-resistant lines, also identify certain exceptions and differences.

Discussion

Cell lines resistant to VCR or VDS may be readily established *in vitro*. In the L5178Y lymphoma subline, this resistance can only be overcome by prolonging the exposure of duration beyond 24 hours, the approximate doubling time of the cells. This contrasts with the neuroblastoma subline in which resistance can be overcome either by increasing the VCR concentration using a 24-hour exposure or by prolonging the duration of exposure. This emphasizes that the way in which a drug is administered can affect the expression of sensitivity or resistance.

Patterns of cross-resistance to the vinca alkaloids also differed within these two cell types. In the lymphoma sublines, cross-resistance between VCR and VDS was *not* invariable and proved highly dose-dependent. In the VCR-resistant neuroblastoma cells, however, complete cross-resistance was noted to VDS. All the resistant lines proved least cross-resistant to vinblastine.

In studies with other antitumor drugs, all three resistant sublines showed broadly similar drug responses. Cross-resistance was expressed to a number of anthracycline derivatives, while full sensitivity was retained to methotrexate, 5-fluorouracil and the two podophyllotoxin derivatives. Again, this was not invariable, since VCR-resistant lymphoma cells proved sensitive to m-AMSA. The other two lines showed resistance.

It is suggested that these variable patterns of response to the vincas noted in these different drug-resistant sublines may be related to the involvement of one or several resistance mechanisms. These observations would also tend to confirm some apparently conflicting clinical evidence, since while a few studies suggest that pretreatment with VCR can reduce subsequent response to VDS,[3] a more extensive literature reports an absence of cross-resistance between the two drugs.[4-7]

Conclusions

These experimental laboratory studies show that: 1) the expression of sensitivity or resistance may be dependent on both exposure duration and drug concentration employed; 2) cross-resistance between the various vinca alkaloids is not invariable; and 3) vindesine may complement the antitumor effectiveness of vincristine and vinblastine.

Summary

Three cell sublines were established *in vitro*, two resistant to vincristine (VCR), derived from L5178Y lymphoblasts or neuroblastoma (MNB/PL) cells and a L5178Y line resistant to vindesine (VDS). These lines exhibit differential responses to vinca alkaloids: 1) resistance in lymphoblasts is more related to exposure duration than drug dose, contrasting with dose- *and* time-dependent resistance in MNB/PL cells, 2) Cross-resistance between VCR and VDS is not absolute in lymphoblasts, but shows dose-dependency, contrasting with complete cross-resistance in MNB/PL cells. However, all three lines exhibit comparable response to 14 other drugs, with m-AMSA proving an exception by effectively killing VCR-resistant lymphoblasts but not MNB/PL cells. Cross-resistance between VCR and VDS is not invariable *in vitro*, reflecting clinical experience.

REFERENCES

1. Hill, B.T. and Whelan, R.D.H.: *J Natl Cancer Inst* 67: 437, 1981.
2. Hill, B.T. and Whelan, R.D.H.: *Cancer Chemother Pharmacol 8: 163, 1982.*
3. Young, C.W.: *Cancer Treat Rev (Suppl) 7: 53, 1980.*
4. Mathé, G., Misset, J.L., De Vassal, F., et al.: *Cancer Treat Rep 62: 805, 1978.*
5. Smith, I.E., Hedly, D.W., Powles, T.J., and McElwain, T.J.: *Cancer Treat Rep 62: 1427, 1978.*
6. Bayssas, M., Gouveia, J., Riboud, P., et al.: *Cancer Chemother Pharmacol 2: 247, 1979.*
7. Krivit, W., Chilcote, R., Pyesmany, A., et al.: *Cancer Chemother Pharmacol 2: 267, 1979.*

CHAPTER 37

In vivo Murine and Human Cross-Resistance or Non-Cross-Resistance: Example of Anthracycline and Vinca Alkaloids

R. Maral, C. Bourut, E. Chenu, and G. Mathé

Introduction

The discrepancies between cross-resistance in experimental animals and in man as studied for anthracyclines and vinca alkaloids are the subject of this paper. Generally speaking, resistance to an agent belonging to one class of compounds does not necessarily imply resistance to all agents of the same class. This is the case, for example, for alkylating agents. Differences in the mode of transport into cells, in activation by cellular enzymes, or in reactive alkylating moieties may occur between compounds of this group. Furthermore, resistant neoplastic cells, which have been induced by alkylating agents, do not show cross-resistance to antimetabolites and vice versa.

On the other hand, treatment with doxorubicin (or adriamycin) in rodent tumors (and perhaps in human therapy) often confers resistance not only to other anthracyclines, but also to very different molecules such as actinomycin D and vinca alkaloids. Experimentally, *in vivo* resistance and cross-resistance are represented schematically by the two theoretical diagrams shown in Figures 1 and 2.

Resistance in a cell population may occur either because some cells are resistant *de novo* to the compound (natural resistance) or because resistant cell lines develop during exposure to the drug (induced resistance). At the cellular level, there are several mechanisms of the drug resistance (Table 1):

1. Insufficient drug uptake by, or increased drug efflux from, the tumor cell, following an alteration of cell membrane glycoproteins, and subsequently an alteration of the cellular transport of compounds.
2. For antimetabolites, deletion of enzymes activating the drug; increased activity of enzymes catabolizing the drug; cross-resistance between antipurines or antipyrimidines when these compounds require the same enzymes for activation; increased concentration of inhibiting enzymes; and increased utilization of an alternative biochemical pathway (salvage process).
3. For alkylating agents, rapid repair of drug-induced lesions.

The compounds to be discussed here are anthracyclines (ATC) and vinca alkaloids. From a chemical point of view they are very different and the mechanisms of action are not the same.

Anthracyclines belong to a very large

Institut de Cancérologie et d'Immunogénétique (INSERM U 50), Hôpital Universitaire Paul-Brousse, Villejuif, France

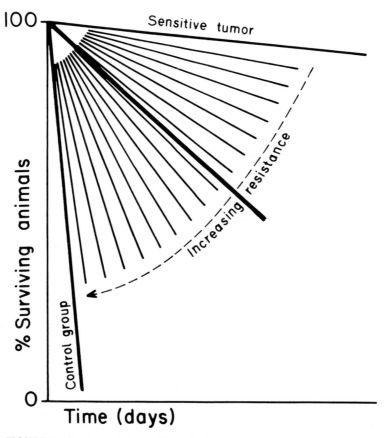

FIGURE 1. *In vivo* resistance (theoretical).

family, the molecules of which contain two parts (Figure 3): a planar anthraquinone nucleus and aminosugar (one or multiple sugars). The modes of action of ATC are numerous and are still explored: intercalation in DNA, interference with the cell respiratory chain, leading to semiquinone radicals, production of free, superoxide, and oxygen radicals which mediate DNA damage, membrane lipid peroxidation, and altered membrane functions. The antitumor activity is related to DNA binding and damage, and also to superoxide radical production. The cardiotoxicity is probably linked to lipid peroxidation and to production of free radicals. The cell uptake of ATC is a passive process and the efflux is an active process.

The vinca alkaloids (Figure 4) are quite different molecules. These dimers bind to tubulin, a dimeric protein found in the soluble fraction of the cytoplasm of all cells. Tubulin exists in equilibrium with a polymerized form, the microtubular apparatus which forms the spindle during mitosis. Furthermore, microtubules play a vital role for the cytoskeleton. The alkaloids, through their binding to tubulin, inhibit the assembly of the microtubules and lead to dissolution of the mitotic spindle and arrest in the metaphase of the mitoses. We know that alkaloids traverse the cell membrane by an active uptake process.

The general methods used for the study of resistance and cross-resistance are: 1) *in vitro:* cell cultures, these studies have been examined by B. Hill and H. Tapiero;[4,5,9,14,27,28] 2) experimentally *in vivo*, usually in mice;[2,6,7,10–12,15,21,23] and 3) in

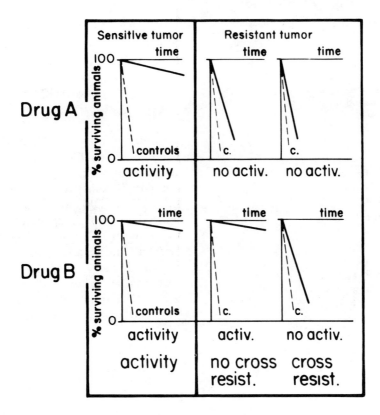

FIGURE 2.   *In vivo* cross-resistance (theoretical).
B may be a compound of the same family (for example, A and B belong to
the anthracycline group or to the vinca alkaloid group), or
B is a compound not related to A (for example, A is an anthracycline and B
is actinomycin D).

human therapy, where the problems encountered are more complicated.

In the laboratory, *in vivo* tumor resistance is induced by suboptimal treatments with the compounds (ATC or alkaloids), followed by repeated passages of the tumor. The treatments are performed at gradually increasing doses. The tumors used are usually the Ehrlich ascitic tumor, the P388 leukemia, and the L5178Y leukemia. With these systems, no great difference in histological appearance, growth speed, or tumorigenicity was observed between the resistant and the original tumors.

In human therapy, clinical observation on differing efficacy of ATC and alkaloids should be evaluated only when such ob-

servations are closely time-related. For example, a positive response to vindesine (VDS) several months after the last (ineffective) dose of vinblastine (VBL) or vincristine (VCR) would not meet this criterium. It is necessary to recall here a well-known phenomenon in human therapy where the tumors encountered are heterogeneous: a tumor refractory to a certain drug may be responsive at a later date when a more sensitive fraction of the tumor has regrown.

In vitro Experimental and Human Studies

We will discuss the cross-resistance between adriamycin (ADM) and aclacino-

TABLE 1. Mechanisms of Drug Resistance

Mechanisms	Examples
Insufficient drug uptake or/and increased drug efflux by the tumor cells (changes in membranes glycoproteins)	DNR, ADM Actinomycin D Alkaloids
Deletion of drug-activating enzymes	6-MP 5-Fu 6-TG
Increased utilization of an alternative biochemical pathway (salvage)	5-Fu
Increased drug catabolizing enzyme activity	ARA-C
Increased concentration of an inhibited enzyme (target enzyme)	MTX
Rapid repair of drug-induced lesions	Alkylating agents

mycin-A (AA) on one hand, and between vincristine (VCR) and vindesine (VDS) on the other.

METHODS

In Mice

Anthracyclines (ADM and AA). The mice used were B6D2F1 male mice, average weight 25–30 g. The tumors were P388 leukemia; 1 sensitive and 1 ADM-resistant line (P388/ADM) was used. They were grafted I.P. (10^6 cells) on day 0. The treatments with ADM or AA, at optimal dose and half the optimal dose, took place on days 1, 5, and 9. There were eight mice in each treated group and 16 in the control group. The index of activity is the ratio of the median survival time of the treated

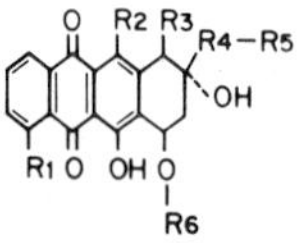

Compound	R1	R2	R3	R4	R5	R6
I Daunorubicin (DNR)	-OCH3	-OH	-H2	-CO-	-CH3	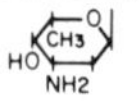 (sugar, HO–CH3, NH2)
II Daunorubicinol	id	id	id	-CHOH-	id	id
III Doxorubicin Adriamycin (ADM)	id	id	id	-CO-	-CH2OH	id
IV Doxorubicinol	id	id	id	-CHOH-	id	id
V Zorubicin Rubidazone	id	id	id	-C(CH3)NNHCOC6H5		id
VI Detorubicin	id	id	id	-COCH2OCOCH(OC2H5)2		id
VII Carminomycin	-OH	id	id	-CO-	-CH3	id
VIII N-L-Leu Daunorubicin	-OCH3	id	id	id	id	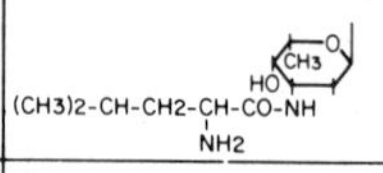 (CH3)2-CH-CH2-CH-CO-NH, HO, NH2
IX 4'Epi-Adriamycin	id	id	id	id	-CH2OH	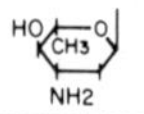 (sugar HO–CH3, NH2)
X AD 32	id	id	id	-COCH2OCO(CH2)3CH3		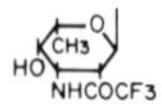 (sugar HO–CH3, NHCOCF3)
XI Aclacinomycin-A	-OH	-H	-CO2CH3	-CH2-	-CH3	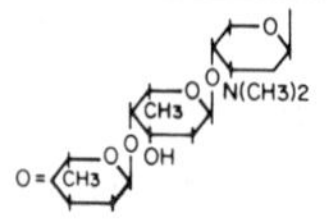 (trisaccharide, N(CH3)2, OH, O=)
XII 4'-O-Tetrahydro pyranyl-Adriamycin (b-isomer)	-OCH3	-OH	-H2	-CO-	-CH2OH	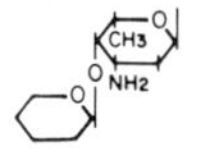 (sugar CH3, O, NH2)

FIGURE 3. Main anthracycline derivatives of clinical use.

Catharanthine moiety	Drug	Vindoline moiety		
		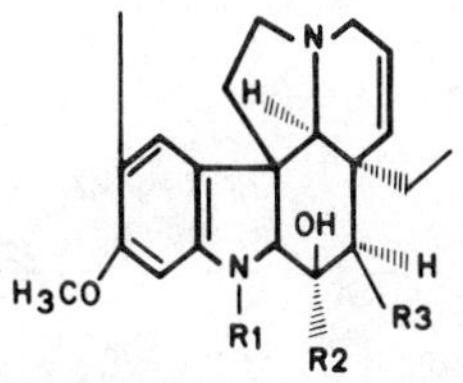		
		R1	R2	R3
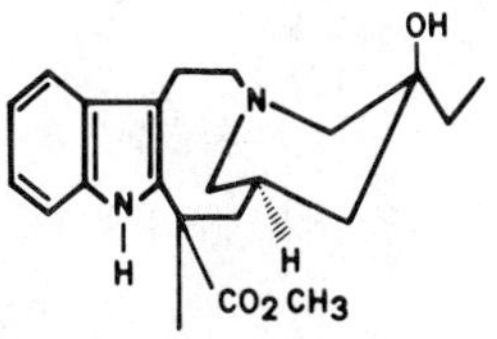	Vincristine (**VCR**)	$-CHO$	$-CO_2CH_3$	$-O-CO-CH_3$
	Vinblastine (**VLB**)	$-CH_3$	$-CO_2CH_3$	$-O-CO-CH_3$
	Vindesine desacetyl amide Vinblastine (**VDS**)	$-CH_3$	$-CONH_2$	$-OH$
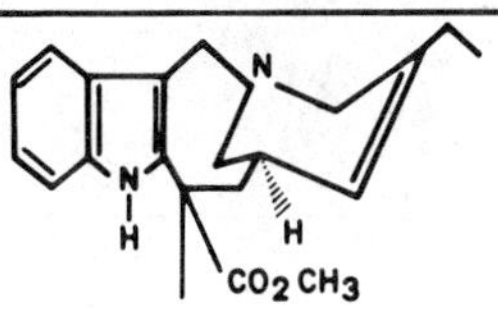	Navelbine 5'-Nor-anhydro Vinblastine (**NAV**)	$-CH_3$	$-CO_2CH_3$	$-O-CO-CH_3$

FIGURE 4.   Vinca alkaloid derivatives.

group over that of the control group. The results were statistically analyzed according to the Wilcoxon's nonparametric test.

Vinca alkaloids (VCR and VDS). We used the same P388 strain of murine leukemia, highly sensitive to VCR and a subline resistant to VCR (P388/VCR). The method was the same as above: B6D2F1 mice were grafted I.P. (10^6) cells on day 0 and treated at optimal dose and half the optimal dose with VCR or VDS.

In Human Therapy

Anthracyclines (ADM and AA). Nineteen patients (acute myeloblastic leukemia or AML) who were clinically resistant to ADM (50 mg/m²) were treated with 10–30 mg AA/m² I.V./day for 10 days with 10-day intervals.

Vinca alkaloids (VCR and VDS). During a clinical phase II study of VDS,[3,16,17] 27 patients (15 acute lymphoblastic leukemia or ALL; five blastic crises in chronic myeloid leukemia or CML; seven non-Hodgkin lymphomas or NHL) were considered clin-

ically resistant to VCR because the neoplasm progressed or remained unchanged during the application of VCR (1.6 mg/m², one treatment each week).

RESULTS

In Mice

ATC (ADM and AA). Table 2 shows typical cross-resistance between ADM and AA. All the compounds are active on P388 (particularly AA) but not on P388/ADM. However, mitoxantrone (an anthracenedione) is active on P388/ADM and consequently not cross-resistant with the other ATCs.

Vinca alkaloids (VCR and VDS). Table 3 shows the results obtained. It is clear that a cross-resistance exists with these compounds. However, there are degrees in this cross-resistance which seem less marked in the case of vinblastine and navelbine.

In Human Therapy

ATC (ADM and AA) (Table 4). Of the 19

TABLE 2.   Anthracyclines—Cross-resistance

		P388			P388/ADM		
Drug	mg/kg I.P. Days: 1, 5, 9	I	No. Surviving Mice on Day 30	S	I	No. Surviving Mice on Day 30	S
Doxorubicin	4	191	2/8	S	120	0	N.S.
(Adriamycin:ADM)	8	266	5/8	S	100	0	N.S.
Carminomycin	0.1	158	0	S	100	0	N.S.
	0.2	158	0	S	116	0	N.S.
THP–ADM	4	216	0	S	112	0	N.S.
	8	300	7/9	S	104	0	N.S.
4′Epi-ADM	4	200	1/8	S	125	0	N.S.
	8	212	2/8	S	116	0	N.S.
Aclacinomycin A	4	125	0/8	S	91	0	N.S.
	8	158	0/8	S	58	0	N.S.
Mitoxanthrone	0.75	283	4/8	S	166	0	S
	1.50	200	2/8	S	166	0	S

Male $B_6D_2F_1$/Olac Mice (25–30g) – 10^6 Cells Grafted I.P. on Day 0

$$I = \frac{\text{Median Survival Time—Treated Mice}}{\text{Median Survival Time—Controls}} \times 100$$

S = Wilcoxon non parametric test; S = significant; NS = not significant.

AML patients who were resistant to ADM, 11 patients responded to the treatment with AA (optimal treatment 15 mg/m²/day I.V., for 10 days followed by a 10-day rest period). More than 50% of the cases showed an apparent absence of cross-resistance between ADM and AA.

Vinca alkaloids (VCR and VDS) (Table 5). We obtained remissions with VDS in seven cases of 15 ALL, two of five CML blastic crises and three of seven NHL, in patients who were clinically VCR-resistant.

Discussion and Conclusion

The evidence of activity of VDS in patients unresponsive to treatments which include VCR was confirmed by others.[1,22,26] The results of the studies on resistance and non-cross-resistance appear to be different according to the method used: *in vitro* (cell cultures), *in vivo* (in animals), and in human therapy. The question is

why agents belonging to the ATC or the alkaloid family are cross-resistant *in vivo* in mice, but not in treated patients? It is suggested that these agents share a common transport pathway, the dysfunction of which might lead to resistance[6,7,10–12,21] and to cross-resistance.[13,19,24] Further studies of the disorders of the common efflux pump mechanism, which is energy-dependent, would be of interest. Furthermore, we know that Tween 80[20] or Verapamyl,[25] known to inhibit the Ca^{++} transport across the membrane, are able to restore the decreased influx or increased efflux of drug in resistant cells. The biochemical lesions in resistant cells have not been adequately defined. Much has to be learned about the molecular mechanisms that determine both sensitivity and cross-resistance with ATC and vinca alkaloids.[8]

In the individual clinical situation, the absence of cross-resistance may have other explanations. Due to differences in pharmacology (lower toxicity) or in phar-

TABLE 3. Activity of Vinca Alkaloids on P388 and P388/VCR Leukemia

Drug	mg/kg I.P.	P388			P388/VCR		
		I.L.S. T/C × 100	P^a	No. Alive D. 30[b]	I.L.S. T/C × 100	P^a	No. Alive D. 30[b]
Vincristine	1.0	283	0.001	7/8	103	NS[d]	0/8
(VCR)	0.5	203	0.001	4/8	103	NS[d]	0/8
Vinblastine	1.0	196	0.001	3/8	130	0.001	0/8
(VLB)	0.5	157	0.001	0/8	123	0.01	0/8
Vindesine	3.0	∞[c]	0.001	7/8	116	NS[d]	0/8
(VDN)	1.5	∞[c]	0.001	7/8	113	NS[d]	0/8
Navelbine	10.0	196	0.001	4/8	123	0.001	0/8
(NAV)	5.0	166	0.001	0/8	120	0.01	0/8

[a]P = statistical analysis in comparison with controls (Wilcoxon's nonparametric test).
[b]Long survivors on day 30.
[c]∞ = when in a treated group 50% or more of the animals are cured.
[d]NS = not significant ($P = 0.05$).

TABLE 4. Apparent Absence of Cross-resistance between Adriamycin (ADM) and Aclacinomycin (A.A.)

Diagnosis	$N°$ of Resistant Patients to ADM	Resmissions with A.A. (CR +PR)
First Trial: AML	11	6
Second Trial: AML	8	5

ADM: 50gm/m²
A.A.: First trial: 10–30mg/m², slow I.V. infusioon for 10 to 30 days, depending on tolerance.
Second trial: 15mg/m²/day, I.V. push during 10 days, followed by a 10-day rest period. These 10-day cycles were repeated two or more cycles–times until remission.

TABLE 5. Apparent Absence of Cross-resistance between Vindesine (VDS) and Vincristine (VCR)

Diagnosis	No. of Patients Resistant to VCR	Resmissions (CR +PR) with VDS
ALL	15	7
CML, blastic crisis	5	2
N.H.L.	7	3
Total	27	12

VDS = 2 mg/m²; VCR = 1,6 mg/m².

macokinetics (higher concentrations in the target cells),[18] one compound may have a better therapeutic index than another compound of the same family. This differential therapeutic activity may be the result of different treatment schedules (doses, timing) resulting in more appropriate blood and tissue concentrations. Moreover, in human therapy the situation is complicated, polychemotherapies are used, and collateral sensitivity phenomena may occur.

REFERENCES

1. Anderson, J., Krivit, W., Thomson, J., Chilcote, R., Pysemany, A., and Hammond, D.: *Proceedings of the 11th International Congress Chemotherapy,* vol. II, 1567, 1980.
2. Barnett, C.J., Cullinan, G.J., Gerzon, K., Hoying, R.C., Jones, W.E., Newlon, W.M., Poore, G.A., Robinson, R.L., Sweeney, M.J., Todd, G.C., Dyke, R.W., and Nelson, R.L.: *J Med Chem 21: 88, 1978.*
3. Bayssas, M., Gouveia, J., Ribaud, P., Musset, M., De Vassal, F., Pico, J.L., De Luca, L., Misset, J.L., Machover, D., Belpomme, D., Schwarzenberg, L., Jasmin, C., Hayat, M., and Mathé, G.: *Cancer Chemother Pharmacol 2: 247, 1979.*
4. Biedler, J.L. and Riehm, H.: *Cancer Res 30: 1174, 1970.*
5. Dan, K.: *Cancer Chemother Rep 55: 133, 1971.*
6. Dano, K.: *Acta Path Microbiol Scand A (Suppl 256) 39: 1976.*
7. Dano, K.: *Cancer Chemother Rep 55: 113, 1971.*
8. Fourcade, A., Farhi, J.J., Bennoun, M., and Tapiero, H.: *Cancer Res 42: 1950, 1982.*
9. Hill, B.T. and Whelan, R.D.H.: *Cancer Chemother Pharmacol 8: 163, 1982.*
10. Inaba, M., Fujikura, R., and Sukurai, Y.: *Biochem Pharmacol 30: 1863, 1981.*
11. Johnson, R.K., Chitnis, M.P., Embrey, W.M., and Gregory, E.B.: *Cancer Treat Rep 62: 1535, 1978.*

12. Kaye, S.B. and Boden, J.A.: *Biochem Pharmacol 29: 1081, 1980.*

13. Kessel, D.: *Molec Pharmacol 16: 306, 1979.*

14. Kessel, D., Botterill, V., and Wodinsky, I.: *Cancer Res 28: 938, 1968.*

15. Maral, R., Bourut, C., Chenu, E., and Mathé, G.: *Cancer Chemother Pharmacol 5: 197, 1981.*

16. Mathé, G., Misset, J.L., De Vassal, F., Gouveia, J., Hayat, M., Machover, D., Belpomme, D., Pico, J.L., Schwarzenberg, L., Ribaud, P., Musset, M., Jasmin, C., and De Luca, L.: *Cancer Treat Rep 62: 805, 1978.*

17. Mathé, G., Bayssas, M., Gouveia, J., De Vassal, F., Ribaud, P., Misset, J.L., Machover, D., Schwarzenberg, L., Hayat, M., Musset, M., and Jasmin, C.: *International Symposium on Vinca Alkaloids,* Washington D.C., 1979.

18. Nelson, R.L., Dyke, R.W., and Root, M.A.: *Cancer Treat Rev (Suppl 7) 17: 1980.*

19. Seeber, S., Meshkov, T., Kading, J., and Schmidt, C.G.: *Twelfth International Congress of Cancer,* Buenos-Aires, vol. 1, 266, 1978, (abstract).

20. Seeber, S., Meshkov, T., and Schmidt, C.G.: *Current Chemother 1249: 1978.*

21. Skovsgaard, T.: *Cancer Res 38: 4722, 1978.*

22. Smith, I.E., Hedley, D.W., Powles, T.J., and McElwain, T.J.: In *Proceedings of the Sixth Vinca Alkaloids Symposium: Vindesine,* Ely Lilly and Co., Ltd., Basingstoke, 1978, p. 11.

23. Sweeney, M.J., Boder, G.B., Cullinan, G.J., Culp, H.W., and Daniel, W.D.: *Cancer Res 38: 2886, 1978.*

24. Tapiero, H., Fourcade, A., Vaigot, P., and Farhi, J.J.: *Cytometry 2: 298, 1982.*

25. Tsuruo, T., Iida, H., Tsukagoshi, S., and Sakurai, Y.: *Cancer Res 41: 1967, 1981.*

26. Valdivieso, M.: *Cancer Treat Rev 7 (Suppl) 31: 1980.*

27. Wilkoff, L.J., and Dulmadge, E.A.: *Proc Amer Soc Cancer Res 19: 37, 1978.*

28. Wilkoff, L.J., and Dulmadge, E.A.: *J Natl Cancer Inst 61: 1521, 1978.*

CHAPTER 38

Cellular Heterogeneity with respect to Clonogenicity and Drug Sensitivity

Y.M. Rustum, Z.P. Pavelic, and H.K. Slocum

Introduction

The lethal action of drugs in target cells depends on numerous factors operating in the whole organism as well as in the target cell itself. Thus, examination of a single parameter may not provide enough information to predict chemotherapeutic sensitivity. A single parameter, such as the lack of drug uptake, however, may indicate intrinsic tumor insensitivity. Target cell determinants may vary among tumor masses obtained from different sites in the same patient[1-7] or from the same patient at different stages of the disease and/or treatment.[8-10] Presumably, increased knowledge of the action of drugs in sensitive and resistant tumors may permit more rational use of drugs in the treatment of human malignancy.

Recent work[11-14] indicates that clonogenicity in semisolid media provides a means for examining drug sensitivity *in vitro* and may be useful for predicting therapeutic responsiveness *in vivo*. Cloning efficiencies, however, are low (usually <1%), implying that only a small subpopulation of tumor cells may be important in determining chemotherapeutic responsiveness. If the biochemical characteristics of the nonclonogenic cells of the tumor are different from those of the clonogenic

Department of Experimental Therapeutics, Grace Cancer Drug Center, Roswell Park Memorial Institute, Buffalo, New York

population, then biochemical measurement in the whole tumor tissues or whole cell suspensions would relate poorly to drug responsiveness. It is important, therefore, to investigate whether clonogenic cells have such unique biochemical characteristics that they must be studied alone in order to identify determinants of drug action, or whether whole cell suspension can be used. Expansion of clonogenic populations to a relatively large number of cells by the use of recloning techniques and transplantation of these colonies into nude mice, would permit their biochemical characterization to identify critical determinant(s) that are responsible for the sensitivity of target cells *in vitro*.

Application of the cloning techniques to human solid tumor cells is associated with a number of problems. Disaggregation of solid tumor mass to form a single-cell suspension is often difficult and reaggregation of cells before plating may also occur. In addition, selection of appropriate or inappropriate cells may occur.[15,16] While mechanical disaggregation yields cells with poor viabilities, enzymatic treatment can yield higher numbers of viable cells and remove "dead" cells already present in the cell suspension. It is not clear, however, what method of disaggregation is most useful for study of the determinants of drug action at the cellular level.

We have recently developed a two-step method for obtaining large numbers of viable cells from human solid tumor specimens,[15,16] employing a mechanical disaggregation step followed by an enzymatic disaggregation step. These suspensions have proven to be suitable for characterization through cytology, culture in semisolid media,[15–18] growth in nude mice,[18] karyology,[19] flow cytometry, determination of ribonucleoside triphosphate pools,[15,16] intactness of DNA,[21] and uptake and metabolism of radiolabeled drugs.

In this study, cloning efficiency and drug sensitivity in soft agar of mechanically and enzymatically released cells from either the whole tumor population or from different parts of the same tumor have been studied in individuals with different solid tumors.

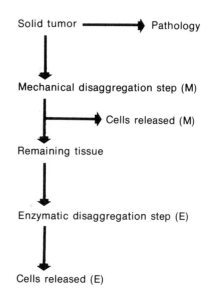

FIGURE 1.   Flow chart for disaggregation of tumor tissues by mechanical and enzymatic means.

Methods

TUMORS

Melanoma, sarcoma, lung, breast, and colon carcinomas were obtained aseptically from the surgical theater and transported on ice into the laboratory for disaggregation. In those cases where more than two grams of tumors were obtained, tumor tissues were divided into several parts and each was subjected to mechanical and enzymatic disaggregation as described below.

DISAGGREGATION OF TUMORS

A two-step disaggregation procedure as described previously[15,16] was employed, and is outlined in Figure 1.

MECHANICAL DISAGGREGATION

Mechanical disaggregation consisted of slicing the tumor tissue into 0.5-mm slices using a Stadie-Riggs microtome,[15] (A.H. Thomas Co., Philadelphia, PA), followed by brief mincing with crossed scalpel blades in ice-cold RPMI 1640 medium with

10% heat-inactivated newborn calf serum. Cells thus freed were separated from the tissue fragments by pouring the mince over a 100-mesh stainless steel screen (C-C Apparatus, St. Petersburg, FL). Remaining tissue was gently returned to the Petri dish and the mincing procedure repeated until cell release was no longer significant (one or two cycles were usually required). Cells obtained in this manner were pooled and considered mechanically released. Remaining tissue was treated enzymatically as described below.

ENZYMATIC DISAGGREGATION

A mixture of 0.8% collagenase II (Worthington Biochemicals, Freehold, NJ) and 0.002% deoxyribonuclease I (Sigma Chemical Co., St. Louis, MO) dissolved in RPMI 1640 medium with 10% inactivated newborn calf serum (Grand Island Biological Co., Grand Island, NY) was employed. The tissue mince was exposed to enzyme for 2 hours at 37° in a humidified atmosphere of 5% CO_2 and 95% air. Freed cells were collected by pouring the mince through a

100-mesh screen as described for mechanical disaggregation.

CLONOGENICITY IN SOFT AGAR

The soft agar assay of Pluznik and Sachs[20] was used to culture tumor cells. Briefly, a 2.5-ml lower layer of 0.5% agar in Eagle's medium with 10% fetal bovine serum was placed in a 35 × 10 mm petri dish and permitted to solidify at room temperature. Cells to be tested for colony formation were suspended in a plating layer (0.85 ml) of 0.3% agar in Eagle's minimal medium with 10% fetal bovine serum. The agar was permitted to solidify at room temperature. Cultures were set up in quadruplicate and incubated at 37° in a humidified incubator in an atmosphere of 5% CO_2 and 95% air.

DRUG SENSITIVITY

Stock solutions of intravenous formulations of standard anticancer agents, including adriamycin (Adr), diamino-dichloro-cis-platinum (DDP), methotrexate (MTX), and 5-fluorouracil (5-Fu) were prepared in sterile saline solution and stored at −70° in aliquots sufficient for individual assays. Tumor cell suspensions were transferred to tubes and adjusted to a concentration of 1.0 × 10⁶ cells/ml mixed with appropriate drug dilutions and agar and plated immediately. Although each drug was tested at three dose levels and growth compared to controls plated without drugs, only the results for the highest drug concentration of

Fu (10 μM), cis-DDP (2.5 μg/ml), MTX (2.8 μg/ml), and adriamycin (0.5 μg/ml) are included herein.

Results and Discussion

YIELD AND VIABILITY OF DISAGGREGATED CELLS

Yield and dye exclusion of cells from 486 human are summarized in Table 1. The highest median cell yield by the mechanical step was in melanoma and the lowest in breast carcinoma. Overall tumors viability ranged between 11 and 16% for cells obtained in the mechanical step. Median cell yield in the enzymatic step was the highest in sarcoma and the lowest in breast carcinoma. Approximately 83% of cells obtained in the enzymatic step were dye-excluding overall tumor types. It is possible that cells released enzymatically which failed to exclude dye are eliminated by enzymatic action. The data in Table 1 also indicate that, assuming 1 g of tumor contains up to 1.0 × 10⁹ cells, the combined mechanical and enzymatic cell yield was approximately 4%. In overall experience, about seven-fold more viable cells were obtained in the enzymatic step as compared to the mechanical disaggregation step. These data suggest that only a small fraction of the total cells present in a given specimen are obtained by this tissue disaggregation method. It is not yet known whether the cells thus obtained accurately represent all cells comprising the solid tumor mass.

TABLE 1. Yield and Dye Exclusion of Cells Obtained in Mechanical and Enzymatic Steps from Human Solid Tumor Specimens

Disaggregation Technique	Tumor Type	N	Median Yield	Median Dye Exclusion(%)
Mechanical	Overall	486	18	16
	Melanoma	40	39	12
	Breast Carcinoma	36	9	11
Enzymatic	Overall	494	21	84
	Sarcoma	53	30	80
	Breast Carcinoma	30	9	87

TABLE 2.   Clonogenicity of Cells Obtained from Human Solid Tumors by Mechanical (M) and Enzymatic (E) Means

Tumor Type	Disaggregation Technique	Median Clonogenicity[a]	Plating Efficiency (Percent Inoculum)
Melanoma	M	130 ± 30	0.026
	E	162 ± 15	0.032
Sarcoma	M	31 ± 11	0.006
	E	74 ± 25	0.015
Lung carcinoma	M	87 ± 40	0.017
	E	56 ± 10	0.011
Breast carcinoma	M	178 ± 20	0.036
	E	85 ± 30	0.017
Colon carcinoma	M	57 ± 16	0.011
	E	224 ± 65	0.045

[a]Colonies of >30 cells/500,000, cells plated, ± standard deviation.

CLONOGENICITY OF HUMAN SOLID TUMOR CELLS RELEASED BY MECHANICAL AND ENZYMATIC MEANS

The data in Table 2 summarize cloning efficiency of human solid tumor cells obtained from melanoma, sarcoma, lung, breast, and colon carcinoma. Each tissue specimen was disaggregated sequentially by mechanical and enzymatic means. The plating efficiency was low (0.006–0.045%) and not significantly different whether cells were obtained mechanically or enzymatically.

Table 3 outlines the overall success in cloning of cells derived by mechanical and enzymatic methods. Success in cloning, whether defined as 5, 25, 50, or 100 colonies was similar with both suspensions, and ranges from 25% if one requires 100 colonies/plates, up to 50% if increase is defined as only 5 colonies/plate. It is surprising, however, that the cloning efficiency in the soft agar used here was independent of cellular viability.

COLONY GROWTH IN SOFT AGAR OF CELLS OBTAINED FROM DIFFERENT PARTS OF THE SAME TUMOR

Intratumor cellular heterogeneity was investigated with respect to the number of colonies obtained from different parts of the same tumor and the results are outlined in Table 4. In spite of wide variability in clonogenicity of a given specimen, it is apparent that differences exist in clonogenicity of cells from different areas of the same tumor in colon carcinoma 1, lung carcinoma 1, the liposarcoma, and possibly lung carcinoma 2. Simply cutting

TABLE 3.   Overall Success in Colony Formation Using Cells of Various Tumor Types Disaggregated by Mechanical and Enzymatic Means

Disaggregation Step	Total Number of Plates Plated	Number of Colonies/ Plate	Frequency of Experience
Mechanical	1259	>5	51%
		>25	44%
		>50	37%
		>100	28%
Enzymatic	3317	>5	56%
		>25	43%
		>50	35%
		>100	25%

TABLE 4. Colony Growth in Soft Agar of Human Solid Tumor Cells Obtained from Different Parts of Same Tumor

Disease	Pieces	Mean number of Colonies per 5 × 10⁵ cells + S.D.		Plating Efficiencies + S.D.
Colon carcinoma #1	A	355 ± 25	400	0.071 ± 0.005
	B	543 ± 17	500	0.109 ± 0.003
Colon carcinoma #2	A	43 ± 15	73	0.009 ± 0.003
	B	93 ± 28	30	0.008 ± 0.002
Lung carcinoma #1	A	532 ± 108	230	0.107 ± 0.022
	B	57 ± 6	69	0.011 ± 0.001
Lung carcinoma #2	A	152 ± 5	140–160	0.031 ± 0.001
	B	415 ± 106	215–615	0.083 ± 0.021
	C	283 ± 142	0–500	0.057 ± 0.028
	D	405 ± 169	100–700	0.081 ± 0.034
	E	342 ± 106	150–550	0.069 ± 0.021
Renal cell carcinoma	A	138 ± 60	20–250	0.028 ± 0.012
	B	502 ± 304	0–800	0.101 ± 0.061
Renal cell carcinoma	A	65 ± 38	0–120	0.013 ± 0.008
	B	95 ± 46	0–120	0.019 ± 0.009
	C	108 ± 52	0–200	0.021 ± 0.008
Liposarcoma	A	90 ± 12	70–120	0.018 ± 0.002
	B	8 ± 9	0–25	0.022 ± 0.002
	C	417 ± 3	350–4701	0.084 ± 0.006
Melanoma	A	125 ± 21	80–160	0.025 ± 0.004
	B	100 ± 32	40–160	0.032 ± 0.002
Fibrosarcoma	A	95 ± 13	70–120	0.030 ± 0.002
	B	120 ± 18	90–150	0.025 ± 0.004

a tumor into random parts without any anatomical clue as to possible segregation of important subpopulations of cells is a very insensitive method. These data may suggest marked heterogeneity within tumor specimens.

DRUG SENSITIVITY

Sensitivity of tumor cells to anticancer drugs were carried out by continuous exposure of cells to the drug in the upper layer. This procedure was chosen due to technical difficulties in maintaining suspensions of single cells through the washing procedure at the end of limited drug exposure time. Furthermore, considerable cell loss was observed when cells were washed by centrifugation. Clumps of cells may appear on the soft agar plate through the initial failure of disaggregation or through reaggregation when either mechanically derived or enzymatically de-rived cells are allowed to settle or are packed through mild centrifugation processes. In either case, simple interpretation of the assay as clonal growth of tumor stem cells is not possible if cell aggregates are present initially.

Drug exposure in the soft agar upper layer was carried out at 100%, 10%, and 1% of the clinically achievable peak plasma values.[14] Overall, 266/310 (84%) tumors tested revealed greater than 30% of control growth of drug-containing plates at every drug concentration used, indicating resistance in vitro. In 15 cases, only mechanically derived cells showed sensitivity in vitro, and in 28 cases, only enzymatically derived cells showed sensitivity in vitro. In theory, any resistant stem cells present in the tumor would imply drug resistance clinically. Only in six cases was sensitivity in vitro seen in both mechanically and enzymatically derived cells

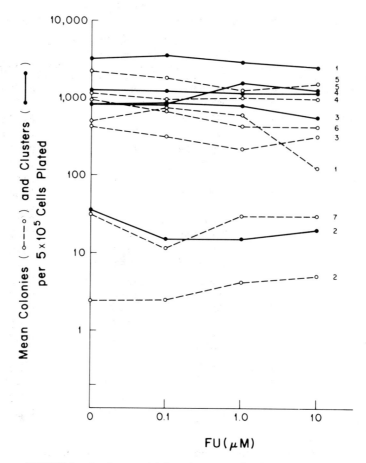

FIGURE 2. *In vitro* sensitivity of tumor cell colonies and clusters (<30 cells) to 5-fluorouracil. Five × 10^5 cells were exposed continuously to the drug in the upper layer of the soft agar system. On day later. 1–7 reflect individual specimen numbers for identification on the plates as cluster (——) or colonies(– – –).

from the same specimen. While continuous drug exposure might be expected to overpredict for sensitivity, the data indicate drug resistance *in vitro*.

The data in Figure 2 outline the results obtained with *in vitro* sensitivity of human tumors to 5-fluorouracil. These data are representative of our experiences with other agents, including adriamycin, *cis*-platinum and its analog diisopropyl-diamino-dichloro-*cis*-platinum; the 5-fluorouracil prodrug 5'-deoxy-5-fluorouridine, dimethyltriazine-imidazole carboxamide (DTIC), and vincristine. The data in Figure 2 clearly demonstrate *in*

vitro resistance at all drug concentrations used.

DRUG SENSITIVITY OF CELLS DERIVED FROM DIFFERENT PARTS OF THE SAME TUMOR

The data in Figure 3 demonstrate the effects of FU, *cis*-DDP, Adr, and MTX on the *in vitro* growth of tumor cells obtained from different parts of the same tumor. Tumors include melanoma (2), colon carcinoma (2), lung carcinoma (2), renal carcinoma (2) and lieomyosarcoma (1). If 70% inhibition of colony formation is consid-

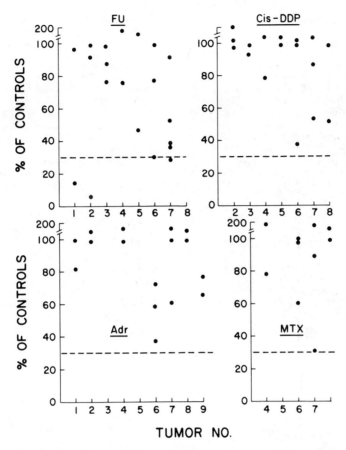

FIGURE 3. *In vitro* drug sensitivity of tumor cells obtained from those outlined in Figure 2. FU = flourouracil; *Cis*-DDp = diiso-propyl-diamino-dichloro-*cis*-platinum; Adr = adriamycin; MTX = methotrexate.

ered the minimum requirement defining sensitivity *in vitro,* it is apparent that cells derived from different areas of the same tumor specimen generally fall on the same side of the sensitivity cut-off line. With 5-fluorouracil, for example, in only two instances did cells from one portion of the tumor show resistance, while those of another portion showed sensitivity *in vitro.* Within the area or resistance, however, a good deal of heterogeneity is apparent in response to 5-fluorouracil (tumors #5–7), *cis*-DDP (#6–8), adriamycin (#6), and methotrexate (#4 and #7). This may indicate different degrees or mechanisms of chemotherapeutic resistance even within the same tumor.

Cellular heterogeneity of response to chemotherapeutic agents may in large measure contribute to the often encountered clinical resistance of solid tumors to chemotherapy. Thus, cellular heterogeneity must be defined and considered to improve the rational design of cancer chemotherapy further.

ACKNOWLEDGMENT

This work was supported in part by project program grant CA-21071 from NCI.

REFERENCES

1. Sibacky, J.: *Br J Cancer 39: 570–577, 1979.*
2. Hakansson, L., and Trope, C.: *Acta Pathol Microbiol Scand, Section A 82: 41–47, 1974.*
3. Weiss, L.: *Pathology Annual 10: 51–81, 1980.*
4. Trope, C., Aspegrem, K., Kullander, S., and Astedt, B.: *Acta Obstet Gynecol Scand, 58: 546, 1979.*
5. Miller, B.E., Miller, F.R., and Heppner, G.H.: *Cancer Res 41: 4378–4381, 1981.*
6. Hakansson, L. and Trope, C.: *Acta Pathol Microbiol Scand, Section A 82: 35–40, 1974.*
7. Biorklund, A., Hankansson, L., Stenstam, B., Tropes, C., and Akerman, M.: *Eur J Cancer 16: 647–654, 1980.*
8. Rustum, Y., and Higby, D.: *Eur J Cancer 14: 5–14, 1978.*
9. Early, A.P., Preisler, H.D., Slocum, H., and Rustum, Y.M.: *Cancer Res 42: 1587–1594, 1982.*
10. Rustum, Y.M., and Preisler, H.D.: *Cancer Res 39: 42–49, 1979.*
11. Buick, R.N., Fry, S.E., Salmon, S.E., and Stanistic, T.H.: *Cancer Res 20: 196, 1979.*
12. Salmon, S.E., Hamburger, A.W., Soehnlen, B.S., Durie, B.G.M., Alberts, D.S., and Moon, T.E.: *N Engl J Med 298: 1321–1327, 1978.*
13. Hamburger, A.W., Salmon, S.E., Kim, M.B., Trent, J.M., Soehnlen, B.J., Alberts, D.S., and Schmidt, H.J.: *Cancer Res 38: 3438, 1978.*
14. Salmon, S.: *Prog Clin Biol Res 48: 1980.*
15. Slocum, H.K., Pavelic, Z.P., and Rustum, Y.M.: In *Cloning of Human Tumor Stem Cells,* S. Salmon. Ed., Alan R. Liss and Co., New York, pp. 339–343, 1980.
16. Slocum, H.K., Pavelic, Z.P., Rustum, Y.M., Creaven, P.J., Karakousis, C., Takita, H., and Greco, W.R.: *Cancer Res 41: 1428–1434, 1981.*
17. Pavelic, Z.P., Slocum, H.K., Rustum, Y.M., Creaven, P.J., Karakousis, C., and Takita, H.: *Cancer Res 40: 2160–2164, 1980.*
18. Pavelic, Z.P., Slocum, H.K., Rustum, Y.M., Creaven, P.J., Nowak, N.J., Karakousis, C., Takita, H., and Mittelman, A.: *Cancer Res 40: 4150–4158, 1980.*
19. Wake, N., Slocum, H.K., Rustum, Y.M., Matsui, S., and Sandberg, A.A.: *Cancer Genet Cytogenet 3: 1–10, 1981.*
20. Pluznik, D., and Sachs, L.: *J Cell Comp Physiol 66: 319–324, 1966.*
21. Slocum, H.K., Pavelic, Z.P., Kanter, P.M., Nowak, N.J., and Rustum, Y.M.: *Cancer Chemother Pharmacol 6: 219–225, 1981.*

CHAPTER 39

Tumor Stem Cell Assay in Pediatric Oncology

Claudio Lombardo, Michela Paganuzzi, Bruno De Bernardi, Tiziana Ruzzon, and Alberto Garaventa

Introduction

Chemotherapy plays an essential role in the multimodal management of most human malignant neoplasms. However, the choice of the antiblastic drugs for the individual patient is made empirically, that is, on the basis of their proved efficacy in previous patients affected by the same disease. This implies the risk of administering ineffective and toxic therapy and may contribute to the failure of treatment as a whole. Clearly, better results could be obtained by knowing in advance the sensitivity of the particular tumors to the available anticancer agents.

The issue has been approached by several investigators utilizing different methodologies. These have evaluated the effect of drugs on tumor cells measuring: 1) morphologic changes;[2,23] 2) inhibition of growth;[4,12] 3) effect on cellular respiration;[6,13] and 4) inhibition of cell metabolism using radiolabeled precursors.[3,5]

None of these techniques,[2-6,12,13,23] however, has become an established guide in planning treatment of cancer patients. In this respect, an increasing interest has recently arisen regarding the tumor stem cell assay (TSCA) proposed by Hamburger and Salmon.[7-9] This method, utilizing a double-layer agar system, permits the selective cloning of tumor cells responsible for the continuous renewal of the tumor itself. When the *in vitro* growth occurs, colonies become visible in a 2–3 week period. The cell sensitivity to a given therapeutic agent is evaluated by adding the drug at proper concentrations to the medium for a brief period of time shortly after plating.

The research, which has explored the clinical applicability of TSCA, has revealed significant correlations between the effects of drugs *in vitro* and the behavior of the tumor treated with the same agents. This has been best documented in ovarian carcinoma and multiple myeloma[17] and, to a lesser degree, in a variety of other cancers.[21]

Scarce data are available regarding pediatric tumors grown in the TSCA. In a recent study of Von Hoff *et al.*,[20] however, a number of neuroblastoma specimens underwent TSCA and the colony cells eventually grown were examined by light and electron microscopy, for catecholamine secretion, and for chromosome analysis. This work did not entail *in vitro*, *in vivo* correlations.

Our paper, following a preliminary one,[15] presents the results of the application of the TSCA in a group of pediatric malignancies observed at the Giannina Gaslini Children's Hospital in a 30-month period.

Multiscreening Laboratory and Department of Pediatric Hematology-Oncology, Giannina Gaslini Children's Hospital, Genoa, Italy

Material and Methods

PATIENT MATERIAL

In the period between December 1979 and June 1982, 51 tumor specimens derived from an equal number of children aged 1–14 years were processed by TSCA. The tumors examined are listed in Table 1.

Of these 51 children, 22 were at diagnosis, the remaining 29 were studied at moment of relapse, and all had received previous antiblastic chemotherapy. The test was performed at least 3 weeks following the last course of tumor chemotherapy.

Main clinical characteristics of the patients, data on the eventual treatment preceding the TSCA, and the positive or negative occurrence of significant *in vitro* growth for each patient are listed in Table 2.

COLLECTION OF SAMPLES

The surgical specimens collected into sterile vessels were immediately placed with a small amount of complete CMRL 1066 medium containing 15% of horse serum (HS) and antibiotics. Bone marrow aspirates were collected into heparinized

TABLE 1. TSCA Applied to Pediatric Malignancies

Period of Study December 1979–June 1982	
No. of cases studied	51
At diagnosis	22
At relapse	29
Patient's age (median, years)	7
Range 1–14 years	
Type of tumors	
Solid neuroblastoma	18
Neuroblastoma (bone marrow)	5
Wilms' tumor	5
Osteogenic sarcoma	7
Rhabdomyosarcoma	5
Non-Hodgkin's lymphoma	4
Teratoma	2
Hepatocarcinoma	1
Malignant histiocytosis	1
Acute promyelocytic leukemia	1
Chorioncarcinoma	1
Medulloblastoma	1

syringe (100 U of preservative-free heparin/ml).[8]

COLLECTION OF CELLS

Bone Marrow Aspirates

Bone marrow was mixed in equal volume of 3% dextran–saline and sedimented at room temperature for 45 minutes or more.[8] The cells in the supernate were collected after centrifugation at 700 rpm for 10 minutes and washed twice in Hank's balanced salt solution (HBSS) with 10% heat-inactivated fetal bovine serum (FBS) (30 minutes at 56°C).

Solid Samples

Cellular suspension from biopsy was obtained by mechanical or enzymatic dissociation.[18]

Mechanical dissociation: The sample, washed in HBSS with 10% heat-inactivated FBS, was minced with a scalpel and filtered through a 100-mesh sterile screen. To remove cellular aggregates, the suspension was passed through a 25-gauge needle and then washed by centrifugation, as described above.

Enzymatic dissociation: The sample, weighted and minced, was incubated for 2 hours at 37°C in a humidified atmosphere of 5% CO_2/95% air in RPMI1640 medium additioned with 10% FBS, 0.8% collagenase II, and 0.002% deoxyribonuclease I; 5 ml of medium was used for up to 2.5 g of tumor tissue.

Cells freed from the tissue were collected by the same filtering and washing procedures described for the mechanically released cells. Tumor cells were counted in hemocytometric chamber, after vital staining with tryptan blue.

Only samples with vitality above 75% were utilized. In case of lower percentages, an attempt to separate live from dead cells was made, using a Ficoll gradient. The cell morphology of the initial suspension was examined by Wright-Giemsa and Papanicolau staining methods.

IN VITRO EXPOSURE OF TUMOR CELLS TO DRUGS

Solutions of drugs at various concentrations were prepared in sterile buffered saline or water (Table 3). Since cyclophosphamide, an important bifunctional alkylating agent, is inactive in vitro, melphalan was used as the index for this antiblastic drug.[17]

Each drug was tested at a minimum of three dose levels, selected on the basis of pharmacokinetic data provided by several sources[1,11] and achievable pharmacologically in vivo. The maximum dosage utilized was 5–10% of plasma concentration time product (cxt), or peak plasma drug concentration.[1] Cells were incubated with appropriate drug dilution or control medium for 1 hour at 37°C in McCoy's 5A medium with 10% FBS; they were then centrifuged at 700 rpm for 10 minutes and washed twice in HBSS.

CULTURE ASSAY

The assay was performed as described by Hamburger and Salmon[7–9,17] with minor modifications. Cells to be tested were suspended in 0.3% agar in enriched CMRL 1066 medium supplemented with 15% HS to yield the final concentration in a range of $2–5 \times 10^5$ cells/ml, depending on the plating indexes of the individual tumors (Table 4).

One ml of the mixture, in triplicate, was pipetted for each drug concentration into a 35-mm plastic petri dish over a 1 ml of agar 0.5% in enriched McCoy's 5A medium. Cultures were incubated at 37°C in 5% CO_2/95% air in humidified incubator. Cultures were examined immediately after plating with an inverted phase microscope to evaluate the eventual presence of cellular aggregates mimicking colonies.

In successful tests, the first clusters composed of 5–10 cells were visible 5–7 days after plating. Colonies (consisting of at least 30 cells) were first observed 7–14 days after plating. Neuroblastoma specimens tended to grow faster than other tumors.

At this time, counting of plates was performed.

The tumoral nature of colonies was verified by Wright-Giemsa and Papanicolau staining methods, performed directly in agar.[16] The cell morphology appeared similar to that of the initial suspension examined before plating.

RESULTS

The in vitro effect of the antitumor compounds tested were assessed on the basis of the reduction of colony numbers in treated plates, compared with the control. Percentage of surviving cells in plates treated with different drug concentrations — compared with the untreated — were plotted on a semilogarithmic scale and the area under survival curves were calculated.

A tumor was defined sensitive, or resistant, to an antiblastic drug when the area under the survival curve was respectively smaller or greater than a "sensitivity index" of this drug.[14]

The "sensitivity index" for the in vitro concentration percent survival curve is defined as the area under the survival curve between 0 and an upper "cut-off" concentration limit, defined by clinical experience and in vivo plasma disappearance kinetic.[14] The sensitivity indexes selected from Salmon et al. have been utilized in this study,[14] since our patient series is inadequate to allow our own statistic elaboration of sensitivity indexes.

The evaluation of the in vivo antitumor efficiency of the compounds tested in vitro was based on: 1) assessment of patient's clinical status; 2) careful measurement of all lesions (i.e., primary mass, lung metastases, and metastatic lymph nodes) utilizing clinical and instrumental tools. These often included, among others, ultrasonographic and CT scan studies and liver and bone scintigraphies.

In the case of neuroblastoma, representing a consistent part of our casuistic, a high excretion of specific tumor markers (vanilmandelic acid, homovanilic acid) was con-

TABLE 2.   Characteristics of 51 Children with Malignant Tumors Cultured in the TSCA

Case No.	Age(years)/Sex	Tumor Type/Primary Site	Source of Material for TSCA	Treatment before TSCA	Significant Growth in vitro
1	12/M	Osteogenic sarcoma/L femur	Lung mets	Surgery, chemotherapy	No
2	2/F	Neuroblastoma/L adrenal	Primary tumor	Chemotherapy	No
3	12/F	Acute myeloid leukemia	Bone marrow	None	No
4	5/M	Neuroblastoma/L adrenal	Metastatic lymph nodes	Chemotherapy	Yes
5	5/M	Wilms' tumor/R kidney	Primary tumor	None	Yes
6	0.6/F	Neuroblastoma/R kidney	Primary tumor	None	No
7	5/F	Neuroblastoma/retroperitoneum	Metastatic lymph nodes	Chemotherapy	No
8	7/M	Hepatocarcinoma/liver	Primary tumor	None	Yes
9	5/M	Neuroblastoma/retroperitoneum	Bone marrow	None	Yes
10	2/F	Neuroblastoma/L adrenal	Bone marrow	Chemotherapy	Yes
11	3/M	Neuroblastoma/R adrenal	Bone marrow	None	No
12	3/F	Neuroblastoma/retroperitoneum	Primary tumor	None	No
13	5/F	Neuroblastoma/retroperitoneum	Primary tumor	None	No
14	3/F	Neuroblastoma/mediastinum	Metastatic lymph nodes	Chemotherapy	No
15	4/F	Osteogenic sarcoma/R tibia	Primary tumor	None	No
16	10/M	Rhabdomyosarcoma/oral flow flow	Epidural mass	Surgery, chemotherapy, radiotherapy	Yes
17	10/M	Medulloblastoma/cerebellum	Primary tumor	None	No
18	10/M	Osteogenic sarcoma/rib	Primary tumor	Chemotherapy	Yes
19	12/F	Wilms' tumor/L kidney	Primary tumor	None	No
20	6/M	Wilms' tumor/L kidney	Primary tumor	None	No
21	7/F	Osteogenic sarcoma/spine	Primary tumor	None	No
22	3/M	Rhabdomyosarcoma/retroperitoneum	Primary tumor	None	No
23	7/F	Rhabdomyosarcoma/retroperitoneum	Primary tumor	Chemotherapy, radiotherapy	Yes
24	1/M	Malignant histiocytosis	Lymph nodes	Chemotherapy, radiotherapy	No
25	13/M	Chorioncarcinoma/mediastinum	Lung mets	None	No
26	3/M	Neuroblastoma/mediastinum	Metastatic lymph nodes	None	Yes

27	4/M	Wilms' tumor/L kidney	Primary tumor	None	No
28	6/M	Wilms' tumor/L kidney	Lung mets	Surgery, chemotherapy, radiotherapy	Yes
29	4/F	Neuroblastoma/R adrenal	Primary tumor	Chemotherapy, radiotherapy, surgery	Yes
30	7/F	Rhabdomyosarcoma/retroperitoneum	Primary tumor	Surgery, chemotherapy, radiotherapy	No
31	13/F	Osteogenic sarcoma/R hip bone	Primary tumor	None	Yes
32	3/M	Neuroblastoma/R adrenal	Bone marrow	Chemotherapy, radiotherapy	Yes
33	4/M	Rhabdomyosarcoma/R hip	Primary tumor	None	No
34	7/M	Lymphoma/laterocervical	Lymph nodes	Chemotherapy, radiotherapy	No
35	0.7/F	Neuroblastoma/retroperitoneum	Primary tumor	None	No
36	10/F	Neuroblastoma/abdomen	Pleural effusion	Chemotherapy	Yes
37	8/M	Neuroblastoma/retroperitoneum	Lymph nodes	Surgery, chemotherapy, radiotherapy	No
38	6/F	Lymphoma laterocervical	Lymph nodes	Chemotherapy	No
39	/F	Teratoma		Chemotherapy	No
40	/F	Teratoma/sacrococcygeal	Primary tumor	None	No
41	7/F	Osteogenic sarcoma/L hip bone	Primary tumor	None	No
42	4/M	Neuroblastoma/abdomen	Bone marrow	Chemotherapy	No
43	6/M	Wilms' tumor/L kidney	Lung mets	Surgery, chemotherapy	No
44	14/F	Neuroblastoma/abdomen	Lymph nodes	Surgery, chemotherapy	Yes
45	2/M	Neuroblastoma/L adrenal	Primary tumor	None	Yes
46	7/M	Sarcoma/L jaw sinus	Primary tumor	None	No
47	7/M	Lymphoma/R axilla	Lymph nodes	None	No
48	0.9/F	Neuroblastoma/retroperitoneum	Primary tumor	None	No
49	3/F	Neuroblastoma/retroperitoneum	Primary tumor	None	No
50	6/M	Lymphoma/ileum	Primary tumor	None	No
51	3/F	Wilms' tumor/L kidney	Primary tumor	None	No

TABLE 3.   Antiblastic Agents and Their Concentrations Used in the TSCA

Melphalan (MPH)	0.1	0.05	0.025
Adriblastine (ADR)	0.2	0.1	0.05
Methotrexate (MTX)	0.2	0.1	0.05
Cis-platinum (Cis-Pl)	0.2	0.1	0.05
Vincristine (VCR)	0.2	0.1	0.05
Aracytin (Ara-C)	0.5	0.25	0.125
Bleomycin (BLC)	0.1	0.05	0.025
Peptichemio (PTC)	0.8	0.4	0.2
m-AMSA	0.2	0.1	0.05
Daunomycin (DAU)	0.2	0.1	0.05
5-fluorouracil (5-Fu)	0.2	0.1	0.05
Vepesid (VP-16)	1	0.5	0.25
Vumon (VM-26)	1	0.5	0.25
DTIC	0.2	0.1	0.05

Drug concentrations are expressed in μg/ml.

sidered evidence of tumor activity and its variation during therapy as expression of drug activity or ineffectiveness. The same can be said for the case of hepatocarcinoma, which produced an abnormal amount of alfa-fetoprotein. Bone marrow invasion (again a frequent event in neuroblastoma), when present, was an easily evaluable parameter of disease.

Patients were considered responsive to a given drug when more than 50% decrease of all tumoral parameters had occurred following administration of an antitumor compound. At the bone marrow level, a response meant the disappearance of all tumor cells, including pseudo-rosettes.

No in vitro/in vivo correlation of drug effect was feasible in patients with no clear tumor lesions at the moment of therapy administration. This was the case in two patients with Wilms' tumor who underwent total resection of their primary.

Results

Of the 51 specimens processed by TSCA, 32 developed visible in vitro colonies; however, effects of the antitumor drugs could be evaluated only in 16 cases. In 14 instances, a total of 35 correlations of in vitro/in vivo sensitivity or resistance were made on the basis of either retrospective or prospective analysis of tumor responses to

TABLE 4.   Colony Growth[a] and Plating Efficiency of 51 Pediatric Tumors Cultured in TSCA

Tumor Type	In vitro Growth/ Case Tested[c]	Colonies/Plates Mean (Range)		Plating efficiency[b] Mean (Range)	
Solid neuroblastoma	13/18	85	(6–267)	0.016	(0.001–0.05)
Neuroblastoma from invaded bone marrow	4/5	88	(15–134)	0.018	(0.003–0.03)
Wilms' tumor	4/5	590	(88–880)	0.12	(0.003–0.2)
Osteogenic sarcoma	4/7	38	(7–89)	0.008	(0.001–0.02)
Rhabdomyosarcoma	2/5	57	(45–68)	0.012	(0.009–0.015)
NDH	2/4	10	(6–14)	0.002	(0.0012–0.003)
Teratoma	1/2	7	(7)	0.0014	(0.0014)
Hepatocarcinoma	1/1	40	(40)	0.03	(0.03)
Malignant histiocytosis	1/1	20	(20)	0.015	(0.015)
Acute promyelocytic leukemia	0/1	—		—	
Coriocarcinoma	0/1	—		—	
Medulloblastoma	0/1	—		—	
Total	32/51	—		—	

[a]Evaluated on 5×10^5 cells/plate.
[b]Number of cases with visible in vitro colonies, including those with 30 colonies/plate.
[c]Plating efficiency: ratio of control colony growth over plated cells.

drugs. In the two remaining instances, no correlation was feasible because of the lack of measurable tumor lesions following the radical excision of the tumor itself.

The accuracy of predicting tumor resistance was 88%. Tumor sensitivity was predicted in 66% of cases (Table 5).

Discussion

A sensitivity test for evaluating the effects of chemotherapeutic agents on malignant tumor cells would be of great help for optimizing treatment of cancer patients. In this respect, the TSCA proposed by Hamburger and Salmon may represent a remarkable achievement. The test deals selectively with the tumoral component responsible for the continuous growth of the tumor itself.[7] In effect, chromosome studies,[19] staining characteristics,[16] and secretion of tumor markers[22] have all confirmed that the cells growing in the TSCA retain the basic characteristics of the original malignant population.

Early results have shown convincingly the clinical usefulness of the test, suggesting that it might play an important role in the selection of adjuvant treatment modalities.[17] In particular, the method seems to be most valuable in defining the lack of activity of a given antitumor compound, with an accuracy rate above 88%.[17] The in vitro predictability of drug sensitivity in the clinical setting is less precise (66%), even though still appreciable.

Data regarding pediatric tumors analyzed by the TSCA are limited to the study of Von Hoff et al. on neuroblastoma specimens derived from either solid masses or bone marrow aspirate.[20] These authors, who also studied chromosome and biochemical patterns of tumor cells, obtained evaluable growths in 30/38 (79%) specimens.

Our contribution deals with a variety of childhood malignancies, although neuroblastoma again was the type of tumor more often encountered. We have been successful in obtaining colony growth in 32/51 cases (63%). However, in only 16 of them was the number of colonies above the limit required for demonstrating suitable evaluations of drug effects.

Neuroblastoma from involved bone marrow, Wilms' tumor, solid neuroblastoma, and osteogenic sarcoma were the neoplasias more susceptible in the agar system. Rhabdomyosarcoma and non-Hodgkin's disease displayed inadequate growth. For the remaining cases (Table 4), an evaluation of cloning capability is not yet available due to the small amount of patients tested.

Thirty-five in vitro/in vivo correlations of sensitivity and resistance were obtained

TABLE 5. *In vitro/in vivo* Correlations: Sensitivity (S) or Resistance (R) of 14 Pediatric Malignancies to Anticancer Drugs

Tumor Type	No. of Cases	No. of Correlations	S/S	S/R	R/S	R/R
Solid neuroblastoma	6	16	6	3	1	6
Neuroblastoma from invaded bone marrow	3	8	2	3		3
Osteogenic sarcoma	2	5	1			4
Rhabdomyosarcoma	2	3	2		1	
Hepatocarcinoma	1	3	1			2
Total	14	35	12	6	2	15
			66% True-positive		88% True-negative	

in the 14 cases with measurable tumor lesions. In accordance with the experience of others,[17,21] the accuracy of the test in predicting tumor resistance *in vivo* has been superior to that of prediction of tumor sensitivity (88% vs. 66%). This difference was, however, less pronounced than that obtained by other authors.

In some instances, the information obtained by the TSCA induced us to make appropriate modifications of the chemotherapeutic regimens and this determined significant tumor regressions. This is demonstrated in the case of the patient shown in Figure 1, who had an initially inoperable hepatocarcinoma that did not respond to conventional chemotherapy. Instead, the *in vitro* sensitivity to pep-

tichemio was confirmed by remarkable clinical response which made the tumor amenable to complete surgical excision.

Our data suggest that the TSCA may provide important information regarding the behavior of various pediatric tumors to the commonly used anticancer agents. The concordance of *in vitro* data with the clinical response to therapy was documented in the majority of instances in which comparison was possible. If confirmed by further data, the TSCA could be of remarkable clinical relevance in the treatment of children with cancer. So far, the value of the test is somewhat limited by the still high rate of inadequate *in vitro* growths. However, the improvement of the dissociation techniques[18] and the use

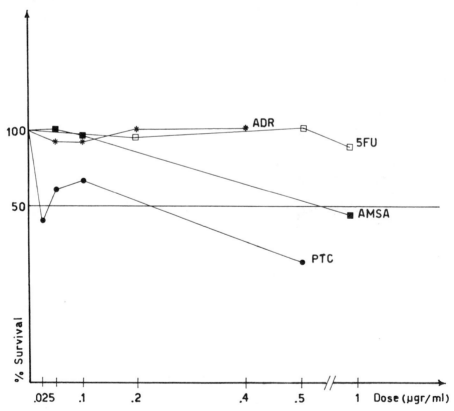

FIGURE 1. Case 8 (see Table 2) — hepatocarcinoma. TSCA was performed before starting therapy. No *in vitro* inhibitory effect was observed after 5-FU, ADR and AMSA; PTC was moderately effective. The administration of PTC, following lack of tumor response to ADR, cyclophosphamide (CPM), VCR, and 5-FU caused remarkable tumor regression; at this time, surgery was attempted and complete tumor excision was possible.

of effective growth factors[10] will probably reduce the number of failures.

REFERENCES

1. Albert, D.S.: In *Cloning of Human Tumor Stem Cells*, S.E. Salmon, Ed., Alan Liss Inc., New York, 1980, p. 197–208.
2. Balconi, G., Bossi, A., and Donelli, M.G., et al.: *Cancer Chemother Rep 57: 115–124, 1973.*
3. Bech-Hansen, N.T., and Sarangi, F., Sutherland, D.J.A., and Ling, V.: *J Natl Cancer Inst 59: 21–27, 1977.*
4. Berry, R.J., Laing, A.H., and Wells, J.: *Br J Cancer 31: 218–227, 1975.*
5. Bickis, I.J., Henderson, I.W.D., and Quastel, J.H.: *Cancer (Phila) 19: 103–113, 1966.*
6. Di Paolo, J.A., and Dowd, J.E.: *J Natl Cancer Inst 27: 807–815, 1961.*
7. Hamburger, A.W., and Salmon, S.E.: *Science 197: 461–463, 1977.*
8. Hamburger, A.W., and Salmon, S.E.: *J Clin Invest 60: 846–854, 1977.*
9. Hamburger, A.W., Salmon, S.E., Kim, M.B., et al.: *Cancer Res 38: 3438–3444, 1978.*
10. Hamburger, A.W.: In *Cloning of Human Stem Cells* S.E. Salmon, Ed., Alan Liss Inc., New York, 1980, pp. 23–42.
11. Hill, B.T., and Whelan, D.H.: *Ped Res 15: 1117–1127, 1981.*
12. Holmes, H.K., and Little, J.M.: *Lancet 2: 985–987, 1974.*
13. Kondo, T.: *Natl Cancer Inst Monogr 34: 251–256, 1971.*
14. Moon, T.E.: In *Cloning of Human Tumor Stem Cells* S.E. Salmon, Ed., Alan Liss Inc., New York, 1980, pp. 209–222.
15. Paganuzzi, M., Ruzzon, T., Lombardo, C., et al.: *Gaslini 13: 48–55, 1981.*
16. Salmon, S.E., and Buick, R.N.: *Cancer Res 39: 1133–1136, 1979.*
17. Salmon, S.E., Hamburger, A.W., Soehnlen, B., et al.: *N Engl J Med 298: 1221–1227, 1978.*
18. Slocum, H.K., Pavelic, Z.P., and Rustum, Y.M.: In *Cloning of Human Tumor Stem Cells*, S.E. Salmon, Ed., Alan Liss Inc., New York, 1980, pp. 339–344.
19. Trent, J.M.: In *Cloning of Human Tumor Stem Cells*, S.E. Salmon, Ed., Alan Liss Inc., New York, 1980, pp. 345–350.
20. Von Hoff, D.D., Casper, J., Bradley, E., et al.: *Cancer Res 40: 3591–3597, 1980.*
21. Von Hoff, D.D., Casper, J., Bradley, E., et al.: *Am J Med 70: 1027–1032, 1981.*
22. Von Hoff, D.D., Johnson, G.E., and Glaubiger, D.L.: *Proc Am Assoc Cancer Res 20: 51, 1979.*
23. Wright, J.C., and Walker, D.A.: *J Surg Oncol 7: 381–393, 1975.*

CHAPTER 40

DNA as a Carrier of Anthracyclines

Gösta Gahrton,[a] C. Paul[a], and C. Peterson[b]

Introduction

The anthracyclines daunorubicin and doxorubicin (adriamycin) are two of the most potent drugs for treatment of acute leukemia. Doxorubicin is effective as well in the treatment of a number of solid tumors. Both drugs have drawbacks in that they induce severe bone-marrow toxicity and cardiotoxicity. Previous work in experimental systems by Trouet[7] suggests that using DNA as a carrier of the anthracyclines may both increase the cytotoxic efficacy and decrease the toxicity of the drugs. The aim with the present work was to study this possibility and its mechanisms in patients with acute nonlymphoblastic leukemia (ANLL).

Materials and Methods

A DNA-saline solution, which had previously been autoclaved at 120°C and passed through a Millipore filter, was mixed with the daunorubicin or doxorubicin solution no more than 12 hours before use as previously described.[7] The pharmacokinetics of the DNA-anthracycline complex thus formed were compared to those of the free drugs in both plasma and leukemic cells in 10 patients with ANLL.[3,5] Two of these patients received first free and later DNA-linked doxorubicin at different treatment courses (interval between the courses 3–4 weeks) (Fig. 1).

High-performance liquid chromatography[1] was used to determine the concentration of the anthracyclines and their reduced metabolites. The area under the drug concentration-versus-time curves was calculated according to the trapezoidal method. The clearance of the drugs was calculated according to the formula

$$\frac{\text{dose}}{\text{AUC}} \quad (\text{AUC} = \text{area under the curve}),$$

the slope of the elimination curve (β) according to the method of least square, and the apparent volume of distribution (Vd) according to the formula

$$Vd = \frac{\text{clearance}}{\beta}.^{6}$$

The efficacy and toxicity of the complex was tested in a randomized clinical trial of 60 patients with ANLL. Twenty-two patients received danorubicin-DNA complex plus ara-C, 18 patients, the same drug combination in exactly the same dose schedules but daunorubicin in the free form substituted for daunorubicin-DNA complex, and 20 patients, daunorubicin plus ara-C in a dose regimen previously used by the Leukemia Group of Central Sweden.[2,4]

[a]Division of Clinical Hematology and Oncology, Department of Medicine, Huddinge Hospital and Karolinska Institute, Huddinge, Sweden
[b]Department of Pharmacology, Karolinska Institute, Stockholm, Sweden

TABLE 1. Pharmacokinetics of DNR and DOX in Plasma and Leukemic Cells from Patients Receiving DNR, DNR-DNA, DOX or DOX-DNA 1.5 mg/kg Body Weight

Patient	Treatment	Plasma			Leukemic Cells		
		AUC$_{DNR (DOX)}$ (μmol × l⁻¹ × hour)	Clearance (l × hour⁻¹ × kg⁻¹)	Vd (l/kg)	AUC$_{DNR (DOX)}$ (nmol × mg⁻¹ × hour)	AUC$_{DOL}$ (nmol × mg⁻¹ × hour)	AUC$_{DNR}$ + AUC$_{DOL}$ (nmol × mg⁻¹ × hour)
I	DNR	1.33	2.00	53.8	5.26	1.48	6.74
II	DNR	3.08	0.86	52.8	6.56	2.35	9.21
III	DNR	2.28	1.16	48.3	2.38	0.71	3.09
IV	DNR	0.58	4.58	30.0	2.97	2.86	5.83
V	DNR	1.34	1.98	20.0	2.88	0.68	3.56
Mean		1.72	2.12	41.0	4.01	1.62	5.69
VI	DNR-DNA	4.76	0.56	10.6	2.98	1.71	4.69
VII	DNR-DNA	2.46	1.08	26.2	2.54	0.57	3.11
VIII	DNR-DNA	1.69	1.57	16.7	4.46	2.13	6.59
Mean		2.97	1.07	17.8	3.33	1.47	4.80
III	DOX	2.10	1.27	54.5	2.73	0	
IX	DOX	2.62	1.02	20.4	2.35	0	
X	DOX	2.21	1.29	26.6	3.85	0	
Mean		2.31	1.19	33.8	2.98		
III	DOX-DNA	10.56	0.25	7.7	6.33	0	
X	DOX-DNA	14.68	0.18	2.7	6.47	0	
Mean		12.62	0.22	5.2	6.40		

DNR   = Daunorubicin
DOX   = Doxorubicin (Adriamycin)
DOL   = Daunorubicinol
DOXOL = Doxorubicinol

Results

The pharmacokinetic studies in the plasma showed that daunorubicin disappeared somewhat more rapidly in the free form than did the complex. The AUC was larger and the Vd smaller when administered as the complex than when administered as the free drug. These differences between the free drug and the complex were much more pronounced for doxorubicin. The AUC was about five times as high when administered as doxorubicin-DNA than when administered as free doxorubicin, and the Vd was six to seven times smaller for the complex (Table 1).

The comparison between the cellular drug uptake after administration of free or complex-bound daunorubicin showed approximately the same uptake when administered as a complex as compared to the free drug as judged by the AUC. A similar comparison between intracellular drug uptake after administration of doxorubicin in the free or DNA-bound form showed that the uptake of doxorubicin was about twice as high when administered in the DNA-carried form (Fig. 1).

The clinical studies showed that the remission induction was similar in patients induced with DNA-bound daunorubicin or daunorubicin in the free form. The frequencies of remission were 68%, 72%, and 70% in the three different groups. Also, the median duration of remission and the median survival were similar, but with a tendency for a somewhat longer survival in daunorubicin-DNA treated patients (median survival with free daunorubicin, 510 days; free daunorubicin, regimen as with daunorubicin-DNA, 495 days; daunorubicin-DNA, 675 days). A study was also made of anthracycline-related cardiac abnormalities. Such abnormalities were less frequent in patients treated with the complex as compared to patients treated with daunorubicin in the free form ($p < 0.05$).

Conclusions

DNA can be used as a carrier of anthracyclines for cancer chemotherapy. Both plasma and intracellular pharmacokinetics

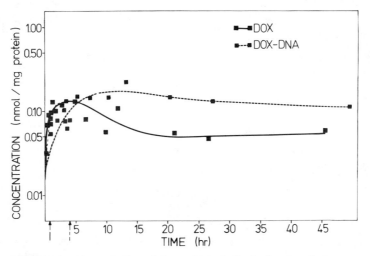

FIGURE 1. Concentration of doxorubicin in the leukemic cells from a patient who on the first course of treatment received doxorubicin 1.5 mg/kg and, at a later time when in relapse, doxorubicin-DNA 1.5 mg/kg. High levels of doxorubicin persist for a longer time when doxorubicin is administered as a DNA complex.

of the anthracyclines are changed by linking to DNA. The plasma is cleared more slowly from the drug, the concentration versus time (area under the curve) is larger, the volume of distribution smaller and the uptake in the leukemic cells higher (doxorubicin) or the same (daunorubicin) if the drugs are administered in complex-bound form as compared to the free form. These results indicate that the tissue affinity of the anthracyclines is reduced by binding to DNA, which in turn might be the reason for decreased cardiotoxicity. The efficacy of daunorubicin-DNA complex in ANLL is as high as for the free drug. Since the pharmacokinetic differences between complex-bound drug and free drug are much larger for doxorubicin than for daunorubicin, it is possible that the clinical efficacy of the doxorubicin-DNA complex is higher and the cardiotoxicity lower as compared to the daunorubicin-DNA complex. This is presently being tested in a randomized trial by the Leukemia Group of Middle Sweden.

REFERENCES

1. Baurain, R., Zenebergh, A., and Trouet, A.: *J Chromatogr 157: 331–336, 1978.*
2. Gahrton, G., Björkholm, M., Brenning, G., Christenson, I., Engstedt, L., Franzén, S., Gullbring, B., Holm, G., Högman, C., Hörnsten, P., Jameson, S., Killander, A., Simonsson-Lindemalm, C., Lockner, D., Lönnqvist, B., Mellstedt, H., Palmblad, J., Paul, C., Pauli, C., Peterson, C., Reizenstein, P., Simonsson, B., Skårberg, K-O., Udén, A-M., and Wadman, B.: *Cancer Chemother Pharmacol 2: 73–76, 1979.*
3. Paul, C., Baurain, R., Gahrton, G., and Peterson, C.: *Cancer Lett 9: 263–269, 1980.*
4. Paul, C., Björkholm, M., Christenson, I., Engstedt, L., Gahrton, G., Hast, R., Holm, G., Killander, A., Lantz, B., Lockner, D., Lönnqvist, B., Mellstedt, H., Palmblad, J., Peterson, C., Simonsson, B., Stalfelt, A-M., Udén, A-M., Wadman, B., and Öberg, G.: *Cancer Chemother Pharmacol 6: 65–73, 1981.*
5. Peterson, C., Paul, C., and Gahrton, G.: In *Controlled Release of Pesticides and Pharmaceuticals.* D.H. Lewis, Ed., Plenum Press, New York, 1981, pp. 49–65.
6. Sjökvist, F., Borgå, O., and Orme, M.: In *Drug Treatment Principles and Practice of Clinical Pharmacology and Therapeutics* 2nd ed., G. S. Avery, Ed., Churchill Livingstone, Einbergh and London, 1980, pp. 1–61.
7. Trouet, A., Deprez-de Campeneere, D., de Smedt-Malengreaux, M., and Atassi, G.: *Eur J Cancer 10: 405–411, 1974.*

CHAPTER 41

Razoxane (ICRF-159; NSC 129,943)

K. Hellmann

Introduction

Razoxane inhibits the growth of a variety of leukemias and solid tumors. It does not seem to kill cells, but merely stops their division, often with multinucleate cell formation. It seems to be a true cytostatic agent.

Pharmacokinetic studies show poor absorption from the gut and at higher doses the amount absorbed is independent of the amount given. Single doses are essentially nontoxic, even at 20 g, but with multiple doses the dose-limiting toxicity of leukopenia is seen at approximately 750 mg/m^2 given in three divided doses at eight hourly intervals over 3 days. No cardiovascular, hepatic, renal, neurotoxicity, or pulmonary toxicity has been described.

Results

The results with razoxane, gathered over a decade, reveal a well-tolerated compound with unusual biological activities that is moderately active clinically and has a broad spectrum of activity. It does not seem to kill cells at doses generally employed and since it is phase-specific in G_2 or G_2/M, it only inhibits division of a small percentage of tumor cells at any one time. It is highly probable that the use of maximum tolerated doses — as has been the case in most clinical trials — is inappropri-

Cancer Chemotherapy Department, Imperial Cancer Research Fund, WC2, and Westminster Hospital, London, England

ate for this drug and the full effectiveness of razoxane has not yet emerged.

Discussion

The decision to test razoxane for antitumor activity arose from the vague speculative notion that intracellular chelation might be useful. Consequently, a nonpolar compound related to EDTA which might penetrate tumor cells and chelate an unknown substance or substances of importance to an unknown enzyme or enzymes and thereby selectively inhibit tumor growth was tested. At the present time, despite considerable work (mostly unpublished), no evidence has emerged that would lend any support to the original notion on the basis of which the compound was tested. There is also no indication of the mechanism actually involved in the inhibitory action of this or any of the other compounds in the series of *bis*dioxopiperazines to which razoxane belongs.

Critical to the issue of the value of razoxane is the meaning and importance of tumor regression. A compound that does not destroy cells but merely stops their division would not be expected to cause regressions. It would be expected to produce an increase of life span. Razoxane has been shown to do this experimentally and to do so without much apparent influence on tumor size. It would follow that such a compound would have to be given on a continuous basis, but most phase II clinical studies have used maximum tolerated doses over short periods interspersed with long bone marrow recovery intervals.

It seems likely that razoxane has not yet been sufficiently closely examined to permit evaluation of the full extent of its clinical utility.

Summary

Razoxane (ICRF-159, NSC 129,943) is a broad spectrum, antimitotic agent blocking cell cycle progression in late G_2 or G_2/M. It selectively inhibits metastases from a number of spontaneously metastasizing tumors, normalizes the development of tumor neovasculature, sensitizes tumor cells to radiation, and is synergistic with a series of other antitumor agents. Razoxane also protects completely against the acute toxicity (mortality) of daunomycin and the chronic myocardial toxicity of adriamycin in a variety of species. In clinical trials, it is effective when given orally in acute leukemia of childhood, blast cell crisis of chronic myeloid leukaemia, Hodgkin's and non-Hodgkin's lymphoma, Kaposi's sarcoma, head and neck cancer, and as adjuvant treatment of resectable (Dukes' B and C) colorectal cancer, and in combination with radiation in soft tissue sarcomas. It is highly effective in psoriasis and psoriatic arthropathy (Table 1). Its dose-limiting side effect is leukopenia, but it is otherwise well tolerated. Partial alopecia and gastrointestinal disturbances occur in less than 10% of patients.

TABLE 1.   Clinical Activity of Razoxane

Malignancy	Reference No.
ALL (childhood)	9,11,14
Acute Leukemia (adult)	2
AML (chronic) blast cell crisis	3
Hodgkin's and non-Hodgkin's disease	15
Kaposi's sarcoma	16
Ca. colon (advanced)	4,6,13,17
Ca. colon (adjuvant)	8
Head & neck	19
Ca. cervix	5
Ca. ovary	7
Psoriasis	1,12
In combination with RTX	
Soft tissue sarcomas	10
Chondrosarcomas	18

REFERENCES

1. Atherton, D.J., Wells, R.S., Laurent, M.R., and Williams, Y.F.: Razoxane (ICRF-159) in the treatment of psoriasis. Br J Dermatol 102: 307–317, 1980.
2. Bakowski, M.T., Prentice, H.G., Lister, T.A., Malpas, J.S., McElwain, T.J., and Powles, R.L.: Limited activity of ICRF-159 in advanced acute leukemia. Cancer Treat Rep 63: 127–129, 1979.
3. Bakowski, M.T., Brearley, R.L., and Wrigley, P.F.M.: Treatment of blast cell crisis of chronic myeloid leukemia with ICRF-159 (Razoxane) Cancer Treat Rep 63: 2085–2087, 1979.
4. Bellet, R.E., Engstrom, P.F., Catalano, R.B., Creech, R.H., and Mastrangelo, M.J.: Phase II study of ICRF-159 in patients with metastatic colorectal carcinoma previously exposed to systemic chemotherapy. Cancer Treat Rep 60: 1395–1397, 1976.
5. Conroy, J., Blessing, J., Lewis, G., Mangan, C., Hatch, K., and Wilbanks, G.: Phase II trial of ICRF-159 in treatment of advanced squamous cell carcinoma of the cervix (meeting abstract). Proc Am Assoc Cancer Res 21: 423, 1980.
6. Douglass, H.O., Kaufman, J., Engstrom, P.F., Klaassen, D.J., and Carbone, P.O.: Single agent chemotherapy of advanced colorectal cancer with ICRF-159, YOSHI-864, piperazinedione (PZD) CCNU, actinomycin D (DACT), L-PAM, or methotrexate (MTX) (meeting abstract). Proc Am Assoc Cancer Res 20: 434, 1979.
7. Edmonson, J.H., Decker, D.G., Malkasian, G.D., and Webb, M.J.: Concomitant phase II studies of pyrazofurin and razoxane in alkylating agent-resistant cases of epithelial ovarian carcinoma. Cancer Treat Rep 65: 1127–1129, 1981.
8. Gilbert, J.M. Cassell, P.C., Ellis, H., Wastell, C., Hellmann, K., Evans, M.G., and Stoodley, B.J.: A controlled prospective trial of adjuvant razoxane in resectable colorectal cancer. Rec Res Cancer Res 79: 48–58, 1981.
9. Hellmann, K., Newton, K.A., Whitmore, D.N., Hanham, I.W., and Bond, J.V.: Preliminary clinical assessment of ICRF-159 in acute leukaemia and lymphosarcoma. Br Med J 1(5647): 822–824, 1969.
10. Hellmann, K., Ryall, R.D., MacDonald, E., Newton, K.A., James, S.E., and Jones, S.: Comparison of radiotherapy with and without razoxane (ICRF-159) in the treatment of soft tissue sarcomas. Cancer 41: 100–107, 1978.

11. Krepler, P., and Pawlowsky, J.: Clinical trials with *bis*-dioxopiperazine propane (ICRF-159: NSC 129,943) in acute leukemias. *Oesterr Z Onkol 2(4): 112–114, 1975.*

12. Leigh, I.M., and Gold, S.C.: Acrodermatitis of Hallopeau. *Br J Dermatol 101 (suppl 17): 41–42, 1979.*

13. Marciniak, T.A., Moertel, C.G., Schutt, A.J., Hahn, R.G., and Reitemeier, R.J.: Phase II study of ICRF-159 (NSC 129,943) in advanced colorectal carcinoma. *Cancer Chemother Rep 59: 761–763, 1975.*

14. Mathé, G., Amiel, J.L., Hayat, M., de Vassal, F., Schwarzenberg, L., Schneider, M., Jasmin, C., and Rosenfeld, C.: Preliminary data on acute leukemia treatment with ICRF-159 *Rec Res Cancer Res 30: 54–55, 1970.*

15. O'Connell, M.J., Begg, C.B., Silverstein, M.N., Glick, J.H., and Oken, M.M.: Randomized clinical trial comparing two dose regimens of ICRF-159 in refractory malignant lymphomas. *Cancer Treat Rep 64: 1355–1358, 1980.*

16. Olweny, C.L.M., Sikyewunda, W., and Otim, D.: Further experience with razoxane (ICRF-159; NSC 129,943) in treating Kaposi's sarcoma. *Oncology 37: 174–176, 1980.*

17. Paul, A.R., Engstrom, P.F., and Catalano, R.B.: Phase III trial of razoxane (ICRF-159) vs. 5-fluorouracil (5-Fu) in advanced metastatic colorectal carcinoma. *Cancer Treat Rep 64: 1047–1049, 1980.*

18. Ryall, R.D., Bates, T., Newton, K.A., and Hellmann, K.: Combination of radiotherapy and razoxane (ICRF-159) for chondrosarcoma. *Cancer 44: 891–895, 1979.*

19. Shah, M.K., Catalano, R.B., Engstrom, P.F., and Bellet, R.E.: Phase II trial of razoxane (ICRF-159) in previously treated patients with head and neck squamous cell carcinoma (meeting abstract). *Proc Am Assoc Cancer Res 20: 366, 1979.*

Index